AF566458

The rapid growth of knowledge in molecular biology during the last decade has had far-reaching implications for the understanding, diagnosis and management of haematological malignant disease. The response of many conditions to treatment, and the ease with which patient material can be repeatedly sampled, have made this a fruitful area of study, and in parallel with the expanding contribution of molecular biology there has been growing awareness of the importance of epidemiology, techniques of drug administration, patient support and the evaluation of treatment results.

Haematological Oncology serves as a regular forum for the evaluation and dissemination of this new information, and the topics selected for review range from basic science to clinical applications.

This series provides a comprehensive and up-to-date review of the current state of research and will be an important source of information and knowledge for oncologists, immunologists, postgraduate trainees and other clinical and laboratory workers in the field.

Cambridge Medical Reviews

Haematological Oncology Volume 4

Cambridge Medical Reviews, a programme of review volumes for the clinical sciences, focuses attention on fields in which rapid and continuing advances in biomedical science have increased significantly our understanding and treatment of disease. Each review series is devoted to a single, clinical discipline. The purpose is to provide a regular evaluation and commentary on the growth of knowledge in that subject. Rigorous standards of selection and editing ensure a reliable and topical series of volumes which will meet the requirements of clinicians and research workers alike.

Haematological Oncology

Series editors

James Armitage
Department of Medicine, University of Nebraska Medical Center, Omaha, Nebraska, USA

Adrian Newland
Department of Haematology, The London Hospital, Whitechapel, London, UK

Armand Keating
Autologous Bone Marrow Transplant Program, The Toronto Hospital, Toronto, Ontario, Canada

Alan Burnett
Department of Haematology, University of Wales College of Medicine Cardiff, UK

Cambridge Medical Reviews

Haematological Oncology

Volume 4

EDITORS

JAMES ARMITAGE
Department of Medicine, University of Nebraska Medical Center
Omaha, Nebraska, USA

ADRIAN NEWLAND
Department of Haematology, the London Hospital
Whitechapel, London, UK

ARMAND KEATING
Autologous Bone Marrow Transplant Program
The Toronto Hospital, Toronto, Ontario, Canada

ALAN BURNETT
Department of Haematology, University of Wales College of Medicine,
Cardiff, UK

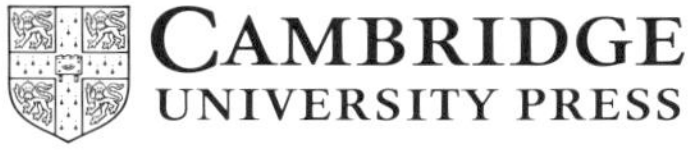

Published by the Press Syndicate of the University of Cambridge
The Pitt Building, Trumpington Street, Cambridge CB2 1RP
40 West 20th Street, New York, NY 10011–4211, USA
10 Stamford Road, Oakleigh, Melbourne 3166, Australia

First published 1995

Printed in Great Britain at the University Press, Cambridge

A catalogue record for this book is available from the British Library

Library of Congress cataloguing in publication data available

ISBN 0 521 46169 3 hardback

WV

Contents

Contributors

AMBINDER, RICHARD F, Department of Oncology, Johns Hopkins University, 418 North Bond Street, Baltimore, MD 21218, USA

AZIZ, DOUGLAS, Specialty Laboratories Inc, 2211 Michigan Avenue, Santa Monica, California 90404, USA

BARATHUR, RAJ R, Vice-President, Specialty Laboratories, 2211 Michigan Avenue, Santa Monica, California 90404, USA

BEZWODA, WERNER R, Department of Medical Oncology, University of Witwatersrand and Johannesburg Hospital, 7 York Road, Parktown, Johannesburg 2193, South Africa

CARBONE, A, Division of Pathology, Centro di Riferimento Oncologico, Via Pedemontana Occidentale, 33081 Aviano, Italy

CASEY, JH, Department of Pathology and Microbiology, University of Nebraska Medical Center, 600 South 42nd Street, Omaha, Nebraska, NE 68198, USA

CATOVSKY, DANIEL, Academic Department of Haematology and Cytogenetics, The Royal Marsden Hospital, Fulham Road, London SW3 6JJ, UK

CHAN, WC, Department of Pathology and Microbiology, University of Nebraska Medical Center, 600 South 42nd Street, Omaha, NE 68198, USA

COHN, R, Department of Paediatrics, University of Witwatersrand, 7 York Road, Parktown, Johannesburg 2193, South Africa

DANSEY, R, Division of Clinical Hematology and Medical Oncology, University of Witwatersrand, 7 York Road, Parktown, Johannesburg 2193, South Africa

FISHER, RICHARD, I, Division of Hematology and Oncology, Loyola University Medical Center, 2160 South 1st Avenue, Maywood, IL 60153, USA

GAYNOR, ELLEN R, Division of Hematology and Oncology, Loyola University Medical Center, 2160 South 1st Avenue, Maywood, IL 60153, USA

GREER, JOHN P, Hematology Division, Vanderbilt University Medical Center, Nashville, TN 37232, USA

GRIGG, ANDREW, Bone Marrow Transplant Service, Department of Medical Oncology and Clinical Haematology, The Royal Melbourne Hospital, Grattan Street, Parkville 3050, Victoria, Australia

KINNEY, MC, Department of Pathology (Hematology), Vanderbilt University Medical Center, Nashville, TN 37232, USA

KOZINER, BENJAMIN, Unidad de Investigaciones Oncohematológicas, Agrelo 3038, 1221–Buenos Aires, Argentina

MACPHAIL, AP, Division of Clinical Hematology and Medical Oncology, Department of Medicine, University of Witwatersrand, 7 York Road, Parktown, Johannesburg 2193, South Africa

MATUTES, ESTELLE, Academic Department of Haematology and Cytogenetics, The Royal Marsden Hospital, Fulham Road, London SW3 6JJ, UK

ORENTAS, RJ, Department of Oncology, Johns Hopkins School of Medicine, 418 North Bond Street, Baltimore, MD 21218, USA

POOLE, J, Department of Paediatrics, University of Witwatersrand, 7 York Road, Parktown, Johannesburg 2193, South Africa

PORTER, BRUCE A, First Hill Diagnostic Imaging, Seattle, Washington, USA

ROBERTSON, KD, Department of Oncology, Johns Hopkins School of Medicine, Baltimore, MD 21231, USA

SEYMOUR, L, Division of Clinical Hematology and Medical Oncology, Department of Medicine, University of Witwatersrand, 7 York Road, Parktown, Johannesburg 2193, South Africa

SHIELDS, ANTHONY F, Department of Medicine and Radiology, University of Washington; the Fred Hutchinson Cancer Research Center, the Veterans Affairs Medical Center, Seattle, WA 98108, USA

SITAS F, National Cancer Registry of South Africa, University of Witwatersrand 7 York Road, Parktown, Johannesburg 2193, South Africa

TIRELLI, UMBERTO, Division of Medical Oncology and AIDS, Centro di Riferimento Oncologico, Via Pedemontana Occidentale, 33081 Aviano, Italy

WHITLOCK, JA, Department of Pediatrics (Division of Hematology and Oncology), Vanderbilt University Medical Center, Nashville, TN 37232, USA

Epstein–Barr virus and Hodgkin's disease

R F AMBINDER, R J ORENTAS
and K D ROBERTSON

Introduction

There is a link between Epstein–Barr virus (EBV) infection and Hodgkin's disease, but the relationship between the two is not a straightforward one. On the one hand, the latent membrane protein-1 (LMP-1), a transforming viral protein, is expressed in Hodgkin's tumour cells, and a history of EBV-infectious mononucleosis or elevated antibody titres against EBV antigens are risk factors for the development of Hodgkin's disease. On the other hand, the virus is present in tumour cells in only about half of the cases of Hodgkin's disease, and while Hodgkin's disease is relatively rare, EBV is ubiquitous, infecting the vast majority of adults worldwide.

In this review, the evidence linking EBV to Hodgkin's disease is discussed in the context of the epidemiology of the lymphoma, the biology of the virus, and the viral association with other tumours. The concluding section of the review discusses therapeutic strategies to target EBV-associated tumours for destruction.

Epidemiology of Hodgkin's disease

Hodgkin's disease has a bimodal age–incidence curve.[1–3] In economically advantaged populations, very few cases occur in children, and the first age–incidence peak is at about age 25. The incidence plateaus in middle age, and then rises in persons over the age of 55. In economically disadvantaged populations, childhood disease is much more common, and young adult disease is rare. These early observations led to proposals that Hodgkin's disease was actually two or three different disease entities with overlapping age distributions. The young adult and childhood diseases were thought to be associated with an infectious process, while the older adult disease was thought to have an aetiology similar to that of other lymphomas.[4–6]

All correspondence to: Professor RF Ambinder, Department of Oncology, Johns Hopkins School of Medicine 418 North Bond Street, Baltimore, MD 21231, USA.

Cambridge Medical Reviews: Haematological Oncology Volume 4

The infectious aetiology hypothesis for young adult disease is supported by observations that social class and childhood environment are important risk factors for the development of Hodgkin's disease.[7,8] Increasing family size, density of childhood housing, number of neighbourhood playmates are all associated with decreasing risk of developing Hodgkin's disease, while higher education, higher social class, and late birth position are all associated with an increasing risk of developing Hodgkin's disease. Early exposure to infectious diseases appears to be protective and delayed exposures to infectious diseases a risk factor. Parallels with other infectious diseases have been noted including paralytic polio and infectious mononucleosis. Early childhood infection with poliovirus or EBV is generally not associated with disease, while infection delayed to young adulthood is commonly associated with disease.[9] Infectious mononucleosis is also recognized as a risk factor for the development of Hodgkin's disease in its own right. Several studies show that infectious mononucleosis and/or elevated EBV titres are associated with a two- to three-fold increased risk of Hodgkin's disease.[7,10–16] Furthermore, increased antibody titres against EBV antigens antedate the diagnosis of Hodgkin's disease by several years.[17]

Direct detection of the EBV in Hodgkin's tumours

The first report of the direct detection of EBV in Hodgkin's disease was in a patient with the apparent direct evolution of infectious mononucleosis to Hodgkin's diseases.[18] Nuclear immunoreactivity in Reed–Sternberg cells was detected using human sera with specificity for EBV nuclear antigens. Subsequently, Southern blot hybridization demonstrated the presence of EBV in unselected series of Hodgkin's patients.[19–22] Motivated by their observation that clonal immunoglobulin gene rearrangements were detected in some cases of Hodgkin's disease, Weiss and colleagues used EBV DNA probes in an attempt to determine whether these clonal immunoglobulin rearrangements might reflect the presence of clonally expanded EBV-infected lymphocytes. Their hybridization studies showed that viral DNA was also present in some cases of Hodgkin's disease, though not consistently associated with the presence of immunoglobulin gene rearrangements. Our investigations at Johns Hopkins were prompted by a survey of B cell lymphomas to detect EBV DNA. DNA from a Hodgkin's tumour, included as a presumed negative control, proved to be the only clinical specimen in which the viral genome was detected. This finding prompted a survey of DNA extracted from 151 lymphoid tissue specimens. EBV DNA was detected in eight of 28 Hodgkin's disease tumours, three of 37 large cell lymphomas, and one case of angioimmunoblastic lymphadenopathy with dysproteinemia.[21] Similar reports of the detection of EBV DNA in Hodgkin's disease were reported by other groups as well.[23–25] With the detection of viral DNA in Hodgkin's tissue by blot hybridization, identifying the locus and character of the viral infection became important. In order to understand the studies addressing these questions, it is necessary to understand something of the biology of the virus and its association with other tumours.

EBV biology

Like other herpes viruses, EBV exists in lytic and latent states distinguished by the presence or absence of virion production, but unlike other herpes viruses, the latent states of EBV predominate in vitro and in most infected tissues in vivo.[26–28] With few exceptions, latent viral infection of tissues appears to play a major role in all diseases associated with EBV. In latent infection, the viral genome is predominantly episomal, although integrated genomes have been recognized in some cell lines and in occasional tumours.[29,30]

Investigation of EBV biology was initially slowed by the absence of a predominantly lytic tissue culture system and by the consequent difficulty in obtaining high titre infectious virus or large quantities of viral DNA. When molecular techniques became available, EBV was the first herpesvirus, and for several years the longest piece of contiguous DNA, to be completely sequenced. The 172 000 base-pair genome encodes approximately 80–100 open reading frames (Fig.1).[31] Repeated sequences punctuate the genome and serve as landmarks. The large internal repeats consist of

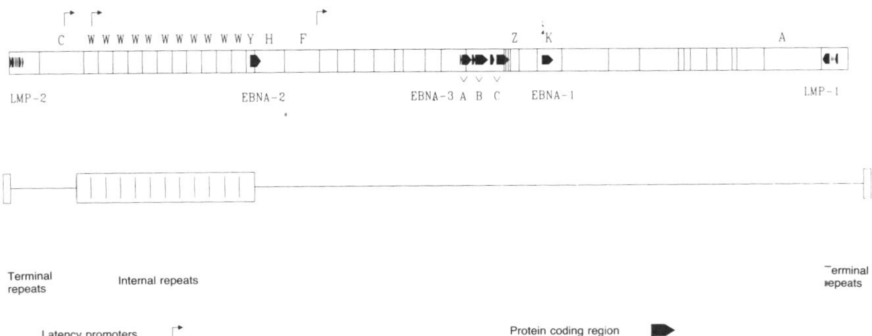

Fig. 1. Map of the EBV genome. Vertical lines indicate *Bam*HI restriction sites. By convention, the restriction fragments are designated alphabetically, with the A fragment being the largest, the B fragment the next largest, and so on. Open reading frames are identified by making reference to the appropriate *Bam*HI restriction fragment. Thus BKRF1 indicates the *Bam*HI-*K* fragment, *r*ightward open reading *f*rame,*1* (EBNA-1). Restriction fragments, latency promoters and coding regions referred to in the text are labelled. (Reprinted with permission of the American Society for Investigative Pathology.)

approximately 12 tandemly reiterated direct repeats of slightly more than 3 kb and divide the genome into unique short and long regions. The ends of the linear genome are bounded by tandem direct repeats of approximately 0.5 kb, referred to as the terminal repeats. The numbers of terminal repeats vary among the viral progeny of a single infected cell.[32] This variation is a consequence of lytic cycle replication which probably involves a rolling circle template and multigenome length concatameric intermediates as illustrated in Fig 2.[33] Upon infection, the ends of the linear genome fuse to form the closed circular (episomal) form of the viral genome. Thus each infectious event results in an episome distinguished by the number of terminal repeats incorporated into its fusion joint. In latent infection, these episomes replicate once with each cell cycle. Episomal replication requires the cellular replication machinery and one viral protein – the EB nuclear antigen-1 (EBNA-1) (Fig.1).[34,35] Neither the viral DNA polymerase nor other viral enzymes involved in nucleic acid metabolism is involved. As a result, latent viral replication is not sensitive to acyclovir or other inhibitors of the viral DNA polymerase. The episomal replication process

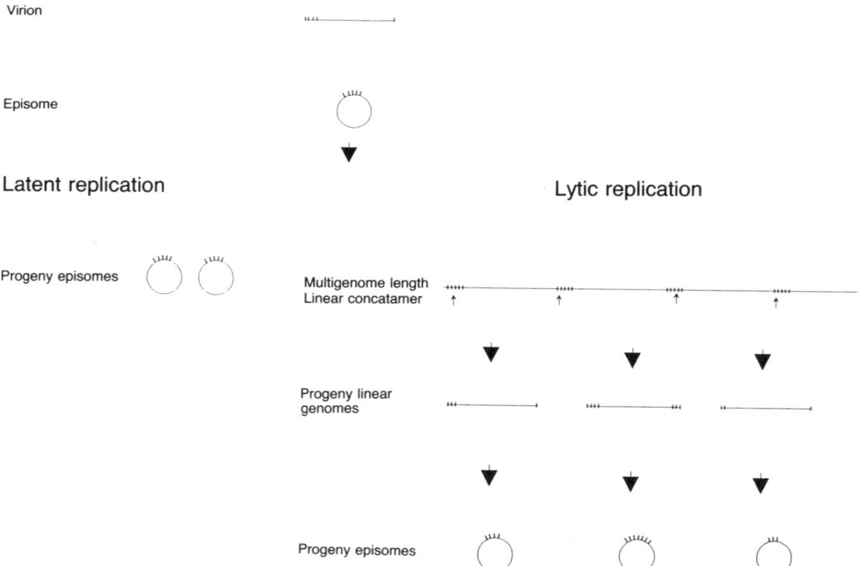

Fig. 2. Latent versus lytic replication. Upon infection, linear virion DNA fuses to form an episome. In latent replication, the numbers of terminal repeats in progeny episomes remain stable over generations. In lytic replication, the numbers of terminal repeats in progeny episomes vary. This variation may result from semi-random cleavage of multigenome length concatamers within the terminal repeats. (Adapted from 28.)

does not involve a linear intermediate and does not lead to variation in the numbers of terminal repeats. Progeny cells carry episomes with the same number of repeats in the fusion joint as the parent cell.

In vitro, infection of peripheral blood lymphocytes or cord blood cells results in the establishment of immortalized B cell lines referred to as lymphoblastoid cell lines. At least 11 EBV genes are expressed in these cell lines (Table 1). Three of these viral genes are well characterized and are essential to lymphocyte immortalization. These are EBNA-1, a sequence-specific DNA-binding protein which binds to the plasmid (or episomal) origin of replication and supplies all the necessary viral functions for replication in latency;[35] EBNA-2, a transcriptional transactivator of cellular and viral genes whose activity is mediated by a cellular DNA binding protein;[36,37] and LMP-1, an integral membrane phosphoprotein that leads directly or indirectly to the upregulation of a variety of cellular genes including lymphocyte activation surface markers, adhesion molecules, and in some circumstances BCL-2.[38,39] LMP-1 is the only EBV protein which is transforming in rodent fibroblast cell lines as manifest by reduced serum requirements, anchorage independence, loss of contact inhibition, and tumourigenicity in nude mice.

Other viral genes expressed in latency are not required for lymphocyte immortalization. These include EBNA-3B; LMP-2A and -2B; and the EBERs -1 and 2.[26,40] Little is known of the function of EBNA-3B. The LMP-2 proteins are related transmembrane proteins.[41,42] LMP-2A binds to the *src* family tyrosine kinases and modulates immunoglobulin-crosslinking mediated transmembrane signalling. The EBERs are two short polymerase III transcripts of approximately 175 bp in length. Although they do not code for protein and their function is entirely unknown, as a result of

Table 1. *EBV latency gene products and the cytotoxic T cell response*

Viral gene product	Latency I	Latency II	Latency III	Cytotoxic T cell response
EBNA-1*	Yes	Yes	Yes	No
EBNA-2*	Yes	No	Yes	Yes
EBNA-3A*	No	No	Yes	Strong
EBNA-3B	No	No	Yes	Strong
EBNA-3C*	No	No	Yes	Strong
EBNA-LP	No	No	Yes	?
LMP-1*	No	Yes	Yes	Yes
LMP-2A, -2B	No	Yes	Yes	Yes, esp HLA-A2
EBERs 1 and 2	Yes	Yes	Yes	Not applicable

* Indicates a gene required for lymphocyte immortalization.

their huge abundance – up to 10^7 copies/cell – they have emerged as important markers of latent infection.[43]

Several different patterns of viral latent gene expression have been recognized.[44,45] The most restricted pattern is termed *latency I*. In this form of latency, EBNA-1 is the only viral protein expressed. Gene expression in *latency II* is less restricted and LMP-1, -2A, and -2B are expressed. In *latency III*, there is unrestricted expression of latency genes including EBNAs -1, -2, -3A, -3B, -3C, -LP, LMP-1, LMP-2A, and 2B. In tissue culture, cell lines may drift from *latency I* to *latency III*. This drift in pattern of viral gene expression is accompanied by concomitant changes in cellular gene expression. These varying patterns of latency viral gene expression reflect alternative patterns of viral promoter usage. In particular, three different promoters are implicated in driving the expression of EBNA-1.[46–48] Shortly after EBV infection of B cells, the EBV genome circularizes and transcription is initiated from a promoter within the large internal repeats, designated W_p. The first transcripts include message for EBNA-2.[49] EBNA-2 interacts with a cellular protein that binds specifically to sequences within the *Bam*HI-C fragment of the genome and in so doing activates an alternative latency promoter, C_p. Thereafter C_p drives expression of all six EBNA genes. C_p is the dominant or exclusive promoter driving transcription of the EBNA genes in established EBV lymphoblastoid cell lines. Exceptions to this generalization are lymphoblastoid cell lines with mutations or deletions of C_p or EBNA-2.[50] A third promoter F_p, drives transcription of EBNA-1 in certain tumour cell lines and in all cell lines characterized to date which are not B lymphoid. In these cells, W_p and C_p are silent and EBNAs other than EBNA-1 are not expressed.

Lytic infection involves the sequential activation of immediate early, early, and late promoters. In tissue culture cells, lytic infection may be initiated by treatment with phorbol esters, superinfection with defective EBV expressing the Z transactivator (ZTA) protein, or in some instances by treating with anti-immunoglobulin. The lytic cascade of viral gene expression involves transactivator proteins, enzymes involved in nucleic acid metabolism including a viral thymidine kinase and DNA polymerase, and production of capsid and other virion proteins.[26,51] Among the proteins expressed in lytic infection are two that warrant special attention because of their homology with cellular proteins. Viral BCL-2 has limited but convincing sequence homology with cellular BCL-2. Preliminary investigations suggest that as with its cellular homologue, viral BCL-2 may protect against apoptotic cell death in certain circumstances. Viral IL-10 is nearly identical with the human IL-10. Both cytokines inhibit production of IL-2, γ-interferon and tumour necrosis factor and are thus potentially powerful modulators of immune response, but their roles in the viral life cycle are still in the early stages of investigation.

Infection of B lymphocytes is mediated by binding of EBV to CD21, the C3b complement receptor.[52] Evidence has been presented that CD21 is expressed at low level on a wide variety of cell types including Reed–Sternberg and epithelial cells. However, the mechanism of entry into non-B cell types is not yet clear. Modes of entry independent of CD21 have been proposed including polymeric IgA mediated transport.[53] Recent studies with cell lines expressing cloned CD21 demonstrate viral adsorption but not infection in many cell lines, suggesting the existence of unidentified determinants of host range.[26]

Clinical EBV infection

EBV infection is generally transmitted in saliva or perhaps in breast milk.[27] Infection in infancy or early childhood is usually asymptomatic or minimally symptomatic. However, primary infection in adolescence or young adulthood is common in affluent populations. In Western countries, infection is commonly associated with infectious mononucleosis.[54] Abundant lytic replication in the pharyngeal epithelium and the cellular response to it are thought to be responsible for the characteristic pharyngitis. Lytic infection in oral epithelium (and probably salivary gland) leads to shedding of virus in the saliva. Lymphadenopathy and atypical lymphocytosis are associated with EBV-infection of lymphocytes and the cellular response to infection. Although initially as many as 10% of peripheral blood lymphocytes may be EBV infected, this percentage very rapidly falls. The atypical lymphocytosis consists mainly of T and natural killer cells. Whether initial infection is or is not symptomatic, intermittent viral shedding and low level infection of lymphocytes is probably maintained for the lifetime of the infected individual. In HIV-infected individuals, and in some other immunocompromised hosts, chronic intense lytic infection of the lingual epithelium is associated with the development of oral hairy leukoplakia.[55]

The addition of exogenous EBV to peripheral blood mononuclear cells from EBV-seronegative individuals, or to fetal cord blood, results in the generation of EBV-immortalized B cell lines. In contrast, the addition of virus to peripheral blood mononuclear cells from EBV-seropositive individuals results in a transient B cell proliferation followed by regression.[56] Regression can be prevented by the physical removal or pharmacological inactivation of T cells. Dilution studies suggest that the T cells which mediate regression occur at a frequency of approximately one in 1000 T cells in healthy seropositive donors.[57,58] Recently, the specificity of cytotoxic T cells for EBV latency antigens from such healthy donors has been determined. Most donors have cytotoxic T cells which recognize EBNA-2, -3A, -3B, or -3C (Table 1).[59–61] A minority of donors have cytotoxic T cells which recognize LMP-1 or LMP-2. LMP-2 is most commonly targeted by donors who are HLA A2.1. Despite efforts in a number of laboratories, no donors have been identified with cytotoxic T cells directed against EBNA-1. The absence of cytotoxic T cells against EBNA-1 is of considerable interest because, as will be discussed later, the only viral antigen expressed by all EBV-associated tumors is EBNA-1 (Table 2). How EBNA-1 circumvents the cytotoxic T cell response is not clear.

Immortalized EBV transformed B cells can also be generated directly from peripheral blood mononuclear cells from EBV-seropositive individuals without the addition of exogenous virus. This is accomplished by suppressing activation of EBV-specific T cells with cyclosporine A. Naturally infected B cells are believed to lyse spontaneously, releasing virus which immortalizes B cells in vitro. The EBV cell lines which result are indistinguishable from those which result from the addition of exogenous virus except for the fact that the associated virus is the patient's own rather than laboratory strain virus. Dilution studies suggest that approximately one in 1 000 000 B cells in peripheral blood carry EBV.[62]

EBV and tumours

EBV was first discovered in cultured endemic Burkitt's lymphoma cells. Early on, the distinctive geographical distribution of Burkitt's lymphoma and its association with particular climatic conditions suggested a possible infectious aetiology for the tumour. However, the hypothesis was challenged by the discovery that the geographic distribution of the lymphoma corresponds to that of holoendemic malaria, whereas EBV infection was seen to be ubiquitous. The complexity of the relationship between the virus and the tumour is further emphasized by the occurrence of Burkitt's lymphoma in North America and Europe. Burkitt's lymphoma in all parts of the world is characterized by a family of chromosomal translocations. Each translocation juxtaposes the *c-myc* locus on chromosome eight with an

Table 2. *EBV latency gene products expressed in cell lines and tumours*

Viral gene product	Immortalized lymphocytes/ post-transplant lymphoma	Hodgkin's disease	Burkitt's lymphoma
EBNA-1	Yes	Yes	Yes
EBNA-2	Yes	No	No
EBNA-3A	Yes	No	No
EBNA-3B	Yes	No	No
EBNA-3C	Yes	No	No
EBNA-LP	Yes	No	No
LMP-1	Yes	Yes	No
LMP-2A, -2B	Yes	Yes	No
EBERs 1 and 2	Yes	Yes	Yes

immunoglobulin locus leading to dysregulated *myc* expression. The histological and karyotypical features of EBV-associated and other Burkitt's lymphomas are grossly indistinguishable. The case for a direct relationship between the virus and tumour is further confounded by the pattern of viral expression associated with the tumour. Early passage Burkitt's lymphoma cells demonstrate a *latency I* phenotype, with EBNA-1 being the only viral protein expressed (Table 2).[63] EBNA-1 has not been shown to have growth regulating properties, and is not transforming in any system. Thus, although EBV was first discovered in Burkitt's lymphoma, and viral DNA is consistently associated with the endemic lymphoma, there is no consensus as to the role of the virus in the pathogenesis of this tumour.[64,65]

In contrast to the situation with Burkitt's lymphoma, the role of EBV in B-cell lymphoma and lymphoproliferative disease occurring in the post-transplant setting, seems much clearer.[56,66–68] Tumours occurring in the setting of therapeutic immunosuppression are usually B cell in origin and EBV-associated. These tumours may represent the in vivo counterpart to spontaneous EBV-driven B cell proliferation in vitro. As noted above, the physical or pharmacological depletion of T cell activity from peripheral blood mononuclear cells in vitro results in the outgrowth of EBV-immortalized B cell lines. Similarly, the depletion of T cell activity in vivo through pharmacological immunosuppression may result in the outgrowth of EBV-immortalized B cells. If a mutation confers an added proliferative advantage on a particular clone, then the proliferation will appear clonal. In support of this hypothesized pathogenesis is the pattern of latent viral antigen expression. The latent viral membrane proteins and all of the EBNAs, including those with growth transforming and immortalizing properties, are expressed just as in spontaneous EBV-transformants in vitro (Table 2). Interestingly enough, when T cell dysfunction is reversed, as when immunosuppressive therapy is withdrawn, these B cell lesions commonly regress. This regression may reflect the broad pattern of viral gene expression, in that the EBNA-2, -3A, -3B, and 3C proteins are the antigens most commonly targeted by cytotoxic T cells.

There are two animal models of EBV-associated tumours that parallel post-transplant lymphoproliferative disease. Multifocal, diffuse large cell, B-cell tumours that express the full range of EBV latency antigens arise following the intravenous administration of virus into cotton top tamarins.[69] The susceptibility of the cottontop tamarin to develop these EBV-driven lymphomas is not well understood but appears to relate to the non-polymorphic nature of the tamarins' major histocompatibility complex class I genes.[70] The second group of model tumours are EBV-associated human B cell lymphomas in mice with severe combined immunodeficiency (SCID).[67,71,72] These tumours may result from the direct injection of EBV-immortalized human lymphoblastoid B-cell lines or may arise following the intraperitoneal injection of human peripheral blood mononuclear cells from EBV-seropositive donors. In the latter instance, it appears that cytotoxic T cell-mediated control of naturally infected EBV-infected B cells eventually wanes allowing proliferation of EBV-infected cells. In parallel with the tamarin tumours, the human tumours in mice are also mutlifocal B-cell tumours expressing the full range of EBV latency antigens in a *latency III* pattern.

EBV-associated lymphomas account for approximately half of the B cell lymphomas arising in immunodeficiency patients.[73–76] Curiously, Burkitt's lymphomas in AIDS patients are usually not EBV associated. Diffuse large cell lymphomas are more commonly associated with EBV, particularly those with immunoblastic features, or those occurring in patients with very low CD4 counts. Primary central nervous system lymphomas occurring in AIDS patients are striking for their uniform EBV association.[77, 78] These tumours arise very late in the course of HIV infection, generally in patients with very low CD4 counts and commonly have immunoblastic features.

A non-lymphoid tumour, nasopharyngeal carcinoma, is also associated with EBV (Table 2).[79, 80] Like Burkitt's lymphoma, the incidence of nasopharyngeal carcinoma shows wide geographical variation. The disease occurs most commonly in men in areas of southern China and in people of southern Chinese extraction. In contrast to Burkitt's lymphoma, the EBV association with nasopharyngeal carcinoma is nearly 100% and seems to be independent of geography, i.e. cases that arise in low incidence areas are non the less EBV associated.

EBV in Hodgkin's disease

The initial studies demonstrating the presence of EBV in a subset of patients with Hodgkin's disease utilized blot hybridization procedures.[19, 21, 22] Blot hybridization procedures also provided evidence that the virus was associated with a monoclonal proliferation of cells. These studies utilized recombinant plasmid clones of the EBV terminal repeats to probe Southern blots of EBV(+) Hodgkin's disease and demonstrated single bands reflecting the presence of unique episomes. As discussed above and illustrated in Fig. 2, the detection of episomes with a fixed number of terminal repeats suggests a clonal expansion of a single latently infected cell. In Hodgkin's disease, this clonal population seemed most likely to be the Reed–Sternberg cells and their variants. Because Reed–Sternberg cells often constitute less than 1% of the cells in a tumour mass, and blotting procedures were at the limits of their sensitivity in detecting 1 copy per cell in 1% of cells, there was the possibility that all Hodgkin's disease was EBV associated but that, in many cases, the viral genome was present at copy numbers below the threshold of Southern blot detections. Polymerase chain reaction amplification overcame these issues of sensitivity and demonstrated conclusively that, in a substantial fraction of specimens, EBV DNA is absent.[81]

The definitive localization of virus in tumour came from in situ hybridization and antigen detection studies. The first in situ hybridization studies used probes containing the large internal repeat to detect viral DNA.[20, 22] These studies demonstrated the presence of EBV in the Reed–Sternberg cells but were relatively insensitive and associated with high background. This was because the viral DNA is present in relatively low copy number in latently infected cells.

With the goal of developing a universal probe for EBV latent infection in tumour specimens, our group targeted the abundant EBER transcripts for detection by in situ hybridization in clinical specimens. The high copy number expression of the EBERs in latently infected B-cell lines in tissue culture had previously been characterized.[82] Although their function was and is unknown, we reasoned that these transcripts must be readily detectable. Single-stranded RNA antisense probes, labelled with ^{3}H, and later with digoxigenin, demonstrated hybridization in cell lines with only two copies of the EBV genome and in the Reed–Sternberg cells of Hodgkin's disease specimens that had been positive by Southern blot (Fig.3).[79, 83, 84]

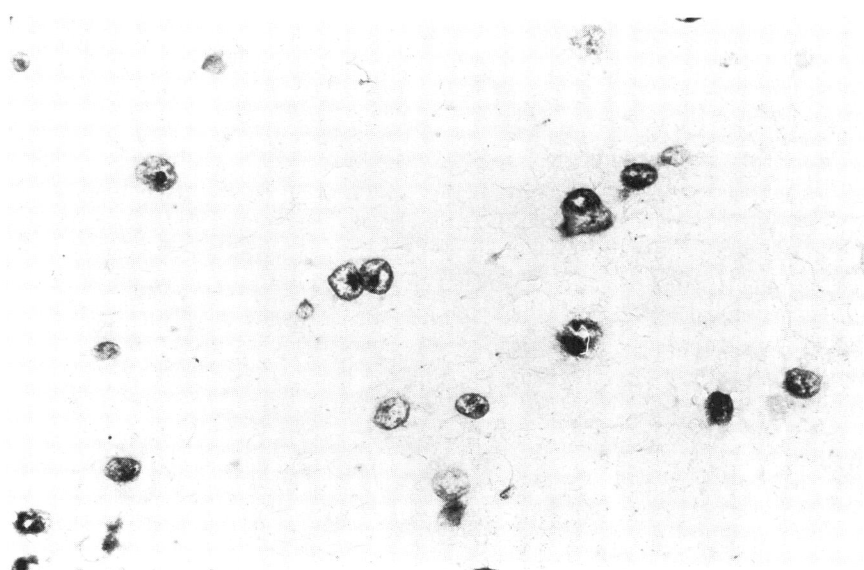

Fig. 3. Hodgkin's disease. In situ hybridization with digoxigenin-labelled EBER1-antisense riboprobe. Hybridization signal is localized to the nucleus of large malignant cells. It characteristically clumps against the nuclear rim and nucleolus and spares areas of the nucleoplasm. (Reprinted with permission of the American Society for Investigative Pathology.)

With technical improvements, it became clear that, in some specimens, occasional small lymphocytes were also EBER positive.[85,86]

Immunohistochemistry to detect LMP-1, has proven to be another useful way to detect latent virus in tumour specimens. Although LMP-1 is not detected in Burkitt's lymphoma and is inconsistently expressed in nasopharyngeal carcinoma, it is readily and consistently detected in the Reed–Sternberg cells of EBV-associated Hodgkin's disease.[87,88] In contrast to the EBERs, LMP-1 is only found in Reed–Sternberg cells and never in small infiltrating lymphocytes. With technical improvements in both hybridization and antigen detection, it became clear and is now generally accepted that there is a nearly perfect correlation between the detection of EBER hybridization signal in Reed–Sternberg cells and the detection of the LMP-1 antigen by immunohistochemisty. The relationship of the variably present infiltrating EBER(+) lymphocytes to the tumour or its pathogenesis is entirely unknown.

The pattern of EBV gene expression in Hodgkin's disease is more restricted than that associated with EBV-immortalized lymphoblastoid cell lines or post-transplant lymphoproliferative disease (Table 2). EBNA-1 but none of the immunogenic EBNAs are expressed, and there is no transcription from the C_p or W_p latency promoters.[89] In this respect, Hodgkin's disease is similar to all EBV-associated tumours that arise in patients that are not profoundly immunocompromised. In Hodgkin's disease as noted above, LMP-1 is expressed. The expression of LMP-1 is very consistent in EBV-associated Hodgkin's disease in contrast to nasopharyngeal carcinoma. Whereas in a substantial fraction of nasopharyngeal carcinoma specimens LMP-1 expression is not detected, the protein is detected in virtually every case of EBV-associated Hodgkin's disease as determined by EBER in situ hybridization signal in malignant cells. The exceptional cases of EBV-associated Hodgkin's disease in which LMP-1 cannot be detected may reflect technical problems rather than the existence of a subset of EBER(+), LMP(−) tumours. LMP-2 RNA has been detected in EBV-associated Hodgkin's disease, but reagents are not yet available to determine whether the viral antigens are expressed. In general, the virus is latent in tumour tissue, but the immediate-early lytic antigen ZTA (also referred to as BZLF1, ZEBRA, or the Z protein) has occasionally been detected in Hodgkin's diseass.[90]

Epidemiology of EBV-tumour association in Hodgkin's disease

The histological subtypes of Hodgkin's disease differ in their EBV associations. Mixed cellularity Hodgkin's disease is highly associated with EBV by EBER1 hybridization and LMP-1 immunohistochemistry in all populations studied.[85,87,88,91–94] This generalization applies to children and adults, males and females, North America, Europe, Latin America, and Asia. In the

United States and Europe, mixed cellularity accounts for about 30% of Hodgkin's disease and occurs most commonly in males. In developing countries, Hodgkin's disease occurs most commonly in childhood, and mixed cellularity histology accounts for a larger percentage of cases. Nodular sclerosis Hodgkin's disease is variably associated with EBV. In North America and Europe, where nodular sclerosis accounts for about 60% of all Hodgkin's disease, EBV is associated with less than 35% of cases. In contrast, in some developing nations, the association is very much stronger. Lymphocyte predominant disease is relatively rare, accounting for approximately 5% of Hodgkin's tumours. It is only occasionally associated with EBV in the largest series.[87,88,93] Lymphocyte depletion is the least common subtype of Hodgkin's disease and, with refinements in the histological diagnosis of Hodgkin's disease, it now appears that some of what was previously classified as lymphocyte depletion Hodgkin's disease is better classified as non-Hodgkin's lymphoma. The EBV association or lack thereof is not yet well characterized.

Some have suggested that there is variation in the fraction of Hodgkin's disease tumours that are EBV associated as a function of age. Younger and older patients are reported to have a higher percentage of EBV-associated tumours.[95] However, younger and older patients are also most likely to have mixed cellularity disease, so there is the potential for some confounding.

Therapeutic implications

The presence of EBV appears not to be associated with an altered prognosis except perhaps in so far as it identifies mixed cellularity histology and thus is more often associated with more advanced disease.[96] On the other hand, EBV may provide a multitude of targets for therapeutic intervention in patients with EBV-associated Hodgkin's disease. Tumour cells carrying the viral genome express, or have the potential to express, 80–100 foreign (viral) genes. Each of these viral proteins carries epitopes that are specific to viral infected cells. Even in patients with EBV-associated Hodgkin's disease, EBV infects very few non-malignant cells, while every tumour cell (identified morphologically or by double labelling with CD30) carries the viral genome. In contrast, mutations of cellular genes associated with malignancy provide relatively few foreign (unique) targets for immunotherapy. In chronic myelogenous leukaemia, for example, unique epitopes that might be targeted by the immune system are limited to those defined by short peptides from the fusion joint of the BCR–ABL protein. In follicular lymphomas, the chromosomal translocation does not result in any epitopes unique to the tumour but rather to dysregulated expression of BCL-2. Even when unique peptide sequences are present in tumour cells, they are not necessarily recognized by the immune system. It is not yet clear, for instance, whether the BCR-ABL protein elicits a cytotoxic T cell response in patients with chronic myelogenous leukaemia. One of the attractions of EBV antigens as targets for immunotherapy is the knowledge that not only are many of these proteins tumour specific in practical terms, but that they are also demonstrably targeted by the immune system in healthy seropositive individuals.

One family of EBV-associated lymphomas is already therapeutically approached immunologically.[97,98] In EBV-associated lymphomas arising in the setting of organ transplantation, viral antigens commonly recognized by cytotoxic T cells are often expressed. Cytotoxic T cell killing of EBV-infected cells is presumably responsible for EBV-lymphoproliferative disease regression that commonly follows withdrawal of immunosuppressive therapy in solid organ transplant recipients or transfusion of donor lymphocytes in allogeneic bone marrow recipients.[97,98] The immunotherapeutic approach to Hodgkin's tumours will be more challenging because the spectrum of viral antigen expression is more limited. Thus the tasks that await us are to define any specific immunological defects in patients with EBV-associated Hodgkin's disease as they relate to EBV, and to find ways to augment the immune response to the viral antigens expressed in tumours in these patients. Possible approaches to targeting viral antigens expressed in Reed–Sternberg cells might include the use of antibodies with or without toxin or radio conjugates; adoptive cellular immunotherapy with cytotoxic T cell lines or clones in the setting of marrow transplantation; or therapeutic vaccines to establish or increase a humoral or cellular immune response.

References

(1) Grufferman S, Delzell E. Epidemiology of Hodgkin's disease. *Epid Rev* 1984; 6: 76–106.

(2) Mueller N. An epidemiologist's view of the new molecular biology findings in Hodgkin's disease. *Ann Oncol* 1991; 2: 23–8.

(3) Glaser SL, Swartz WG. Time trends in Hodgkin's disease incidence. The role of diagnostic accuracy. *Cancer* 1990; 66: 2196–204.

(4) MacMahon B. Epidemiology of Hodgkin's disease. *Cancer Res.* 1966; 26: 1189–200.

(5) MacMahon B, Cole P. Hodgkin's disease: one entity or two? *Lancet* 1971; 1: 240–1.

(6) Correa P, O'Conor GT. Epidemiologic patterns of Hodgkin's disease. *Int J Cancer* 1971; 8: 192–201.

(7) Evans AS, Gutensohn NM. A population-based case-control study of EBV and other viral antibodies among persons with Hodgkin's disease and their siblings. *Int J Cancer* 1984; 34: 149–57.

(8) Gutensohn N, Cole P. Childhood social environment and Hodgkin's disease. *N Engl J Med* 1981; 304: 135–40.

(9) Newell G. Etiology of multiple sclerosis and Hodgkin's disease. *Am J Epidemiol* 1970; 91: 119–22.

(10) Mueller N. Epidemiologic studies assessing the role of the Epstein–Barr virus in Hodgkin's disease. *Yale J Biol Med* 1987; 60: 321–7.

(11) Johansson B, Klein G, Henle W, Henle G. Epstein–Barr virus (EBV) associated antibody patterns in malignant lymphoma and leukemia. I. Hodgkin's disease. *Int J Cancer* 1970; 6: 450–62.
(12) Levine PH, Ablashi DV, Berard CW, Carbone PP, Waggoner DE, Malan L. Elevated antibody titers to Epstein–Barr virus in Hodgkin's disease. *Cancer* 1971; 27: 416–21.
(13) Miller RW, Beebe GW. Infectious mononucleosis and the empirical risk of cancer. *J Natl Cancer Inst* 1973; 50: 315–21.
(14) Rosdahl N, Larsen SO, Clemmesen J. Hodgkin's disease in patients with previous infectious mononucleosis: 30 years' experience. *Br Med J* 1974; 2: 253–6.
(15) Munoz N, Davidson RJL, Witthoff B, Ericsson JE, de-The G. Infectious mononucleosis and Hodgkin's disease. *Int J Cancer* 1978; 22: 1–3.
(16) Hesse J, Andersen E, Levine PH, Ebbesen P, Halberg P, Reisher JI. Antibodies to Epstein–Barr virus and cellular immunity in Hodgkin's disease and chronic lymphatic leukemia. *Int J Cancer* 1973; 11: 237–43.
(17) Mueller N, Evans A, Harris N et al. Hodgkin's disease and Epstein–Barr virus: altered antibody patterns before diagnosis. *N Engl J Med* 1989; 320: 689–92.
(18) Poppema S, van Imhoff G, Torensma R, Smit J. Lymphadenopathy morphologically consistent with Hodgkin's disease associated with Epstein–Barr virus infection. *Am J Clin Pathol* 1985; 84: 385–90.
(19) Weiss LM, Strickler JG, Warnke RA, Purtilo DT, Sklar J. Epstein–Barr viral DNA in tissues of Hodgkin's disease. *Am J Pathol* 1987; 129: 86–91.
(20) Weiss LM, Movahed LA, Warnke RA, Sklar J. Detection of Epstein–Barr viral genomes in Reed–Sternberg cells of Hodgkin's disease. *N Engl J Med* 1989; 320: 502–6.
(21) Staal SP, Ambinder R, Beschorner WE, Hayward GS, Mann R. A survey of Epstein–Barr virus DNA in lymphoid tissue: frequent detection in Hodgkin's disease. *Am J Clin Pathol* 1989; 91: 1–5.
(22) Anagnostopoulos I, Herbst H, Niedobitek G, Stein H. Demonstration of monoclonal EBV genomes in Hodgkin's disease and Ki−1 positive anaplastic large cell lymphoma by combined Southern blot and in situ hybridization. *Blood* 1989; 74: 810–16.
(23) Libetta CM, Pringle JH, Angel CA, Craft AW, Malcolm AJ, Lauder I. Demonstration of Epstein–Barr viral DNA in formalin-fixed, paraffin-embedded samples of Hodgkin's disease. *J Pathol* 1990; 161: 255–60.
(24) Boiocchi M, DeRe V, Dolcetti R, Carbone A, Scarpa A, Menestrina F. Association of EBV genome with mixed cellularity and cellular phase nodular sclerosis Hodgkin's disease subtypes. *Ann Oncol* 1992; 3: 307–10.
(25) Armstrong AA, Alexander FE, Paes RP et al. Association of Epstein–Barr virus with pediatric Hodgkin's disease. *Am J Pathol* 1993; 142: 1683–8.
(26) Liebowitz D, Kieff E. Epstein–Barr virus. In: Roizman B, Whitley RJ, Lopez C, eds. *The human Herpesviruses*. New York: Raven Press; 1993: 107–72.
(27) Miller G. Epstein–Barr virus. Biology, pathogenesis, and medical aspects. In: Fields BN, Knipe DM, eds. *Virology. 3rd ed* New York: Raven Press; 1990: 1921–58.

(28) Ambinder RF, Mann RB. Detection of Epstein-Barr virus in clinical specimens. *Am J Pathol* 1994; 145: 239–52.
(29) Gulley ML, Raphael M, Lutz CT, Ross DW, Raab-Traub N. Epstein–Barr virus integration in human lymphomas and lymphoid cell lines. *Cancer* 1992; 70: 185–91.
(30) Hurley EA, Agger S, McNeil JA et al. When Epstein–Barr virus persistently infects B–cell lines, it frequently integrates. *J Virol* 1991; 65: 1245–54.
(31) Baer B, Bankier A, Biggin MD, et al. DNA sequence and expression of the B95–8 Epstein–Barr virus genome. *Nature* 1984; 310: 207–11.
(32) Raab-Traub N, Flynn K. The structure of the termini of the Epstein–Barr virus as a marker of clonal cellular proliferation. *Cell* 1986; 47: 883–9.
(33) Sato H, Takimoto T, Tanaka S, Tanaka J, Raab-Traub N. Concatameric replication of Epstein–Barr virus: structure of the termini in virus-producer and newly transformed cell lines. *J Virol* 1993; 64: 5295–300.
(34) Yates JL, Warren N, Sugden B. Stable replication of plasmids derived from Epstein–Barr virus in various mammalian cells. *Nature* 1985; 313: 812–5.
(35) Chen MR, Middeldorp JM, Hayward SD. Separation of the complex DNA binding domain of EBNA-1 into DNA recognition and dimerization subdomains of novel structure. *J Virol* 1993; 67: 4875–85.
(36) Ling PD, Rawlins DR, Hayward SD. The EBV immortalizing protein EBNA-2 is targeted to DNA by a cellular enhancer-binding protein. *Proc Natl Acad Sci USA* 1993; 90: 9237–41.
(37) Zimber-Strobl U, Kremmer E, Grasser F, Marschall G, Laux G, Bornkamm GW. The EBV nuclear antigen 2 interacts with an EBNA2 responsive *cis*-element of the terminal protein 1 gene promoter. *EMBO J* 1993; 12: 167–76.
(38) Moorthy RK, Thorley-Lawson DA. Biochemical, genetic, and functional analyses of the phosphorylation sites on the EBV-encoded oncogenic latent membrane protein LMP-1. *J Virol* 1993; 67: 2637–45.
(39) Kaye KM, Izumi KM, Kieff E. Epstein–Barr virus latent membrane protein-1 is essential for B-lymphocyte growth transformation. *Proc Natl Acad Sci USA* 1993; 90: 9150–4.
(40) Swaminathan S, Huneycutt BS, Reiss CS, Kieff E. Epstein–Barr virus-encoded small RNAs (EBERs) do not modulate interferon effects in infected lymphocytes. *J Virol* 1992; 66: 5133–6.
(41) Longnecker R, Miller CL, Tomkinson B, Miao X, Kieff E. Deletion of DNA encoding the first five transmembrane domains of Epstein–Barr virus latent membrane proteins 2A and 2B. *J Virol* 1993; 67: 5068–74.
(42) Longnecker R, Miller CL, Miao XQ, Tomkinson B, Kieff E. The last seven transmembrane and carboxy-terminal cytoplastic domains of Epstein–Barr virus latent membrane protein 2 (LMP2) are dispensable for lymphocyte infection and growth transformation in vitro. *J Virol* 1993; 67: 2006–13.
(43) Ambinder R, Mann R. EBER in situ hybridization. *Hum Pathol* 1994; 25: 602–5.
(44) Rowe M, Rowe DT, Gregory CD. et al. Differences in B cell growth phenotype reflect novel patterns of Epstein–Barr virus latent gene expression in Burkitt's lymphoma cells. *EMBO J* 1987; 6: 2743–51.

(45) Rowe M, Lear AL, Croom-Carter D, Davies AH, Rickinson AB. Three pathways of Epstein–Barr virus gene activation from EBNA1-positive latency in B lymphocytes. *J Virol* 1992; 66: 122–31.
(46) Sample J, Brooks L, Sample C et al. Restricted Epstein–Barr virus protein expression in Burkitt lymphoma is due to a different Epstein–Barr nuclear antigen 1 transcriptional initiation site. *Proc Natl Acad Sci USA* 1991; 88: 6343–7.
(47) Smith PR, Griffin BE. Transcription of the Epstein–Barr virus gene EBNA-1 from different promoters in nasopharyngeal carcinoma and B-lymphoblastoid cells. *J Virol* 1992; 66: 706–14.
(48) Schaeffer BC, Woistschlaeger M, Strominger JL, Speck SH. Exclusive expression of Epstein–Barr virus nuclear antigen 1 in Burkitt lymphoma arises from a third promoter, distinct from the promoters used in latently infected lymphocytes. *Proc Natl Acad Sci USA* 1991; 88: 6550–4.
(49) Rooney CM, Brimmell M, Buschle M, Allan G, Farrell PJ, Kolman JL. Host cell and EBNA-2 regulation of EBV latent-cycle promoter activity in B lymphocytes. *J Virol* 1992; 66: 496–504.
(50) Yandava CN, Speck SH. Characterization of the deletion and rearrangement in the BamHI C region of the X50-7 Epstein–Barr virus genome, a mutant viral strain which exhibits constitutive BamHI W promoter activity. *J Virol* 1992; 66: 5646–50.
(51) Flemington EK, Boras AM, Lytle JP, Speck SH. Characterization of the Epstein–Barr virus BZLF1 protein transactivation domain. *J Virol* 1992; 66: 922–9.
(52) Birkenbach M, Tong X, Bradbury LE, Tedder TF, Kieff E. Characterization of an Epstein–Barr virus receptor on human epithelial cells. *J Exp Med* 1992; 176: 1405–14.
(53) Sixbey JW, Yao Q. Immunoglobulin A-induced shift of Epstein–Barr virus tissue tropism. *Science* 1992; 255: 1578–80.
(54) Evans A, Niederman J. Epstein–Barr virus. In: Evans A, ed. *Viral infections of humans*. Plenum Medical Book Company; 1991: 265–92.
(55) Young LS, Lau R, Rowe M et al. Differentiation-associated expression of the Epstein–Barr virus BZLF1 transactivator protein in oral hairy leukoplakia. *J Virol* 1991; 65: 2868–74.
(56) Moss DJ, Burrows SR, Khanna R, Misko IS, Sculley TB. Immune surveillance against Epstein–Barr virus. *Semin Immunol* 1992; 4: 97–104.
(57) Bourgault I, Gomez A, Gomard E, Levy JP. Limiting-dilution analysis of the HLA restriction of anti-Epstein–Barr virus-specific cytolytic T lymphocytes. *Clin Exp Immunol* 1991; 84: 501–7.
(58) Carmichael A, Jin X, Sissons P, Borysiewicz L. Quantitative analysis of the human immunodeficiency virus type 1 (HIV-1)-specific cytotoxic T lymphocyte (CTL) response at different stages of HIV-1 infection: differential CTL responses to HIV-1 and Epstein–Barr virus in late disease. *J Exp Med* 1993; 177: 249–56.
(59) Murray RJ, Kurilla MG, Brooks JM et al. Identification of target antigens for the human cytotoxic T cell response to Epstein–Barr virus (EBV): implications for the immune control of EBV-positive malignancies. *J Exp Med* 1992; 176: 157–68.

(60) Khanna R, Burrows SR, Kurilla MG et al. Localization of Epstein–Barr virus cytotoxic T cell epitopes using recombinant vaccinia: implications for vaccine development. *J Exp Med* 1992; 176: 169–76.
(61) Kurilla MG. Target antigens of EBV and the implications for immune control of EBV-associated disease. *Semin Virol* 1993; 4: 95–100.
(62) Yao QY, Rowe M, Martin B, Young LS, Rickinson AB. The EBV carrier state: dominance of a single growth transforming isolate in the blood and in the oropharynx of healthy virus carriers. *J Gen Virol* 1991; 72: 1579–90.
(63) Rowe M, Gregory C. Epstein-Barr virus and Burkitt's lymphoma. In: Klein G, ed. *Advances in viral oncology, Volume 8, Tumorigenic DNA viruses.* New York: Raven Press; 1989: 237–58.
(64) Shiramizu B, Barriga F, Neequaye J et al. Patterns of chromosomal breakpoint locations in Burkitt's lymphoma: relevance to geography and Epstein–Barr virus association. *Blood* 1991; 77: 1516–26.
(65) Jain VK, Judde JG, Max EE, Magrath IT. Variable IgH chain enhancer activity in Burkitt's lymphomas suggests an additional, direct mechanism of c-myc deregulation. *J Immunol* 1993; 150: 5418–28.
(66) Gratama JW, Zutter MM, Minarovits J et al. Expression of Epstein–Barr virus-encoded growth-transformation-associated proteins in lymphoproliferations of bone-marrow transplant recipients. *Int J Cancer* 1991; 47: 188–92.
(67) Rowe M, Young LS, Crocker J, Stokes H, Henderson S, Rickinson AB. Epstein–Barr virus (EBV)-associated lymphoproliferative disease in the SCID mouse model: implications for the pathogenesis of EBV-positive lymphomas in man. *J Exp Med* 1991; 173: 147–58.
(68) Young L, Alfieri C, Hennessy K et al. Expression of Epstein–Barr virus transformation-associated genes in tissues of patients with EBV lymphoproliferative disease. *N Engl J Med* 1989; 321: 1080–5.
(69) Young LS, Finerty S, Brooks L, Scullion F, Rickinson AB, Morgan AJ. Epstein–Barr virus gene expression in malignant lymphomas induced by experimental virus infection of cottontop tamarins. *J Virol* 1989; 63: 1967–74.
(70) Watkins DI, Chen ZW, Hughes AL, Evans MG, Tedder TF, Letvin NL. Evolution of the MHC class I genes of a New World primate from ancestral homologues of human non-classical genes. *Nature* 1990; 346: 60–3.
(71) Cannon MJ, Pisa P, Fox RI, Cooper NR. Epstein–Barr virus induces aggressive lymphoproliferative disorders of human B cell origin in SCID/hu chimeric mice. *J Clin Invest* 1990; 85: 1333–7.
(72) Mosier DE, Gulizia RJ, Baird SM, Wilson DB. Transfer of a functional human immune system to mice with severe combined immunodeficiency. *Nature* 1988; 335: 256–9.
(73) Shibata D, Weiss LM. Hernandez AM, Nathwani BN, Bernstein L, Levine AM. Epstein–Barr virus-associated non-Hodgkin's lymphoma in patients infected with the human immunodeficiency virus. *Blood* 1993; 81: 2102–9.
(74) Hamilton-Dutoit SJ, Pallesen G, Franzmann MB et al. AIDS-related lymphoma: Histopathology, immunophenotype, and association with Epstein–Barr virus as demonstrated by in situ nucleic acid hybridization. *Am J Pathol* 1991; 138: 149–63.
(75) Subar M, Neri A, Inghirami G, Knowles DM, Dalla-Favera R. Frequent

c-myc oncogene activation and infrequent presence of Epstein–Barr virus genome in AIDS-associated lymphoma. *Blood* 1988; 72: 667–71.
(76) Hamilton-Dutoit SJ, Rea D, Raphael M et al. Epstein–Barr virus latent gene expression and tumor cell phenotype in AIDS-related non-Hodgkin's lymphoma. *Am J Pathol* 1993; 143: 1072–85.
(77) MacMahon EME, Glass JD, Hayward SD et al. Epstein–Barr virus in AIDS-related primary central nervous system lymphoma. *Lancet* 1991; 338: 969–73.
(78) Chang KL, Flaris N, Hickey WF, Johnson RM, Meyer JS, Weiss LM. Brain lymphomas of immunocompetent and immunocompromised patients: study of the association with Epstein–Barr virus. *Mod Path* 1993; 6: 427–31.
(79) Wu T, Mann RB, Epstein J et al. Abundant expression of EBER1 small nuclear RNA in nasopharyngeal carcinoma: A morphologically distinctive target for detection of Epstein–Barr virus in formalin-fixed paraffin-embedded carcinoma specimens. *Am J Pathol* 1991; 138: 1461–9.
(80) de-The G, Ho JHC, Muir CS. Nasopharyngeal carcinoma. In: Evans AS, ed. *Viral infections of humans–epidemiology and control*. 3rd ed. New York: Plenum Publishing Corporation; 1991: 737–67.
(81) Ambinder RF, Wu T, Lambe B et al. Absence of EBV in Reed–Sternberg cells in many cases of Hodgkin's disease. In: Ablashi DV, ed. *Epstein–Barr virus and human disease*. New Jersey: Humana Press; 1991: 277–81.
(82) Howe JG, Steitz JA. Localization of Epstein–Barr virus-encoded small RNAs by in situ hybridization. *Proc Natl Acad Sci USA* 1986; 83: 9006–10.
(83) Wu T, Mann RB, Charache P et al. Detection of EBV gene expression in Reed–Sternberg cells of Hodgkin's disease. *Int J Cancer* 1990; 46: 801–4.
(84) Wu T, MacMahon EME, Zhang J et al. EBER1 small nuclear RNA in malignancy: a morphologically distinctive target for detection of EBV in formalin-fixed paraffin-embedded specimens. In: Ablashi DV, Huang AT, Pagano JS, Pearson GR, Yang CS, eds. *Epstein–Barr virus and human disease*. New Jersey: Humana Press; 1991: 163–7.
(85) Ambinder RF, Browning PJ, Lorenzana I et al. Epstein–Barr virus and childhood Hodgkin's disease in Honduras and the United States. *Blood* 1993; 81: 462–7.
(86) Lee M, C. K, Cabanillas F, Freireich EJ, Trujillo JM, Stass SA. *Science* 1987; 237: 175–8.
(87) Pallesen G, Hamilton-Dutoit SJ, Rowe M, Young LS. Expression of Epstein–Barr virus (EBV) latent gene products in tumour cells of Hodgkin's disease. *Lancet* 1991; 337: 320–2.
(88) Delsol G, Brousset P, Chittal S, Rigal-Huguett F. Correlation of the expression of Epstein–Barr virus latent membrane protein and in situ hybridization with biotinylated BamH1-W probes in Hodgkin's disease. *Am J Pathol* 1992; 140: 247–53.
(89) Deacon EM, Pallesen G, Niedobitek G et al. Epstein–Barr virus and Hodgkin's disease: transcriptional analysis of virus latency in the malignant cells. *J Exp Med* 1993; 177: 339–49.
(90) Pallesen G, Sandvej K, Hamilton–Dutoit SJ, Rowe M, Young LS. Activation of Epstein–Barr virus replication in Hodgkin and Reed–Sternberg cells. *Blood* 1991; 78: 1162–5.

(91) Khan G, Norton AJ, Slavin G. Epstein–Barr virus in Hodgkin's disease – relationship to age and subtype. *Cancer* 1993; 71: 3124–9.
(92) Weiss LM, Chen YY, Liu XF, Shibata D. Epstein–Barr virus and Hodgkin's disease: a correlative in situ hybridization and polymerase chain reaction study. *Am J Pathol* 1991; 139: 1259–65.
(93) Murray PG, Young LS, Rowe M, Crocker J. Immunohistochemical diagnosis of the EBV-encoded latent membrane protein in paraffin sections of Hodgkin's disease. *J Pathol* 1992; 166: 1–5.
(94) Chang KL, Albújar PF, Chen YY, Johnson RM, Weiss LM. High prevalence of Epstein–Barr virus in the Reed–Sternberg cells of Hodgkin's disease occurring in Peru. *Blood* 1993; 81: 496–501.
(95) Jarrett RF, Gallagher A, Jones DB et al. Detection of Epstein–Barr virus genomes in Hodgkin's disease: relation to age. *J Clin Path* 1991; 44: 844–8.
(96) Vestlev PM, Pallesen G, Sandvej K, Hamilton-Dutoit SJ, Bendtzen SM. Prognosis of Hodgkin's disease is not influenced by EBV latent membrane protein. *Int J Cancer* 1992; 50: 670–1.
(97) Papadopoulos E, Ladanyi M, Emanuel D et al. Infusions of donor leukocytes to treat Epstein–Barr virus-associated lymphoproliferative disorders after allogeneic bone marrow transplantation. *N Engl J Med* 1994; 33: 1185–91.
(98) Lieberman J, Buchsbaum R. Using T cells to treat B-cell cancers. *N Engl J Med* 1994; 330: 1231–3.

Hodgkin's disease and its treatment in sub-Saharan Africa

W R BEZWODA, A P McPHAIL, R DANSEY, L SEYMOUR, F SITAS, R COHN and J POOLE

Introduction

The title begs the question as to whether either Hodgkin's disease (HD) or its treatment in sub-Saharan Africa is sufficiently different to warrant separate consideration. The aim of this chapter will be to show that, while the features of HD as seen in Africa fall recognizably within the ambit of the the clinico-pathologic complex that we have come to recognize as constituting Hodgkin's disease, the emphasis, including therapeutic emphasis, is somewhat different in Africa as compared to the developed countries.

Epidemiology and pathology

Ethnic (? genetic/lifestyle), geographical and/or socioeconomic-based variations of the incidence, age at presentation and frequency distribution of specific histological subtypes as well as therapeutic outcomes of Hodgkin's disease have been noted in a number of publications.[1–6]

Hodgkin's disease appears to increase in frequency from the equatorial to the more temperate zones south of the equator. Age-standardized rates for males and females reported from Uganda during the period 1964–1968 (for which fairly complete statistics are available) were far below those reported for Europe and North America.[6,7] Reports from other African countries within the tropical zone are based largely on single institution reports from academic centres or from large regional hospitals and are mostly characterized by a low frequency of Hodgkin's disease relative to other malignancies, except in the childhood age group. While a substantially higher incidence, approaching that seen in the Northern hemisphere was reported from the Ibadan Province of Western Nigeria,[8] this experience

All correspondence to: Professor WR Bezwoda, Department of Medicine, University of Witwatersrand Medical School, York Road, Parktown 2193, Johannesburg, South Africa.

Cambridge Medical Reviews: Haematological Oncology Volume 4

appears to have been unique and may reflect intra-regional variation owing to undefined specific local factors. Relatively low frequencies of HD are reported from Zambia,[8] Kenya[10] and Zimbabwe.[11] Age-adjusted incidence rates for HD reported from other sub-Saharan countries with cancer registries such as Mali, Uganda and The Gambia are generally < 0.8 per 100 000 population.[12]

Data from the National Cancer registry in South Africa[13] show the age-adjusted incidence (world standard) rates for Hodgkin's disease (HD) to be 0.81 for black females as compared to 1.42 for white females and 0.95 and 3.37 for black and for white males respectively, apparently confirming a lower frequency of HD in the black population. The low rates in the black population may, however, be partly due to underreporting as this is a pathology-based registry.

The age distribution of Hodgkin's disease in developing countries also appears to be different as compared to Europe and North America. World-wide, four epidemiological patterns of occurrence have been suggested.[14,15] Type 1 is characterized by high rates in children and predominance of histological subtypes associated with a poor prognosis with little Hodgkin's disease occurring in older age groups. The type III pattern is characterized by high rates in young adults and predominance of features such as favourable histological subtype associated with better outcome.

Type II is intermediate between types I and III.

Type IV is a low incidence at all ages and is the pattern encountered in Asia. The Type I pattern appears to be the dominant pattern described from hospital-based registries and studies from north–central and central Africa. A study from Zambia,[9] for example, showed that Hodgkin's disease accounted for some 18.6% of malignant lymphomas with 44% of cases occurring in the first two decades of life. The patients were predominantly of more advanced stage and the majority had either mixed cellularity or lymphocyte depleted subtypes. Similar clinical presentations are reported from Nigeria,[8] Kenya,[10,16,17] Uganda[7,17] and Zimbabwe[11,19] although a single series from Uganda, which again may represent intraregional variation, does report a bimodal age-specific incidence curve approximating the type III pattern.

Childhood Hodgkin's disease has previously been reported to be relatively frequent among black children in South Africa.[21] More recent data suggest that, although there may be a peak of incidence of Hodgkin's disease occurring around age 15–19 amongst black children,[13] the overall frequency of HD is lower in blacks of all ages, including the childhood years, as compared to whites (Fig. 1).[13] Hodgkin's disease in the southern part of the African continent (Table 1) appears to be predominantly of the intermediate or type II pattern and more closely approximates the epidemiology seen in the North American black population during the 1950s and 1960s,[22]

(*a*)

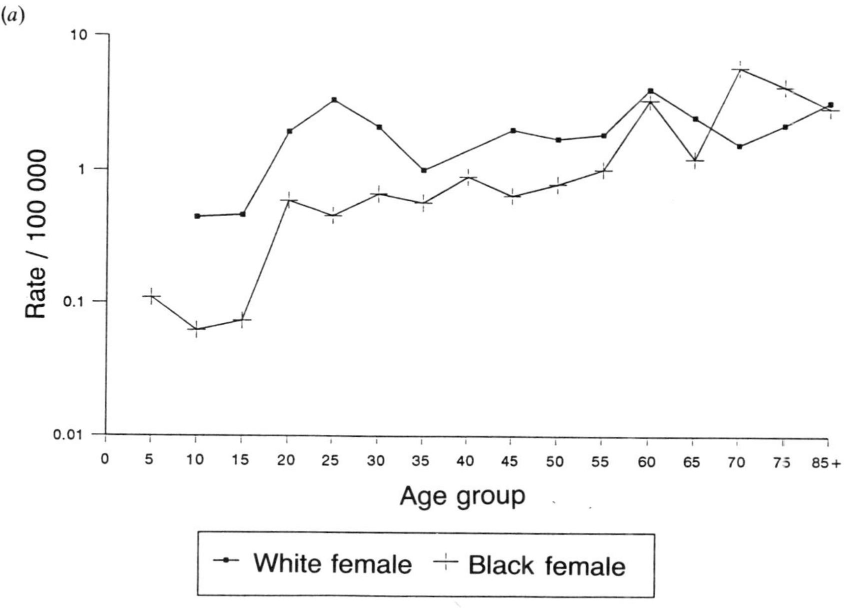

(*b*)

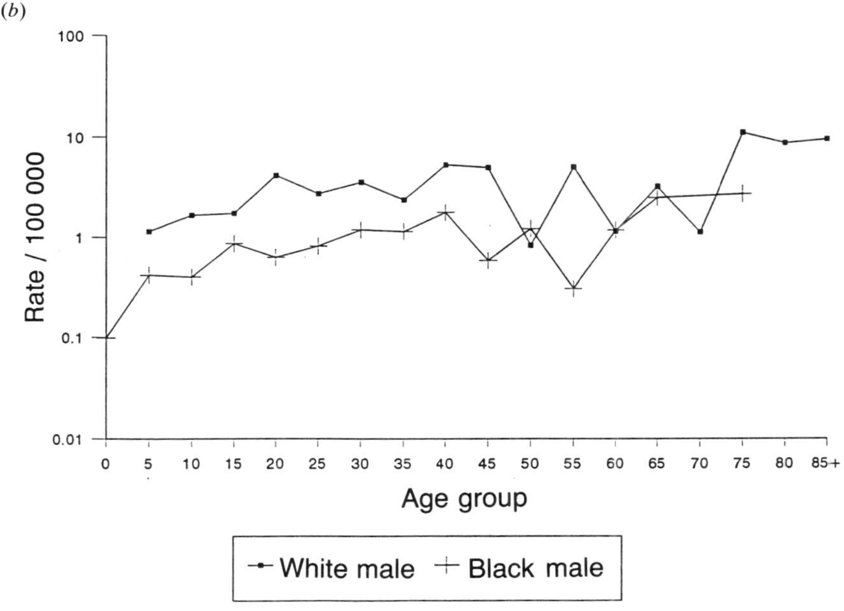

Fig. 1 Distribution of Hodgkin's disease by age in black and white South Africans (*a*) females (*b*) males.

Table 1. *Distribution of Hodgkin's disease by age group and histological subtype in black and white patients in South Africa: crude rates based on pathological diagnosis: data from National Cancer Registry of South Africa*

Histological subtype	Ethnic group: black							Ethnic group: white						
	Age range							Age range						
	10–14	15–24	25–34	35–44	45–54	>55	Total	10–14	15–24	25–34	35–44	45–54	>55	Total
LP	1	0	1	1	4	0	7	0	2	2	2	0	0	6
NS	2	4	7	6	2	7	28	2	6	5	3	0	5	21
MC	5	4	1	4	2	2	18	3	1	1	1	4	3	13
LD	1	5	4	2	1	4	17	0	1	0	1	1	4	7
NOS	9	15	20	17	6	15	82	3	8	16	10	9	18	64
Totals	18	28	33	30	15	28	152	8	18	24	17	14	30	111

LP =Lymphocyte predominant.
NS =Nodular sclerosis.
MC =Mixed cellularity.
NOS=Not otherwise specified.

where HD occurred less frequently as compared to whites, but when it did occur it tended to be with more aggressive histology and of more advanced stage. This epidemiological pattern has been attributed to socio-economic rather than to genetic factors. In this regard there appears to have been a shift, during the last 25–30 years, amongst the North American black population[23] to a pattern more closely approximating the Type I epidemiological pattern. Based on similar inferential reasoning, one may conclude that the intermediate pattern seen in South Africa represents a transitional phase in the epidemiology of Hodgkin's disease. However, these inferences require to be confirmed by direct investigation to establish whether HLA or immune-response linked gene frequencies or other genetic factors might still not play a significant role.

It might also be remarked that it is a moot point as to whether a shift in epidemiological pattern from a lower overall frequency to a higher incidence, albeit with a shift towards better prognostic features, represents a step forward in cancer control. Epidemiological studies have not as yet provided any real clues to suggest a strategy for prevention of Hodgkin's disease in any population group.

Hodgkin's disease and AIDS in Africa

Although the characteristic and most frequent AIDS related malignancy is Kaposi's sarcoma (KS) a number of recent publications have suggested an increased incidence of HD in HIV-infected individuals.[23–25] Most of these cases of HD have occurred in homosexual men with HIV infection or in intravenous drug abusers and have been associated with significant evidence of HIV immune deficiency. Since it is agreed that HIV infection and clinical AIDS is a significant and increasing problem in Africa, the question arises as to whether this epidemic will lead to an increase in cases of HD in Africa.

In a series of 923 HIV positive patients attending the AIDS clinic of the Johannesburg Hospital, only two cases of HD have been recorded (D. Spencer, personal communication). One patient was a white homosexual male and the other a black heterosexual male. Both had mixed cellularity Hodgkin's disease, and in both instances $CD4^+$ lymphocyte counts were $< 400 \times 10^9/l$.

Little other systematic information is available on the relationship of malignancy and HIV in Africa except to comment that, from the hospital-based experience in Southern Africa, epidemic KS appears to be by far the predominant HIV-related malignancy.

Treatment of Hodgkin's disease in sub-Saharan Africa

Radiation therapy

The frequency of advanced stage at presentation, coupled with the high capital costs required to set up radiotherapeutic centres capable of delivering adequate radiation treatment as well as the relatively sophisticated staging investigations required for optimum results with this treatment modality are probably the major factors responsible for the dearth of information regarding the use of radiation therapy for HD in Africa.

In an analysis of cases seen at the Lymphoma clinic of the Johannesburg Hospital and treated by total nodal irradiation (TNI; mantle plus inverted Y field) to standard doses following intensive staging (including laparotomy) for Stage I–IIIA HD in black patients, results were disappointing in all but those few with stage IA disease (Fig. 2(*a*)). However, when patients with poor prognostic features (Table 2) such as presence of B-symptoms high ESR, bulky disease and total lymphocyte count < 1500 × 10^9/l were excluded from analysis, outcome following nodal radiotherapy was significantly better (Fig. 2(*b*)) and was not different to results of radiation therapy in white patients of similar stage. These results suggest that treatment decisions should be based on additional considerations rather than on anatomical stage alone.

(*a*)

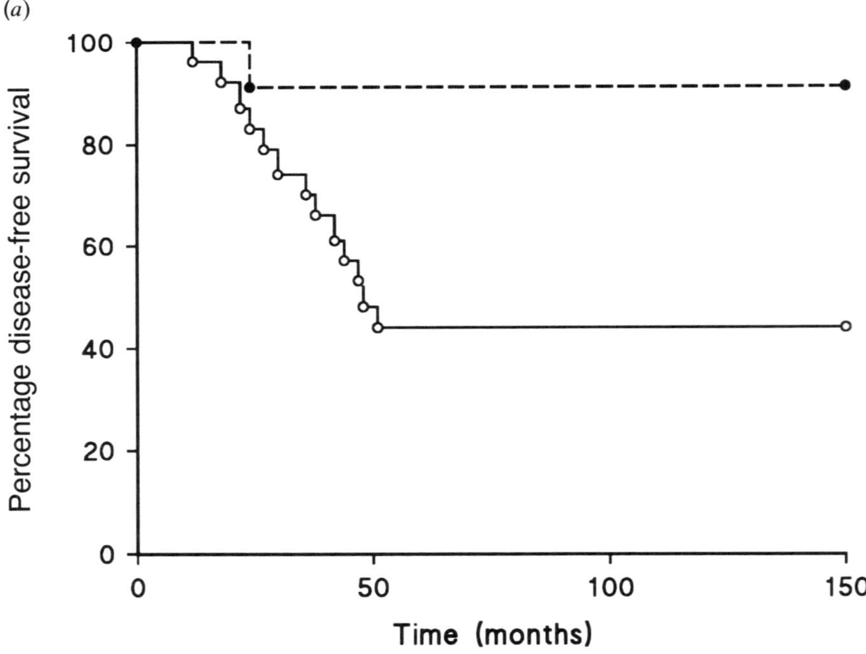

Fig. 2(*a*) Disease-free survival (DFS) following TNI for laparotomy staged, Stage I–IIIA HD in black patients: ● patients with Stage IA disease; ○ patients with Stage II–IIIA disease. 11 patients with laparotomy staged IA disease had DFS comparable to that of HD patients in developed countries. Patients with Stage II–IIIA disease had a significantly poorer survival ($p < 0.005$).

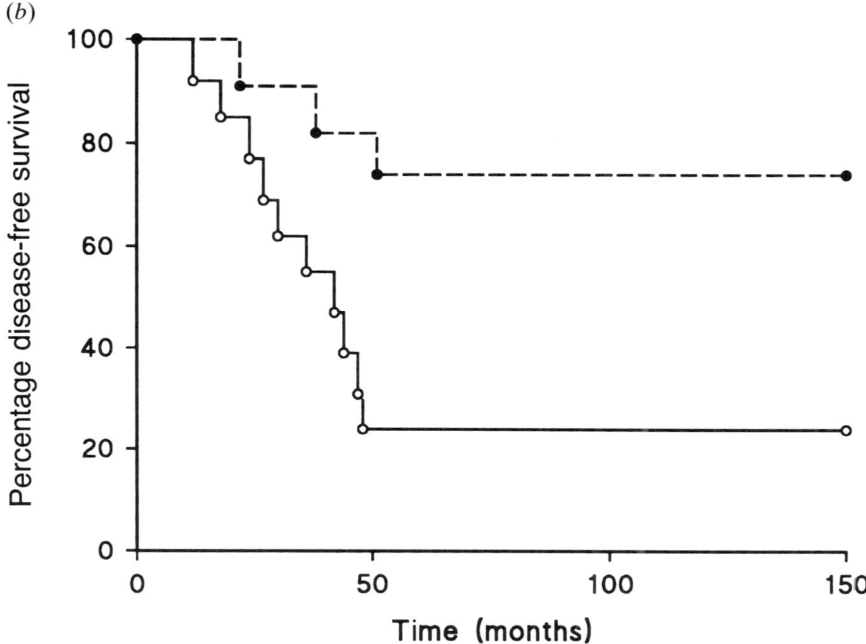

Fig. 2(*b*) Disease-free survival of laparotomy staged Stage II–IIIA HD, treated with nodal irradiation. According to presence (○) or absence (●) of non-stage related adverse prognostic features.

Since black patients, even those with limited stage disease, appear to have a higher frequency of poor prognostic features, the place for extensive and intensive radiation treatment for Hodgkin's disease in the African context would appear to be limited.

Chemotherapy for Hodgkin's disease

Chemotherapy based on conventional combination chemotherapeutic regimens (MOPP or its variants) appears to have been the mainstay of treatment of Hodgkin's disease in Africa.

With few exceptions, the response rate of adult HD in black Africans appears to be significantly less than the response rate seen with similar treatment regimens given in other parts of the world.[27–29] However, while the reported series are small, the results of chemotherapy for childhood Hodgkin's disease in Africa, despite the differences in epidemiological pattern appear to be exceptionally good with an initial complete remission rate approaching 100%.[16, 30–33] These results are probably significantly better

Table 2. *Non-anatomical stage-related prognostic features in black and in white patients with surgically staged Stage II–IIIA Hodgkin's disease treated by means of total nodal radiation therapy*

	Black		White		
	Number	(%)	Number	(%)	
B symptoms*	4	(17)	11	(15)	
Bulky disease (>5 cm or >50% thoracic diameter)	12	(52)	58	(11)	$p<0.001$
Lymphocyte count $<1.0\times10^9$/l	9	(39)	5	(7)	$p<0.001$
ESR >30 mm/h	9	(39)	4	(5)	$p<0.001$

* Patients with Stage IIB disease.

than those achieved in adult Hodgkin's disease treated with the same therapeutic regimens.

Apart from this data, relatively little information is extant regarding the influence of prognostic factors on survival after treatment for HD in Africa.

A retrospective analysis of adult patients with HD seen at the Johannesburg hospital and treated with MOPP or MOPP/ABVD-based chemotherapy (Table 3) demonstrated significant differences in the distribution of histological subtypes between black and white patients (p=0.02), the major differences being in the relative distributions of nodular sclerosis (NS) and mixed cellularity (MC) Hodgkin's disease. Black patients also had significantly more advanced stage and also a higher frequency of non-stage related prognostic factors such as low haemoglobin level and bulky disease (Table 4). When these factors were combined in order to examine the utility of the Newcastle prognostic index,[34] the distribution was not, however, found to be significantly different when comparing the two ethnic groups, probably because of the different weighting factors used to generate this index. Furthermore, while the Newcastle Index clearly differentiated between good and poor prognosis groups amongst the white patients (Fig. 3(*a*); p = 0.0001), no such differentiation was shown for this index amongst black patients with HD (Fig. 3(*b*)). It should also be pointed out that the disease-free survival of black patients, overall, appeared similar to that of poor prognosis whites. These findings led us to examine the prognostic significance of the individual components of the Newcastle prognostic index. In univariate analyses, only stage grouping (Fig. 4) and possibly age (Table 5) were found be predictive. In a multivariate analysis (Table 6), only stage grouping was found to be of prognostic significance in black patients.

Among children with Hodgkin's disease, a similar distribution of clinical and pathological features was seen when black and white ethnic groups were compared (Table 7). Black children had more advanced stage as well as a greater frequency of B symptoms, a lower haemoglobin level and more bulky disease. The survival of black children with HD was also significantly poorer than that of white children (Fig. 5). In a multivariate analysis, the significant factors influencing prognosis among black children were disease bulk (p=0.025) and stage (p=0.028). It should be noted, however, that although the prognosis of black children was poorer than that of whites, black children with HD did significantly better than their adult counterparts.

These findings suggest considerable differences in prognosis and prognostic features between the two race groups. The predominant influence of stage recalls an earlier era of treatment outcome in HD. One possible reason for this difference might be the distribution of histological subtype which was found to be significantly different in the two ethnic groups.

Table 3. *Distribution of histological subtype amongst 413 adult black and white patients with Hodgkin's disease treated with combination chemotherapy (MOPP or MOPP/ABVD)*

	Lymphocyte predominant		Nodular sclerosis		Mixed cellularity		Lymphocyte depleted		
Age (Decile)	Black	White	Black	White	Black	White	Black	White	p-value
10–19	1	2	11	24	9	10	1	0	NS
20–29	2	8	12	41	20	12	3	5	=0.001
30–39	0	6	17	24	17	22	4	2	NS
40–49	1	2	12	18	8	10	2	2	NS
50–59	1	3	3	33	3	12	2	1	<0.03
60–69	–	–	0	9	4	8	1	1	NS
>70	–	1	–	10	–	10	–	3	NS
Totals	5	22	55	159	61	84	13	14	
	NS		p=0.01		p<0.02		NS		

Table 4. *Relative distribution of factors considered to be important in predicting outcome of Hodgkin's disease amongst adult black and white patients treated with combination therapy*

	Black		White		
	Number	(%)	Number	(%)	p-value
Stage					
I and II	26	(19)	151	(54)	0.001
III and IV	108	(81)	128	(46)	
Symptoms					
A	28	(21)	89	(32)	0.02
B	106	(79)	190	(68)	
Age					
<50	129	(90)	197	(71)	0.001
>50	15	(10)	82	(29)	
Haemoglobin g/dl					
>10	107	(74)	255	(91)	0.001
<10	27	(26)	24	(9)	
Disease bulk					
Bulky (>10 cm)	62	(46)	98	(35)	0.05
Non-bulky (<10 cm)	72	(54)	181	(65)	
Lymphocyte count					
$<1.0\times10^9/l$	58	(43)	85	(30)	0.010
$>1.0\times10^9/l$	76	(57)	194	(70)	
Newcastle index					
≤0.5	109	(76)	212	(76)	NS
>0.5	35	(24)	67	(24)	

However, no significant difference in treatment outcome between so-called 'good prognostic' subtypes (LP and NS) and 'poor prognostic' types (MC and LD) could be demonstrated.

Another factor may be treatment related

Treatment effects, particularly the achievement of CR probably override many of the pretreatment prognostic variables such as histological subtype and stage. A potent factor influencing not only CR rate but also long-term treatment outcome is dose intensity.[35–37] Delivery of the optimum dose of chemotherapy on schedule depends not only on haematological reserve and absence of other treatment-related toxicities but also on patient compliance.

(a)

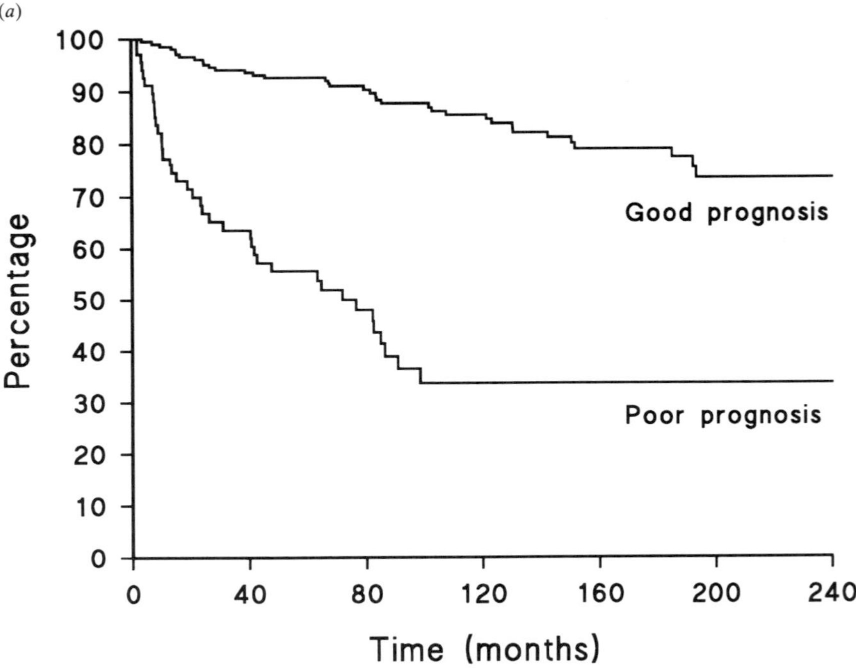

Fig. 3(*a*) Disease-free survival of chemotherapy treated (MOPP or MOPP/ABVD) *white patients* with Hodgkin's disease stratified according to Newcastle Prognostic Index (p = 0.001).

Our own experience has been that a considerable proportion of adult black patients (Table 8) entered on to a chemotherapy treatment programme fail to complete therapy on schedule despite intensive efforts to ensure compliance. Treatment delays were also found to be significantly more frequent in black children with HD than was the case among white children. Factors associated with poor compliance include long distances and travelling times to treatment centres as well as adverse socio-economic factors including loss of employment (60% lost employment subsequent to diagnosis of Hodgkin's disease) which appeared to be responsible, at least in part, for the poor overall prognosis. While some of these factors can, and must, be addressed by suitable adjustments of public policy that must recognize not only the moral responsibility for providing access to treatment but also the economic desirability of providing potentially curative therapy for a predominantly younger group of patients, these factors may not be the only relevant ones. Paradoxically, the rapidity with which even limited

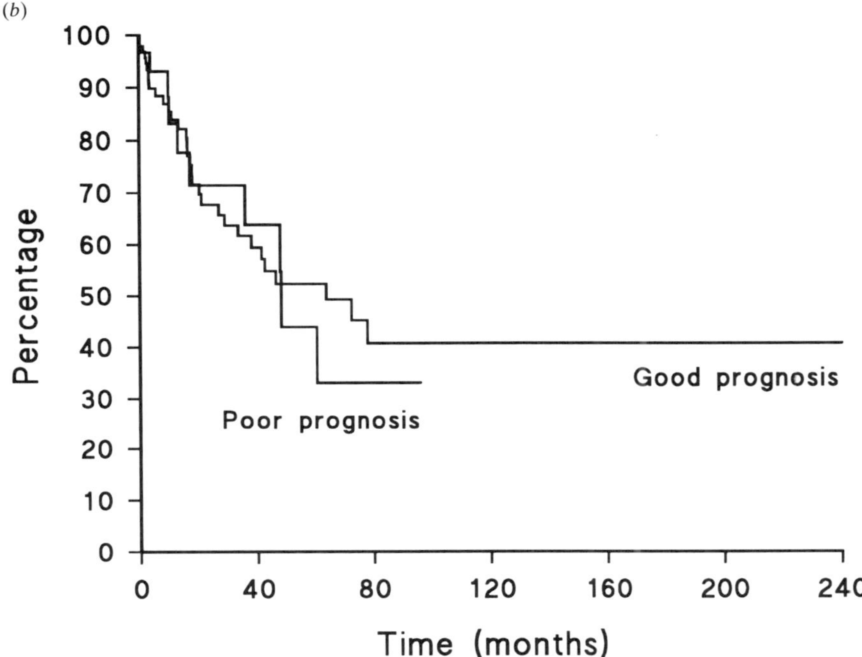

Fig. 3(*b*) Disease-free survival of chemotherapy treated (MOPP or MOPP/ABVD) *black patients* with Hodgkin's disease stratified according to Newcastle Prognostic Index.

treatment results in alleviation of symptoms and perceptible evidence of the disease may mitigate against compliance with demanding treatment schedules in a relatively unsophisticated patient population. It should be pointed out that most black patients who did not fully comply with the treatment programme were not completely lost from follow-up. The majority re-present either after a delay (usually exceeding the duration of two cycles (median delay in treatment time 9 weeks in a projected 24-week total treatment regimen) or even later on with recurrent disease.

While the provision of decentralized treatment facilities will no doubt help to create additional treatment opportunities, other approaches need also to be explored in view of the high frequency of significant adverse prognostic factors among black patients.

A significant dose–response relationship has been shown for Hodgkin's disease.[38,39] High dose chemotherapy with autologous bone marrow rescue (HDC–ABMT) has been applied successfully to the treatment of recurrent

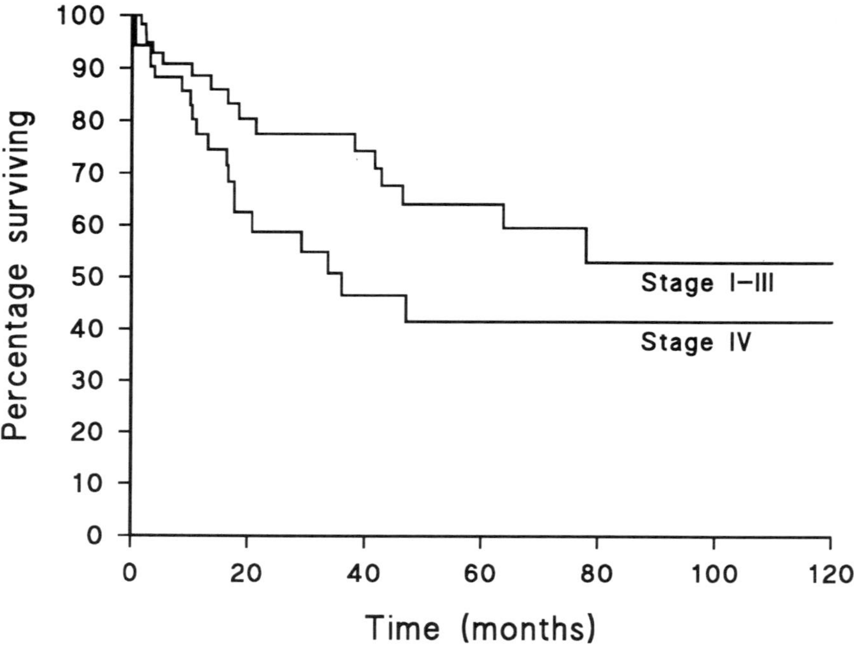

Fig. 4 Disease-free survival of *black patients* with Hodgkin's disease treated with MOPP or MOPP/ABVD: influence of stage. Survival of patients with Stage II–IIIB compared as patients with Stage IV disease ($p < 0.05$).

Table 5. *Univariate factors predicting for disease-free survival in adult black and in white patients with Hodgkin's disease*

	Black p-value	White p-value
Stage grouping	p<0.04	p=0.0001
Age	p=0.059	p=0.0001
Hb level	NS	p<0.04
Lymphocyte count	NS	p=0.0001
Disease bulk	NS	p<0.04

Hodgkin's disease in black patients. In a series of 11 patients with refractory and relapsed HD treated by high dose chemotherapy and autologous bone marrow rescue,[40] three-fifths of the successfully treated patients were black. This study subsequently has been expanded to 48 patients including 22 blacks and 26 whites. The CR rate was 45/48, (90%) with no difference in outcome by population group (Table 9).

Table 6. *Multivariate analysis of factors predicting for disease-free survival in adult black and in white patients with Hodgkin's disease*

	Black p-value	White p-value
Stage grouping	$p<0.02$	NS
Age	NS	$p=0.0001$
Hb level	NS	$p=0.0001$
Lymphocyte count	NS	$p=0.0001$
Disease bulk	NS	$p=0.01$

Factors entered into these analyses were as defined by Proctor and co-workers[34] and are generally known as the Newcastle index where:

Clinical stage (Ann Arbor)	*CS grouping*
IA, IIA, IIA	1
IB, IIB	2
IIIB	3
IV	4

Absolute lymphocyte count ($\times 10^9$/l)	*LC score*
<1.0	1
1.0–1.5	2
1.5–2.0	3
>2.0	4

Index=1.5858−0.0363 Age+0.0005 (Age^2)+0.0683 CS−0.086 LC−0.058 Hb.
Hb (g/dl) is entered as an absolute figure in the equation.
Bulk disease (>10 cm) – index score add 0.3.

One approach to the complex of problems enumerated above, which include not only adverse physical but also psychosocial factors, may be to intensify initial therapy so as to maximize the chance of rapid cure. In a pilot investigation, seven black patients with significant adverse prognostic features have been treated with a regimen consisting of high dose melphelan (140 mg/m^2) plus VP 16 (2.5 g/m^2 over 12 hours) given either as initial treatment or following one to two cycles of conventional MOPP/ABVD debulking therapy. In this treatment, programme, haematological rescue is effected by non-cyropreserved autologous bone marrow, making the whole procedure as simple and as inexpensive as possible.[41] Of the seven patients so treated, all have achieved haematological reconstitution in a median time of 23 days with six of seven achieving CR with a single course of high dose therapy while one patient required a second course of HDC–ABMT to achieve CR. In addition, a number of patients who never had adequate initial therapy and who had recurrent relapses after

Table 7. *Clinical and pathological features amongst 91 children with Hodgkin's disease*

	Black		White		
	Number	(%)	Number	(%)	p-value
Sex					
Male	47	(52)	22	(24)	
Female	14	(15)	8	(9)	
Histological subtype					
LP	1	(1)	3	(3)	
NS	20	(22)	12	(13)	
MC	39	(43)	14	(16)	
LD	1	(1)	1	(1)	
Stage					
I and II	18	(20)	19	(21)	0.001
III and IV	43	(47)	11	(12)	
Symptoms					
A	25	(27)	20	(21)	<0.03
B	36	(40)	10	(12)	
Haemoglobin g/dl					
≥10	24	(26)	18	(20)	0.06
<10	37	(41)	12	(13)	
Lymphocyte count $\times 10^9/l$					
≥1.0	50	(55)	18	(19)	<0.03
<1.0	11	(12)	12	(12)	
Disease bulk					
Bulky	31	(34)	5	(5)	<0.03
Non-bulky	30	(33)	25	(27)	
Age					
Mean±SD	8.2±3.1		9.4±4.1		

defaulting repeatedly, usually after one or two courses of treatment) have also been treated in this fashion with CR in six of seven. Although these patients had relapsed, the incomplete and inadequate therapy they had previously received probably places them in a separate category from other relapsed patients. Treatment-related mortality in the overall group was 1/14 (7%) and that was in a patient with extensive visceral involvement including bone marrow liver and lung involvement with a performance status of 4.

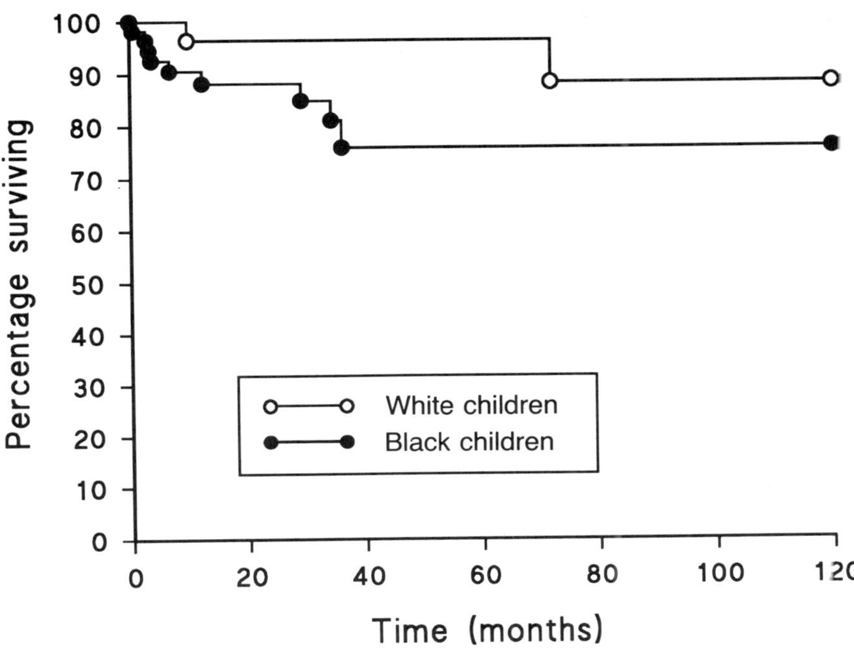

Fig. 5 Disease-free survival of children with Hodgkin's disease (○) white (●) black children. The survival difference was statistically significant (p = 0.03).

Table 8. *Treatment compliance among adult black patients with Hodgkin's disease: first line MOPP or MOPP/ABVD chemotherapy*

	Number of treatment cycles		
	⩽3	4–6	>6
Percentage	31	39	30
Median cycle delay[a] weeks	4[b]	2.5	2.5

[a] Based on optimum treatment cycle time of 4 weeks.
[b] Delay calculated for patients receiving >1 but <4 treatment cycles.

While it is too early as yet to assess long-term cure with this programme, we hope that this treatment approach will make an impact on the relatively poor prognosis that has been demonstrated for black patients with Hodgkin's disease. Although even this simplified HDC–ABMT schedule may not be within reach of all sub-Saharan countries, the new spirit of co-operation with the region may well make it possible to establish a number

Table 9. *Treatment of Hodgkin's disease with single course high dose Melphelan plus Etoposide and non-cryopreserved autologous bone marrow: factors determining outcome*

Treatment outcome	Number	(%)
CR	45	(90)
PR	1	(2)
NR	3	(6)
NE[a]	1	(2)

Prognostic determinants
Response to treatment

	Univariate analyses		Multivariate analysis	
	Chi-square	p-value	Chi-square	p-value
Performance status[b]	14.61	0.003	9.12	0.01
Liver involvement	11.58	0.02		

Survival

	Univariate analyses		Multivariate analysis	
	Chi-square	p-value	Chi-square	p-value
Relapse status[c]	9.12	0.01	12.92	0.02
Liver involvement	3.76	0.05		

[a] NE: Not evaluable (early death).
[b] Performance status: ECOG.
[c] Relapse status: Relapsed after prior response versus primary refractory disease.
Other factors examined and found not to be predictive included race, sex and presence or absence of marrow involvement.

of regional centres where patients, identified as likely to have a poor prognosis with conventional dose treatment, could be referred for definitive treatment.

References

(1) Anderson RE, Ishida K, Li Y et al. Geographic aspects of malignant lymphoma and multiple myeloma. *Am J Pathol* 1970; 61: 85.
(2) Burkitt DP. Distribution of Cancer in Africa. *Proc Roy Soc Med Med* 1973; 66: 312.
(3) Burn C, Davies JNP, Dodge OG, Nias BG. Hodgkin's disease in English and African children. *J Natl Cancer Inst* 1971; 46: 37.
(4) Colonna P, Belhadi–Mezoug K, Henni T, Andrieu J–M. Changes in patterns

of Hodgkin's disease in Algeria, 1966–1985: Influence of health care delivery system. *Acta Hematol* 1988; 80: 227.
(5) Cook PJ, Burkitt DP. Cancer in Africa. *Br Med Bull* 1971; 27: 14.
(6) Jacobs P. The malignant lymphomas in Africa. *Hem Onc Clin North Am* 1991; 5: 953.
(7) Wright DH. Epidemiology and histology of Hodgkin's disease in Uganda. *Natl Cancer Inst Monographs* 1973; 36: 25.
(8) Edington GM, Hendrickse M. Incidence and frequency of lymphoreticular tumours in Ibadan and the Western State of Nigeria. *J Natl Cancer Inst* 1972; 50: 1623.
(9) Naik KG, Bhagwandeen SB. Hodgkin's disease in Zambia. *E Afr Med J* 1976; 53: 459.
(10) Kung'u A. Hodgkin's disease in Kenya. A histopathological and epidemiological study. *E Afr Med J* 1980; 57: 769.
(11) Emmanuel DJ, Gelfand M. A survey into the clinical presentation of Hodgkin's disease at Harare Hospital, Salisbury, Rhodesia. *J Trop Med Hyg* 1975; 78: 44.
(12) Els E, Parkin DM, Mair CS, Whilan SL, Gao YT, Ferlay J, Powel J. Cancer incidence in five contents, Vol VI. *IARC Publication No. 120*. International Agency for Research on Cancer. Lyon 1992.
(13) Sitas F. Cancer in South Africa 1988. *National Cancer Registry of South Africa Annual Statistical Report for 1988. Incidence of Histologically Diagnosed Cancer in South Africa*. Johannesburg: SA Institute for Medical Research, 1992; pp 46–51.
(14) Correa P, O'Connor GT. Epidemiologic patterns of Hodgkin's disease. *Int J Cancer* 1971; 8: 192.
(15) Correa P, O'Connor GT. Geographic pathology of lymphoreticular tumours: summary of survey from Geographic Pathology Committee of the International Union Against Cancer. *J Natl Cancer Inst* 1973; 50: 1609.
(16) Kinuthia DMW, Kasili EG. Hodgkin's disease in Kenya children. A six year report on management. *E Afr Med J* 1992; 60: 416.
(17) Riyat MS. Hodgkin's disease in Kenya. *Cancer* 1992; 69: 1047–1051.
(18) Dhru R, Templeton AC. Post mortem findings in Ugandans with Hodgkin's disease. *Br J Cancer* 1972; 26: 331.
(19) French TJ, Ross M. Hodgkin's disease at Harare Hospital. *Cent Afr J Med* 1976; 22: 237.
(20) Ansel S, Nabembezi JS. Two year survey of hematologic malignancies in Uganda. *J Natl Cancer Inst* 1974; 52: 1397.
(21) Cohen C, Hamilton DG. Epidemiologic and histologic patterns of Hodgkin's disease: comparison of the black and white populations of Johannesburg South Africa. *Cancer* 1980; 46: 186.
(22) Vianna NJ, Thind IS, Louria DB et al. Epidemiology and histology patterns of Hodgkin's disease in blacks. *Cancer* 1977; 40: 133.
(23) Glaser SL. Black – white differences in Hodgkin's disease incidence in the United States by age, sex, histologic subtype and time. *Int J Epidemiol* 1991; 20: 68.
(24) Hessol NA, Katz MH, Liu JY, Buchbinder SP, Rabino CJ, Holmberg SD.

Increased incidence of Hodgkin's disease in homosexual men with HIV infection. *Ann Int Med* 1992; 117: 309.

(25) Tirelli U, Vaccher E, Rezza G, Brochia G, Fassio PG, Gobbi M. Hodgkin's disease and infection with the human immunodeficiency virus in Italy. *Ann Int Med* 1988; 112: 309.

(26) Tirelli U, Serraino D, Carbone A. Hodgkin's disease and HIV. *Ann Int Med* 1993; 118: 4; 313.

(27) Olweny CLM, Ziegler JL, Berard CW, Templeton AC. Adult Hodgkin's disease in Uganda. *Cancer* 1971; 25: 1295.

(28) Williams CKO. Prospective studies on Hodgkin's disease in Ibadan – a preliminary report. *Afr J Med Med Sc* 1985; 14: 3.

(29) Oluboyede OA, Esdu GJF. The therapy of Hodgkin's disease in Nigeria: a five year study. *Afr J Med Med Sc* 1976; 5: 201.

(30) Olweny CLM, Katangole-Mbidde E, Kiite C et al. Childhood Hodgkin's disease in Uganda. A ten year experience. *Cancer* 1978; 42: 787.

(31) Ziegler H, Blumming AZ, Fass I et al. Chemotherapy of childhood Hodgkin's disease in Uganda. *Lancet* 1972; 2: 679.

(32) Jacobs P, King HS, Karabus C et al. Hodgkin's disease in children. A ten year experience in South Africa. *Cancer* 1984; 53: 210.

(33) Jacobsen RJ, Klappenbach RS, Clinton C et al. Hodgkin's disease in South African children. *S Afr Med J* 1981; 53: 133.

(34) Proctor SJ, Taylor P, Mackie MJ, Donnan P, Boys R, Lennard A, Prescott RJ with members of the Scotland and Newcastle Lymphoma Group (SNLG) Therapy Working Party. A numerical prognostic, index for clinical use in identification of poor-risk patients with Hodgkin's disease at diagnosis. *Leukemia and Lymphoma* 1992; 75: 17.

(35) Carde P, Mackintosh FR, Rosenberg SA. A dose and time response analysis of the treatment of Hodgkin's disease with MOPP chemotherapy. *J Clin Oncol* 1982; 1: 146.

(36) Longo DL, Young RC, Wesley M, Habbard SM, Duffey PC et al. Twenty years of MOPP therapy for Hodgkin's disease. *J Clin Oncol* 1986; 4: 1295.

(37) Bezwoda WR, Dansey R, Bezwoda MA. Treatment of Hodgkin's disease with MOPP chemotherapy: effect of dose and schedule modifications on treatment outcome. *Oncology* 1990; 47: 29.

(38) Jagannath S, Armitage JO, Dicke KA et al. Prognostic factors for response and survival after high dose cyclophosphamide, carmustine, and etoposide with autologous bone marrow transplantation for relapsed Hodgkin's disease. *J Clin Oncol* 1989; 7: 179.

(39) Kessinger A, Nademanee A, Forman SJ, Armitage JO. Autologous bone marrow transplantation for Hodgkin's and non-Lymphoma. *Bone Marrow Transplantation* 1990; 4: 577.

(40) Bezwoda WR, Dansey R. High dose chemotherapy with bone marrow rescue for treatment of relapsed and refractory Hodgkin's disease. *Leukemia and Lymphoma* 1989; 1: 71.

(41) Seymour L, Dansey RD, Bezwoda WR. Single high dose etoposide and melphelan with non-cryopreserved autologous marrow rescue as primary therapy for relapsed refractory and poor prognosis Hodgkin's disease. (In press).

AIDS-related non-Hodgkin's lymphoma: clinico-pathological features

U TIRELLI and A CARBONE

Introduction

Since the beginning of HIV epidemic, HIV-related non-Hodgkin's lymphomas (NHL) have been associated with poor outcome. This was mainly due to the adverse clinicopathological features[1] and the underlying HIV disease with its opportunistic infections. HIV-related NHL are distinguished from NHL in the general population by high percentage of high-grade subtypes, frequent extranodal sites of disease, high percentage of advanced in disease, therefore lower response rate to chemotherapy and higher mortality rates have been observed. Moreover, toxicity is much higher also because of the immunosuppression caused by HIV. However, the availability of more efficacious anti-HIV and anti-opportunistic infectious agents, the concomitant use of bone marrow growth factors, a better definition of prognostic risk factors associated with HIV infection and related NHL,[2–9] seem to have improved the prognosis of systemic HIV-related NHL.

Therapy of HIV-related NHL remains quite controversial, in that it is not clear whether treatment with intensive chemotherapy is able to modify the natural history of these malignancies in HIV setting. Levine et al, in fact, employing low dose chemotherapy, observed the same results as with intensive chemotherapy.[10] Overall, 1–2% of patients with AIDS present with primary central nervous system (CNS) lymphoma and both systemic NHL and primary CNS lymphoma are recognized as AIDS defining diseases by Centers for Disease Control. Therapy of CNS lymphoma has not been investigated in large trials, in that usually CNS lymphoma occurs in the late stage of HIV disease, rendering therefore intensive chemotherapy quite difficult. In this setting, usually palliative radiation therapy has been

All correspondence to: Dr U Tirelli, Div di Oncologia Medica AIDS, Centro di Riferimento Oncologico, Via Pedemontana Occidentale, 33081 Aviano (PN), Italy

Cambridge Medical Reviews: Haematological Oncology Volume 4

delivered with no impact on the overall survival. CNS lymphoma should be considered for prospective trials in order to improve its very poor survival.

The aim of the manuscript is to review the pathological and clinical aspects of HIV-related NHL, with emphasis on a new proposed clinico-pathological classification of HIV-related NHL, on the use of bone marrow growth factors in association with chemotherapy of HIV-related NHL and of the possibility of obtaining long-term survival and also cure in a subgroup of such patients.

Pathology

While approximately half of adult NHL are follicular, this pattern is almost never observed in patients with HIV infection; moreover, 80 to 90% of HIV-infected patients with NHL are diagnosed with high-grade B-cell tumours, which would normally be expected in approximately 10% to 15% of individuals.[11]

Low-grade B-cell lymphomas are occasionally reported in HIV-infected patients,[12] while young HIV-infected individuals with multiple myeloma or solitary plasmacytoma have also been reported.[13] These cases are not considered to be AIDS defining.

T-cell lymphomas have also been described in HIV-infected individuals, including cutaneous T-cell lymphoma, lymphoblastic lymphoma, HTLV-1 associated T-cell leukaemia, peripheral T-cell lymphoma.[12] Once again, these cases are not considered to be AIDS defining, and their incidence has not increased since the start of the AIDS epidemic.

On the other hand, it has recently been documented in the European and North-American literature that anaplastic large cell (ALC) CD30/Ki-1$^+$ lymphomas, a heterogeneous group of high-grade lymphomas[14–15] at the borderline between HD and NHL, can occur also in HIV-infected patients.[13,16–21] HIV-related ALC CD30/Ki-1$^+$ lymphomas represent a clinically heterogeneous group of T-cell, B-cell and null-cell malignant lymphomas, distinct from the previously described categories of AIDS-associated NHL, that may expand the spectrum of lymphoid neoplasias associated with HIV-infection.[21] Interestingly, molecular studies showed that in HIV-infected patients ALC CD30/Ki-1$^+$ lymphomas (of non T-cell phenotype) and HD (mostly of non-nodular sclerosing subtype) display almost complete association with Epstein–Barr virus (EBV) in clonal and episomal form.[21–23]

From a morphological point of view, it must be stressed that most high grade lymphomas in HIV-infected patients exhibit pleomorphic features as well as some overlap between NHL histological subtypes,[16,18] thus emphasizing the difficulties in their precise classification with the use of the classic NHL classifications, which were proposed before the AIDS epidemic.

To obtain a detailed and specific histopathologic description of HIV-associated lymphomas, a pathology study group involving 12 French Institutions reviewed a series of 113 cases of HIV-associated NHL, collected and registered at the Pitié-Salpêtrière Hospital, Paris, France.[16] The WF,[11] the updated Kiel Classification,[15] and a recent description of the morphologic variants of the high grade B-cell NHL[24] were used. By using a quite similar pathological approach another study, based on a single Institution 9-year experience, was independently performed on a series of 114 HIV-associated systemic NHL seen at the Centro di Riferimento Oncologico, Aviano, Italy. The latter study expanded a previous published analysis based on 87 patients.[18] Pathological review focused on the recognition of the morphological variants described by Hui and Colleagues,[24] for the small non-cleaved cell lymphomas, and the frequency of lymphoma cases exhibiting overlap between NHL histological subtypes. From the combined results of the French and Italian studies it can be drawn that most systemic HIV-associated NHL have a 'blastic' cell morphology (Table 1). Many of them consist of (a) small non-cleaved cells of typical Burkitt's lymphoma (Fig. 1) and their variants with plasmablastic differentiation,[24] (Fig. 2(b)) or immunoblasts usually polymorphic with plasmacytic features (Fig. 3(c)),

Table 1. *Pathological categories of HIV-associated lymphomas*

(*a*) *'Blastic'*[a] *cell lymphomas*
- centroblastic (G – WF) monomorphic, polymorphic, multilobated, centrocytoid
- immunoblastic (H – WF)
  with or without plasmacytic differentiation
- small non-cleaved cell (J – WF)
  with or without plasmablastic differentiation
- plasmablastic (plasmacytoma)
- blastic cells with intermediate features

(*b*) *'Anaplastic'*[b] *cell lymphomas*
- anaplastic large cell (CD30/Ki-1$^+$)
- ?Hodgkin's lymphoma
  (mixed cellularity and lymphocyte depletion)

(*c*) *Others (rare types)*

WF=International Working Formulation for non-Hodgkin's lymphomas.[11]
[a] The term 'blastic' is used in analogy with the suffix 'blastic' used in the Kiel Classification.[15]
[b] The term 'anaplastic' is used in analogy with the term used in the definition of the CD30/Ki-1$^+$ ALC lymphoma;[14,15] it indicates undifferentiated cells which display marked pleomorphism, with giant cells possessing bizarre and irregular nuclei and large nucleoli.

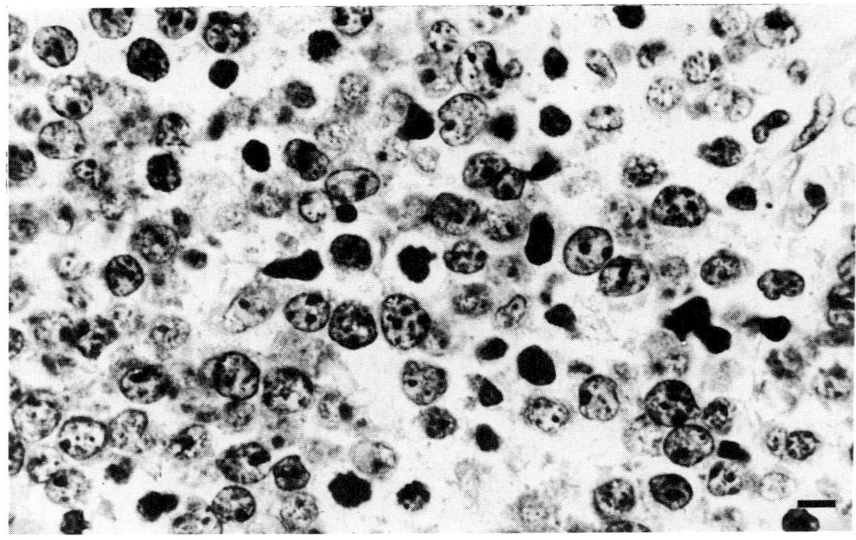

Fig. 1. Burkitt's lymphoma (small non-cleaved cell lymphoma). Medium-sized tumour cells have a monotonous appearance; they show round nuclei containing multiple centrally located nucleoli (haematoxylin–eosin stain; paraffin-embedded tissue section; Bar = 5 μm, oil immersion).

or centroblasts along with their morphologic variants.[24] In addition, lymphomas composed by plasmablasts[13] or by 'blastic' cells exhibiting intermediate features (Fig. 4) between small non-cleaved cells with plasmablastic differentiation and immunoblastic–plasmacytoid cells could be observed;[16,18] moreover, a relatively high occurrence of the ALC CD30/Ki-1$^+$ lymphomas and 'putative histiocytic' lymphoma[18] (Fig. 5) was found in the Italian series.[18] (Table 1)

In contrast to the heterogeneity of systemic HIV-associated NHL, NHL arising in the CNS represent a more uniform group, and in the majority of cases tend to display histological features consistent with immunoblastic–plasmacytoid lymphomas[12,16].

The biological bases and the molecular genetics underlying the pathogenesis of these tumours are still largely unclear.

The lymphomas arising in the setting of AIDS involve multiple factors, including underlying immunosuppression; chronic B-cell proliferation, stimulation, and differentiation (due to HIV, cytokine release, and/or EBV); possible expression of certain latent EBV viral proteins associated with cellular transformation; occurrence of recombinase errors, leading to DNA rearrangements; and subsequent dysregulation of *c-myc* and/or other onco-

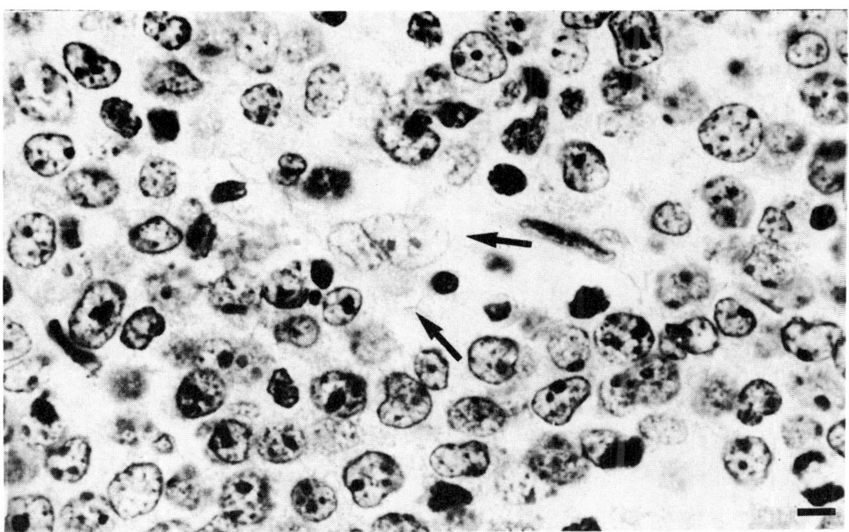

Fig. 2. Burkitt's lymphoma (small non-cleaved cell lymphoma) with plasmablastic differentiation. Several tumour cells are medium sized with abundant cytoplasm; one or two large nucleoli are evident within the nuclei of tumour cells. The nuclei are equal to, or smaller in size than, histiocyte nuclei (arrows) (haematoxylin–eosin stain; paraffin-embedded tissue section; Bar = 5 μm, oil immersion).

genes, as well as the inactivation of tumour suppressor gene(s). While some of these factors may occur in the majority of cases, heterogeneity has already been encountered, indicating that distinct mechanisms of lymphomagenesis may occur in different pathological types, or sites of disease.[12]

A pathogenetic role for EBV in a proportion of HIV-associated lymphomas has been supposed on the basis of EBV genome demonstration in a variable fraction (usually higher than 50%) of NHL cases, depending on the techniques employed (Southern blot, polymerase chain reaction(PCR), and in situ hybridization(ISH), and case selection. Furthermore, a higher frequency (83–100%) of EBV association has been shown in HD tissue from patients with HIV-positive serology.[25,26] Applying small non-polyadenylated EBV RNAs (EBER) ISH to 21 cases of CNS lymphoma in AIDS patients MacMahon and Colleagues[27] found evidence of EBV infection of the malignant cells in every case. Furthermore, EBV genomes associated with HD and ALC CD30/Ki-1$^+$ NHL arising in HIV-1-positive patients have been shown to be episomal and clonal,[22] even when detected in metachronous multiple biopsies,[23] indicating that EBV-infected cells have arisen from a single infectious agent.

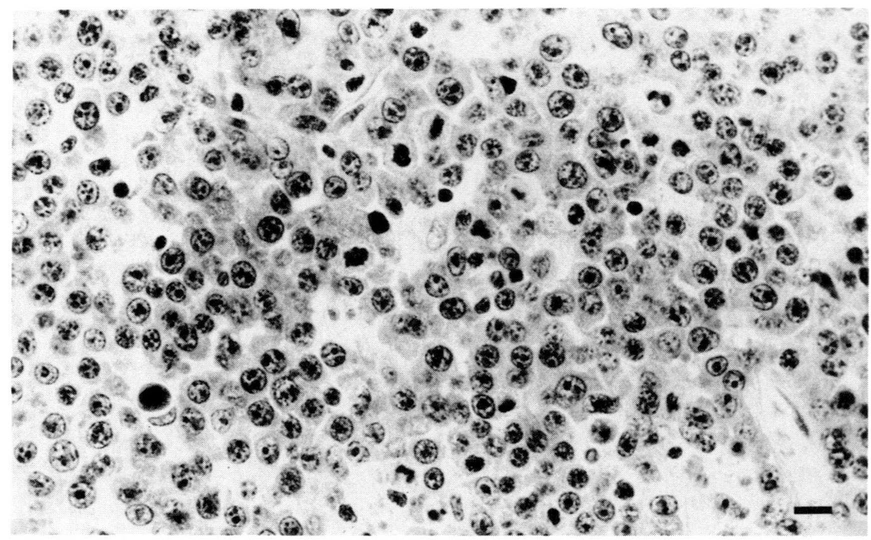

Fig. 3. Immunoblastic lymphoma. Immunoblasts with plasmablastic features are medium sized, but there are several larger forms as well. They have abundant cytoplasm and several medium-sized nucleoli. Some cells have large, solitary nucleoli. Mitotic activity is high. (haematoxylin–eosin stain; paraffin-embedded tissue section; Bar = 12.5 μm).

Recent reports have demonstrated the existence of two EBV subtypes, originally based on the organization of their BamHI–WYH gene region, which codes for the EBV nuclear antigen 2 (EBNA2).[28] Type 1 EBV virus is a more potent transformer of lymphocytes than type 2. However, while type 2 virus does not seem to play an important role in inducing both lymphocyte transformation and the development of lymphoproliferative diseases in immunocompetent hosts, this virus strain may be pathogenetically involved in HIV-associated NHL[29] and in HD.[30,31]

In a previous study,[18] combined ISH studies for viral DNA and EBER revealed EBV in 10 of 12 (83%) ALC CD30/Ki-1$^+$ (Fig. 6) and in three of seven immunoblastic lymphomas; the association of EBV, as detected by ISH studies and immunohistological demonstration of latent membrane protein-1 (LMP-1) (Figs. 7 and 8), with both ALC CD30/Ki-1$^+$ and immunoblastic lymphomas occurring in HIV-infected patients, supports the view that both entities may be different from other HIV-associated lymphomas. In particular, there were differences in viral latent gene expression between ALC CD30/Ki-1$^+$ or immunoblastic lymphomas (LMP-1$^+$) and EBV-infected cells of small non-cleaved cell lymphomas (J group) which did not express LMP-1,[18] as is the case for endemic and

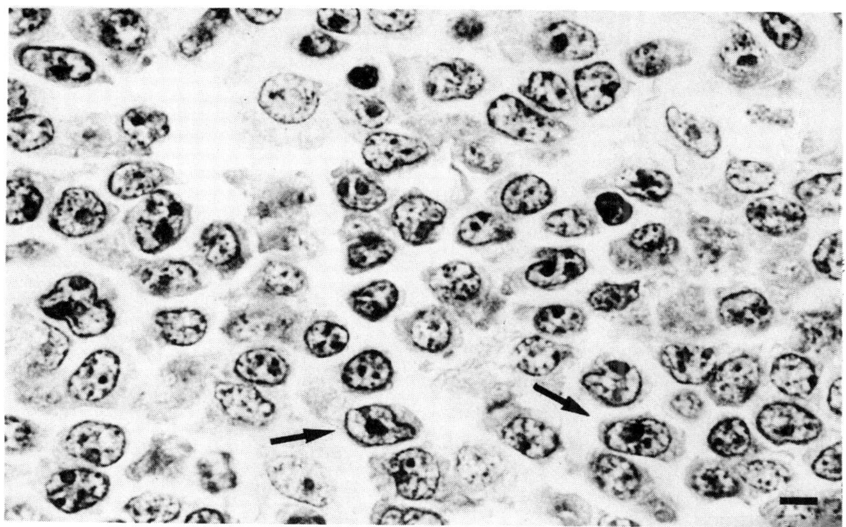

Fig. 4. Unclassified non-Hodgkin's lymphoma with intermediate features between small non-cleaved cells with plasmablastic differentiation and immunoblasts. A majority of the tumour cells are medium sized with several small or medium-sized nucleoli. Some larger cells (arrows) have large solitary nucleoli, being indistinguishable from immunoblasts. (haematoxylin–eosin stain; paraffin-embedded tissue section; Bar = 5 μm, oil immersion).

sporadic Burkitt's lymphoma.[17,32] Interestingly, EBV association (without LMP-1 expression) was also found in two of three plasmacytomas.[18] The presence of EBV genomes, as detected by DNA ISH studies in a plasma cell tumour occurring in a HIV-infected patient has been previously reported.[33] In conclusion, the demonstration of EBV-encoded LMP-1 expression, that is evidence for an active role of EBV in the disease,[34] was restricted to ALC CD30/Ki-1$^+$ lymphomas and a proportion of immunoblastic lymphomas;[18] this finding supports a causal role for the virus in the pathogenesis of only a specific group of HIV-associated systemic lymphomas. Immunoblastic lymphomas, however, seem to be a rather heterogeneous category based on the presence of a fraction of LMP-1 negative cases. HD occurring in HIV-infected patients shows a frequency of EBV association and an EBV latent antigenic phenotype similar to that seen in HIV-associated ALC CD30/Ki-1$^+$ lymphomas.[18,19] Therefore, both these disorders seem to be associated with the transforming properties of EBV.

The role of other viruses in AIDS lymphomagenesis has also been tested; however, numerous studies failed to detect the presence of several herpes viruses (cytomegalovirus, human herpes virus-6) or retroviruses (human T-cell lymphoma virus-1, HIV) within the tumour clone.[35,37]

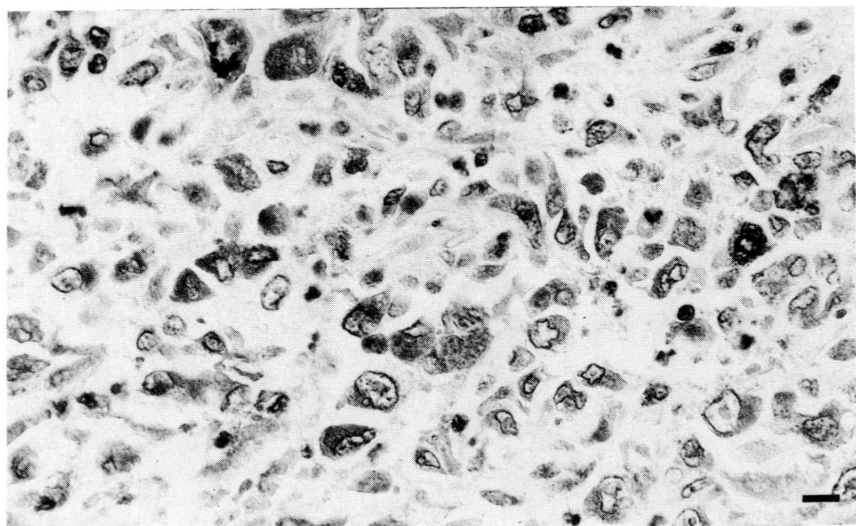

Fig. 5. 'Putative histiocytic' lymphoma. Paraffin-embedded section immunophenotyping shows cytoplasmic staining of the large neoplastic cells with the KP1/CD68 histiocytic-associated marker. (Avidin–biotin–peroxidase complex; haematoxylin counterstain; paraffin-embedded tissue section; Bar = 12.5 μm).

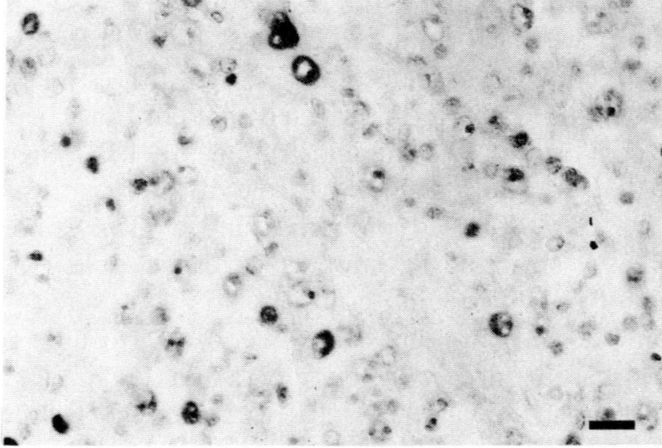

Fig. 6. EBER in situ hybridization signal is present as dense grains over the nuclei of tumour cells of an anaplastic large cell (CD30/Ki-1^+) lymphoma. (In situ hybridization; nuclear fast red counterstain; Bar = 20 μm.)

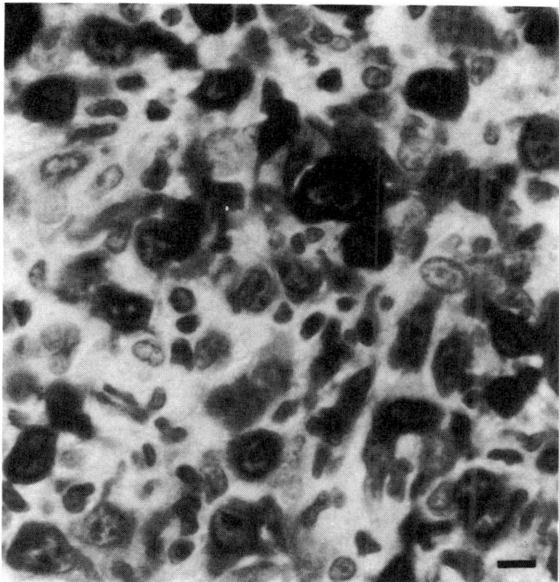

Fig. 7. Anaplastic large cell (CD30/Ki-1$^+$) lymphoma showing many tumour cells strongly stained with the anti LMP-1 monoclonal antibody. (APAAP method; haematoxylin counterstain; paraffin-embedded tissue section; Bar = 12.5 μm.)

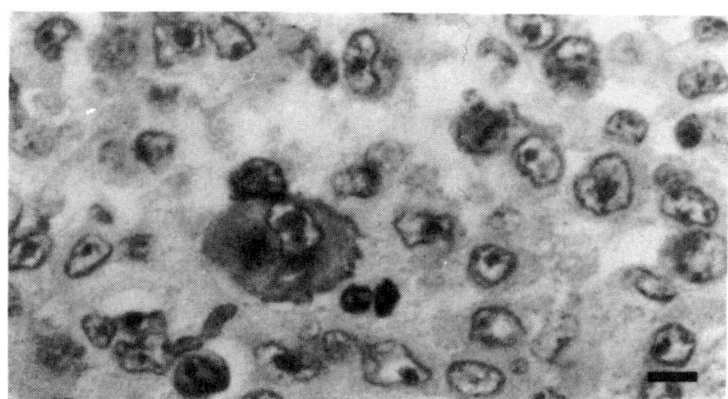

Fig. 8. A Reed–Sternberg-like cell of an anaplastic large cell (CD30/Ki-1$^+$) lymphoma shows staining for LMP-1 with a dot cytoplasmic pattern. (Alkaline phosphatase anti-alkaline phosphatase; haematoxylin counterstain; paraffin-embedded tissue section; Bar = 12.5 μm.)

Regarding additional genetic events contributing to the development of HIV-associated NHL, several reports have pointed to an association of NHL with chromosomal traslocations involving the *c-myc* oncogene. Activation of the *c-myc* oncogene has been detected in 100% of AIDS-small non-cleaved cell lymphomas, whereas in large non-cleaved cell lymphomas and immunoblastic–plasmacytoid lymphomas it is restricted to a minority of tumours.[35,38] The molecular mechanisms leading to *c-myc* activation in AIDS–NHL are similar to sporadic Burkitt's lymphoma, as opposed to endemic Burkitt's lymphoma in many respects, including the analogous breakpoint location in both chromosomes 8 and 14, as well as comparable frequency of association between *c-myc* activation and EBV infection.[35,38]

Another genetic lesion associated with AIDS-NHL concerns p53 inactivation; it is specifically associated with Burkitt's lymphoma (Fig. 9), while consistently negative in all other types of NHL.[38–40] The frequent association of *c-myc* deregulation and p53 inactivation in small non-cleaved cell lymphomas may underlie a synergistic effect of these two lesions in small noncleaved cell lymphomas pathogenesis.[38]

Other oncogenes commonly involved in the pathogenesis of lymphomas in the immunocompetent host (e.g. bcl-1, bcl-2) do not seem to be relevant for AIDS-associated lymphomagenesis. On the other hand, mutations of the *Ras* genes, which are never detected in B-cell NHL of the immunocompetent host,[41] are present in AIDS-NHL, although at low frequency.[38]

Therefore, AIDS–lymphomagenesis seems to be associated with multiple genetic lesions (*c-myc* activation, *Ras* mutation, EBV infection, p53 inactivation), however, the repertoire of genetic lesions differs substantially in different histological types of AIDS–NHL, suggesting that AIDS–lymphomagenesis may be associated with distinct molecular pathways.[42] At least two independent patterns of genetic lesions are observed in these tumours. On one side, NHL displaying small non-cleaved cell histology are strictly associated with *c-myc* deregulation and p53 inactivation, while EBV infection is limited to a subset of these tumours. On the other side, a monoclonal EBV infection is consistently associated with systemic ALC CD30/Ki-1^{+} NHL, a subset of large cell-immunoblastic–plasmacytoid lymphomas, HD and central nervous system AIDS–NHL.

As a consequence of these morphological and biological data, a pathological classification of HIV-associated systemic lymphomas based on the recognition of two main groups, i. e. 'blastic' cell and 'anaplastic' cell lymphomas, which include specific cytomorphologic subtypes and possibly HD, may be formulated (Table 1). This classification, which use the terminology of the WF[11] and the updated Kiel classification,[15] acknowledges morphologic variants of the high-grade B-cell NHL described by Hui and colleagues.[24] Some categories, such as small non-cleaved cell and immunoblastic lymphomas, are more precisely distinguished, the cases with

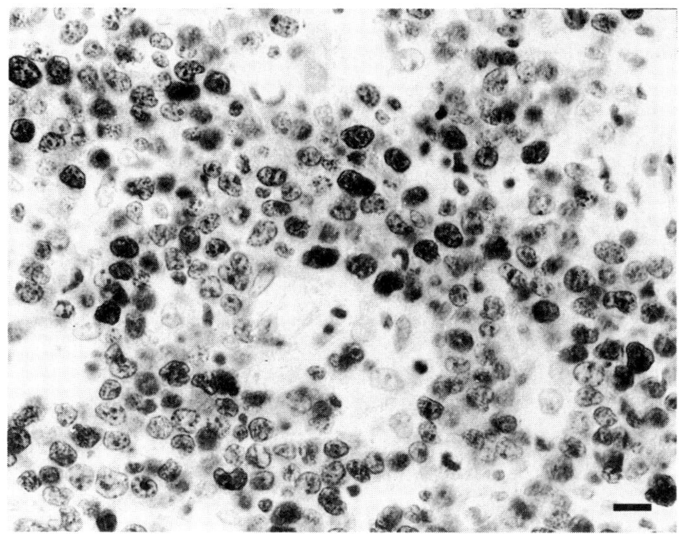

Fig. 9. Small non-cleaved cell lymphoma stained with DO-7, which recognizes wild and mutant p53 protein. Positively stained cells are diffusely distributed in the tumour cellularity. The nuclear staining (brown) of cells is of variable intensity. (Avidin–biotin–peroxidase complex; haematoxylin counterstain; paraffin-embedded tissue section; magnification Bar = 12.5 μm.)

intermediate features being classified separately. Moreover, the clear-cut separation of anaplastic cell lymphomas, including ALC CD30/Ki-1$^+$ lymphomas and possibly a proportion of HD cases, should stimulate the consideration of these entities in the differential diagnosis with immunoblastic polymorphic lymphomas in these patients.

This proposal represents a pragmatic attempt to indicate precise morphological categories within a heterogeneous group of disorders with possible differences in their pathogenesis. The grouping of the different pathologic categories based on the morphological features and their association with genetic lesions (Table 2) may provide a reliable basis for further biologically oriented investigations on the pathogenesis of HIV-associated lymphomas.

Whether this classification might be useful for the clinical management of patients with HIV-associated lymphomas, should be tested in patients treated within large prospective studies.

Clinical findings

The majority of patients with AIDS-related NHL present with B-symptoms, widespread disease and extranodal involvement at presentation, the most

Table 2. *Classification schema for systemic lymphomas occurring during HIV-1-induced immunosuppression (based on morphologic features and the association with genetic lesions)*

(*a*) *'Blastic' cell lymphomas* (which are not associated with EBV encoded LMP-1 expression)
- centroblastic
- small non-cleaved cell (associated with *c-myc* deregulation+p53 inactivation)
- plasmablastic
- blastic cells with intermediate features

(*b*) *'Blastic' cell lymphomas* (which may be associated with EBV encoded LMP-1 expression)
- immunoblastic[a]

(*c*) *'Anaplastic' cell lymphomas* (associated with monoclonal EBV infection and LMP-1 expression
- anaplastic large cell (CD30/Ki-1^+)
- Hodgkin's lymphoma

[a] Immunoblastic lymphomas were included as a separate entity because they are different in Epstein–Barr viral latent gene expression from other 'blastic' cell systemic lymphomas.

common sites being the CNS, gastrointestinal tract, bone marrow and liver. Any site of the body is, however, at risk of involvement.[1,43] On account of the unfavourable presentation of NHL and the prevalence of high-grade subtypes, in addition to the underlying HIV infection with associated opportunistic infections, the overall outcome of these malignancies is poor. However, some prognostic factors for survival have been identified recently and some patients with AIDS-related NHL can obtain long-term survival and possibly cure with appropriate therapy. Levine et al identified Karnofsky performance status less than 70%, AIDS diagnosis prior to the diagnosis of NHL, bone marrow involvement and low CD4 counts as prognostic factors associated with a poorer prognosis.[6] Those patients who presented one or more of these factors had a significantly lower survival than those patients without any of these factors (4 months vs 11 months of median survival).[6] Kaplan et al identified CD4 less than 100 cells/dl as the most significant factor in predicting the survival but also performance status, development of AIDS prior to the lymphoma and presence of advanced disease were also significant prognostic factors.[4] Also Gisselbrecht et al identified low performance status, CD4 less than 100 and AIDS diagnosis prior to NHL as prognostic factors predicting survival, with 50% of those patients without any of these factors being alive after 2 years from diagnosis of NHL.[44]

Patients with primary CNS NHL had a significantly shorter median survival in comparison with patients with peripheral systemic lymphomas,[6] perhaps related to the significantly lower CD4 counts and consequent more severe immunosuppression. It is important to stress that leptomeningeal disease is not related to a poorer survival, but it is not unusual to find asymptomatic leptomeningeal lymphomas during the staging procedures of these patients. Therefore, lumbar punctions should be performed routinely in the staging of these patients. On account of the aggressive course of NHL, intensive chemotherapy regimens should be employed. The risk of severe side effects, in particular bone marrow toxicity, is of special concern in these patients with such aggressive NHL. It has recently been demonstrated that HIV-positive patients in a low risk category, i.e. without opportunistic infections and AIDS diagnosis and with good performance status can be treated with an intensive chemotherapy approach such as LNH 84.[45] Complete response (CR) have been obtained in 64% of the 141 patients, that is not significantly different from that obtained with HIV-negative NHL (75%). 14% of patients died during treatment, half due to the toxicity and half to the progression of the disease.[44] For patients with CD4<100/cells/dl and PS <2 the probability of survival at 2 years was 50%. Levine et al[10] have evaluated a low dose of Metotrexate, Bleomycin, Doxorubicin, Cyclophosphamide, Vincristine, Dexametazone (M-BACOD) regimen in a prospective trial of patients with and without adverse prognostic factors, showing that the less intensive regimens of combination chemotherapy with early CNS prophylaxis may be comparable to more intensive regimens, which have been associated with high rate of opportunistic infections. Others have shown that high risk patients respond poorly to low dose chemotherapy with a CHOP (Cyclophosphamide, Doxorubicin, Vincristine and Prednisone)-like regimen in association with zidovudine with complicating opportunistic infections and with disappointing overall survival.[46] However, the use of the bone marrow growth factors could overcome some of these problems.[47,48] The recently activated EORTC AIDS and Tumour Study Group has undertaken a multicentre European study on NHL in order to compare chemotherapy regimens at different intensity in patients with low, intermediate and high risk category. High risk was defined as the presence of one or more of the following prognostic factors: CD4 less than 100 cells/dl, PS $\geqslant$ 2 and diagnosis of AIDS. G–CSF will be given to all of these patients and zidovudine will be given after the induction of chemotherapy.

Role of G–CSF

Primary haematopoietic failure combined with the myelotoxicity of anti-viral, antiinfective and antineoplastic therapies often complicate the treatment of the acquired immunodeficiency syndrome (AIDS).[49–51]

Haematopoietic growth factors that affect granulocytopoiesis (granulocyte–acrophage colony stimulating factor, GM–CSF and granulocyte colony stimulating factor, G–CSF) have been investigated extensively in clinical trials of patients of general population,[52–62] but to a lesser extent in HIV setting.[47,63–66] In patients with HIV infection treated with Zidovudine (AZT) and consequent neutropenia, G–CSF has been shown to elevate and to maintain high neutrophil levels.[66] There are no data reported in literature on the use of G–CSF in HIV-related malignant tumours. Kaplan et al reported an improvement of the chemotherapy related bone marrow toxicity in patients with HIV-related non-Hodgkin lymphoma (NHL) treated with chemotherapy and GM–CSF versus those treated with chemotherapy alone. In this study, however, GM–CSF has increased the p24 antigen level in the majority of patients, although without a clinical stimulation of the HIV infection.[47]

Treatment of HIV-related NHL with chemotherapy regimens is associated with a substantial risk of side effects, in particular bone marrow toxicity, that precludes therapy in the majority of patients.[10,67] With the availability of CSFs and in particular of G–CSF, we thought it logical to evaluate in a prospective study the prophylactic use of G–CSF, that is not associated as GM–CSF with the potential stimulation of HIV replication, in association with chemotherapy in patients with HIV-related NHL.[68]

New medical technology might offer significant benefits as well as higher cost. In the present economic climate, the evaluation of the cost-effective balance is becoming increasingly important. The cost of G–CSF is high, but its use theoretically could reduce the cost of the overall treatment in that it could substantially decrease antibiotical therapy required for treatment of infectious complications related to bone marrow toxicity and the days of hospitalization required for the bone marrow toxicity as well. For these reasons, in addition to the evaluation of the clinical effects, the economic evaluation of G–CSF in this setting seems worthy to being undertaken.

This study reports the monoistitutional experience of treatment of HIV-related NHL with chemotherapy and prophylactic G–CSF, as far as toxicity, in particular bone marrow toxicity, and the cost of the overall treatment, comparing 37 consecutive patients treated with intensive chemotherapy regimens, 19 without and 18 with G–CSF.

In July 1991, G–CSF was available at the Division of Medical Oncology and AIDS of the Centro di Riferimento Oncologico, Italy, for treatment of HIV-related NHL. Eighteen consecutive patients from July 1991 to September 1992 were therefore submitted to chemotherapy and G–CSF 5 mcg/kg subcutaneously per day starting 24 after chemotherapy for 13 days in all cycles. The group of control was a comparable group of 19 patients consecutively treated from July 1989 to June 1991 with chemotherapy but without G–CSF, not yet available.

All patients had evidence of HIV infection, as determined by the presence of HIV antibodies by Elisa and confirmed by Western Blot. All patients had a diagnosis of HIV-related NHL. All patients were diagnosed and treated at our Institution. None of the patients had previously received chemotherapy or radiotherapy.

We have analysed 37 consecutive patients treated with intensive chemotherapy regimens, 19 patients from July 1989 to June 1991 without G–CSF and 18 patients from July 1991 to September 1992 with G–CSF, 5 mcg/kg/day s.c. starting 24 hours after chemotherapy for 13 days in all cycles. The chemotherapy regimens employed were the LNH84 regimen (Coiffier et al. JCO 1989, 8: 1018–26) composed by Adriamycin, Cyclophosphamide, Vindesine, Bleomycin and Prednisone and CHOP-like regimen CHVmP/VCR-BLM (Carde et al. *Ann Oncol* 1991, 2: 431–436) given for 3–6 cycles. The analysis was performed only for the first three cycles of chemotherapy. The cost of one day of hospitalization in our Division is about 450 US dollars. G–CSF has significantly reduced the duration of nadir to a mean of 8.4 days compared to 10.8 days in the control groups ($p = 0.006$), while among patients with lymphocyte CD4+ count $\geqslant 200/mm^3$ the nadir WBC as well was significantly higher in the G–CSF group than in the control group ($p = 0.009$). The events rates for fever with neutropenia and for culture confirmed infections were comparable among the two groups. The mean duration of delays between cycles of chemotherapy was reduced from 9 days in the control group to 4 days in the G–CSF treated patients ($p = 0.01$). In conjunction with an overall reduction of the duration of nadir in the G–CSF group, there was also a significant decrease in the mean duration of hospitalization for toxicity per patient compared to the control group. Therefore, by contrast to what one might have expected, the cost of chemotherapy plus G–CSF vs chemotherapy alone did not increase, actually it decreased. The relative dose intensity (RDI) and the overall response rates were similar in the two groups. Surprisingly, the median survival time was higher in the control group than in the G–CSF treated patients, although the clinico-pathological characteristics of NHL in this relatively small series of patients were apparently comparable. This could be explained by the lower CD4 count/mm^3 in the G–CSF treated patients than in the control group (120 vs 235).

In conclusion, the prophylactic use of G–CSF in patients with HIV-related NHL receiving intensive chemotherapy is associated with a significant reduction of treatment-related myelosuppression, without an increase in the cost.

Are some Aids-related NHL potentially curable malignancies?

Although it is clear from the literature that some patients with HIV-related NHL may survive in complete remission for two years, these data are insufficient to determine whether these patients are actually cured because of lack of further follow-up.[1–9,44,46,69–73] For this reason we reviewed our monoinstitutional experience at the Aviano Cancer Institute, Italy, with emphasis on the clinico-pathological characteristics of a subgroup of patients with long-term survival after treatment of HIV-related NHL.

From April 1985 to February 1993, 91 HIV-infected patients with peripheral NHL were identified through pathology and clinical records at the Centro di Riferimento Oncologico, Aviano, Italy. Eighteen of these patients were excluded from the current analysis, because 15 were treated elsewhere and 3 patients received no treatment. Therefore 73 patients constitute the basis for this study in that data are available for analysis of their clinicopathological features and therapeutic outcome. Clinicopathological features and EBV association findings of subgroups of our patients with HIV-related NHL have been previously reported.[13,17,18,22]

To evaluate the possibility of cure, we reviewed our monoinstitutional experience at the Centro di Riferimento Oncologico, Italy, with emphasis on the clinico-pathological characteristics of a subgroup of 13 patients with long-term survival, observed between April 1985 and February 1993.

We have identified arbitrarily two groups of patients, the first one (group A) including patients with a CR lasting for at least two years and the other comprising all remaining patients (group B).

Comparing the two groups we found that the 13 patients of group A differed significantly from the other patients in terms of better CD4+ cell count and performance status (PS) at the time of diagnosis of NHL, while there was no significant difference in the histological subtypes. The overall survival of the 73 patients was 8 months. Four prognostic factors influenced survival: younger patients, those who had a better PS, those with CD4+ cell count $\geqslant 100/mm^3$ and patients without B symptoms had a significantly longer survival period. The median survival in patients of group A was 42 months (range 24–72), but none of these patients relapsed after up to 6 years of observation.

Thus a subgroup of patients can be cured from HIV-related NHL, with some being alive without evidence of disease 3 to 6 years after therapy, and others who died of causes related to underlying HIV infection, in particular opportunistic infections, but without relapse of NHL.

In conclusion, it is clear that HIV-related NHLs are highly aggressive malignancies associated with a poor prognosis per se, as well as from the underlying HIV infection. However, it is possible to cure a subgroup of these patients, who have better PS and less advanced immune dysfunction related to HIV infection. These patients should therefore be considered for chemotherapy with curative intent, although it is not clear from our data whether conventional aggressive chemotherapy like LNH84 is superior to lower intensive chemotherapy regimens in inducing long-term survival of such a favourable subgroup of patients. Further improvements of therapy of HIV infection and of its opportunistic infections are needed in order to increase significantly the chances of cure of patients with HIV-related NHL.

Acknowledgement

Supported by grants of Istituto Superiore di Sanità, AIDS Project 1993 and AIRC 1993.

References

(1) Ziegler JL, Beckstead JA, Volberding PA et al. Non-Hodgkin lymphoma in 90 homosexual men. Relation to generalized lymphadenopathy and the acquired immunodeficinecy syndrome. *N Engl J Med* 1984; 311: 565–70.

(2) Knowles DM, Chamulak GA, Subar M et al. Lymphoid neoplasia associated with the acquired immunodeficiency syndrome (AIDS). The New York University Medical Center experience with 105 patients (1981–2086). *Ann Intern Med* 1988; 108: 744–53.

(3) Lowenthal DA, Straus DJ, Campbell SW et al. AIDS-related lymphoid neoplasia. The Memorial Hospital experience. *Cancer* 1988; 61: 2325–37.

(4) Kaplan LD, Abrams DI, Feigal E et al. AIDS-associated non-Hodgkin's lymphoma in San Francisco. *JAMA* 1989; 261: 719–24.

(5) Roithmann S, Toledano M, Tourani JM et al. HIV-associated non-Hodgkin's lymphomas: clinical characteristics and outcome. The experience of the French Registry of HIV-associated tumors. *Ann Oncol 1991*; 2: 289–95.

(6) Levine AM, Sullivan-Halley J, Pike MC et al. Human immunodeficiency virus-related lymphoma-prognostic factors predictive of survival. *Cancer* 1991; 68: 2466–72.

(7) Pedersen C, Gerstoft J, Lundgren JD et al. HIV-associated lymphoma-histopathology and association with Epstein–Barr virus genome related to clinical, immunological and prognostic features. *Eur J Cancer* 1991; 27: 1416–23.

(8) Gill P, Levine A, Krailo M et al. AIDS-related malignant lymphoma: results of prospective treatment trials. *J Clin Oncol* 1987; 5: 1322–8.

(9) Monfardini S, Tirelli U, Vaccher E et al. Malignant lymphomas in patients with or at risk for AIDS. *J Natl Cancer Inst* 1988; 80: 855–60.

(10) Levine AM, Wernz JC, Kaplan L et al. Low-dose chemotherapy with central nervous system prophylaxis and zidovudine maintenance in AIDS-related lymphoma. A prospective, multi-instutional trial. *JAMA* 1991; 266: 84–8.

(11) The non-Hodgkin's lymphoma pathologic classification project. National Cancer Institute sponsored study of classification of non-Hodgkin's lymphomas. Summary and description of a Working Formulation for clinical usage. *Cancer* 1982; 49: 2112–35.

(12) Levine AM. AIDS-related malignancies: the emerging epidemic. *J Natl Cancer Inst* 1993; 85: 1382–97.

(13) Carbone A, Tirelli U, Vaccher E et al. A clinicopathologic study of lymphoid neoplasias associated with human immunodeficiency virus infection in Italy. *Cancer* 1991; 68: 842–52.

(14) Stein H, Mason DY, Gerdes J et al. The expression of the Hodgkin's disease associated antigen Ki-1 in reactive and neoplastic lymphoid tissue: evidence that Reed–Sternberg cells and histiocytic malignancies are derived from activated lymphoid cells. *Blood* 1985; 66: 848–58.
(15) Stansfeld AG, Diebold J, Kapanci Y et al. Updated Kiel classification for lymphomas. *Lancet* 1988; i: 292–3.
(16) Raphael M, Gentilhomme O, Tulliez M, Byron PA, Diebold J, and the French Study Group of Pathology for Human Immunodeficiency Virus-Associated Tumors. Histopathologic features of high-grade non-Hodgkin's lymphomas in acquired immunodeficiency syndrome. *Arch Pathol Lab Med* 1991; 115: 15–20.
(17) Carbone A, Gloghini A, Zanette I, Canal B, Volpe R. Demonstration of Epstein–Barr viral genomes by in situ hybridization in AIDS-related high-grade and anaplastic large cell $CD30^+$ lymphomas. *Am J Clin Pathol* 1993; 99: 289–97.
(18) Carbone A, Tirelli U, Gloghini A, Volpe R, Boiocchi M. Human immunodeficiency virus-associated systemic lymphomas may be subdivided into two main groups according to Epstein–Barr viral latent gene expression. *J Clin Oncol* 1993; 11: 1674–81.
(19) Carbone A, Gloghini A, Volpe R, Boiocchi M, Tirelli U, and the Italian Cooperative Group on AIDS & Tumors. High frequency of Epstein–Barr virus latent membrane protein-1 expression in AIDS-related Ki-1 (CD30) – positive anaplastic large cell lymphomas. *Am J Clin Pathol* 1994; 101: 768–72.
(20) Gonzalez–Clemente JM, Ribera JM, Campo E, Bosch X, Montserrat E, Grau JM. Ki-1+ anaplastic large-cell lymphoma of T-cell origin in an HIV-infected patient. *AIDS* 1991; 5: 751–5.
(21) Chadburn A, Cesarman E, Jagirdar J, Subar M, Mir NM, Knowles DM. CD30 (Ki-1) positive anaplastic large cell lymphomas in individuals infected with the human immunodeficiency virus. *Cancer* 1993; 72: 3078–90.
(22) Boiocchi M, De Re V, Gloghini A et al. High incidence of monoclonal EBV episomes in Hodgkin's disease and anaplastic large cell Ki-1-positive lymphomas in HIV-1-positive patients. *Int J Cancer* 1993; 54: 53–9.
(23) Boiocchi M, Dolcetti R, De Re V, Gloghini A, Carbone A. Demonstration of a unique Epstein–Barr virus-positive cellular clone in metachronous multiple localizations of Hodgkin's disease. *Am J Pathol* 1993; 142: 33–8.
(24) Hui PK, Feller AC, Lennert K. High-grade non-Hodgkin's lymphoma of B-cell type. 1. Histopathology. *Histopathology* 1988; 12: 127–43.
(25) Uccini S, Monardo F, Ruco LP et al. High frequency of Epstein–Barr virus genome in HIV-positive patients with Hodgkin's disease. *Lancet* 1989; i: 1458.
(26) Audouin J, Diebold J, Pallesen G. Frequent expression of Epstein–Barr virus latent membrane protein-1 in tumor cells of Hodgkin's disease in HIV-positive patients. *J Pathol* 1992; 167: 381–4.
(27) MacMahon EME, Glass JD, Hayward SD et al. Epstein–Barr virus in AIDS-related primary central nervous system lymphoma. *Lancet* 1991; ii: 969–73.
(28) Adldinger HK, Delius H, Freese UK, Clarke J, Bornkamm GW. A putative transforming gene of Jijoye virus differs from that of Epstein–Barr virus prototypes. *Virology* 1985; 141; 221–34.

(29) Boyle MJ, Sewell WA, Sculley TB et al. Subtypes of Epstein–Barr virus in human immunodeficiency virus-associated non-Hodgkin's lymphoma. *Blood* 1991; 78: 300–11.
(30) Boyle MJ, Vasak E, Tschuchnigg M et al. Subtypes of Epstein–Barr virus (EBV) in Hodgkin's disease: association between B-type EBV and immunocompromise. *Blood* 1993; 81: 468–74.
(31) De Re V, Boiocchi M, De Vita S et al. Subtypes of Epstein–Barr virus in HIV-1-associated and HIV-1-unrelated Hodgkin's disease cases. *Int J Cancer* 1993; 54: 895–8.
(32) Gaidano G, Dalla-Favera R. Biologic aspects of human immunodeficiency virus-related lymphoma. *Curr Opin Oncol* 1992; 4: 900–6.
(33) Voelkerding KV, Sandhaus LM, Kim HC et al. Plasma cell malignancy in the acquired immune deficiency syndrome. Association with Epstein–Barr virus. *Am J Clin Pathol* 1989; 92: 222–8.
(34) Herbst H, Dallenbach F, Hummel M et al. Epstein–Barr virus latent membrane protein expression in Hodgkin and Reed–Sternberg cells. *Proc Natl Acad Sci USA* 1991; 88: 4766–70.
(35) Subar M, Neri A, Inghirami G, Knowles DM, Dalla-Favera R. Frequent *c-myc* oncogene activation and infrequent presence of Epstein–Barr virus genome in AIDS-associated lymphoma. *Blood* 1988; 72: 667–71.
(36) Karp JE, Broder S. Acquired immunodeficiency syndrome and non-Hodgkin's lymphomas. *Cancer Res* 1991; 51: 4743–56.
(37) Pelicci P-G, Knowles DM II, Arlin ZA et al. Multiple monoclonal B cell expansions and *c-myc* oncogene rearrangements in acquired immune deficiency syndrome-related lymphoproliferative disorders: implications for lymphomagenesis. *J Exp Med* 1986; 164: 2049–76.
(38) Ballerini P, Gaidano G, Gong JZ et al. Multiple genetic lesions in acquired immunodeficiency syndrome-related non-Hodgkin's lymphoma. *Blood* 1993; 81: 166–76.
(39) Gaidano G, Ballerini P, Gong JZ et al. P53 mutations in human lymphoid malignancies: associations with Burkitt lymphoma and chronic lymphocytic leukemia. *Proc Natl Acad Sci USA* 1991; 88: 5413–17.
(40) De Re V, Carbone A, De Vita S et al. p53 protein overexpression and p53 gene abnormalities in HIV-1-related non-Hodgkin's lymphomas. *Int J Cancer* 1994; 56: 662–7.
(41) Gaidano P, Dalla Favera R. Proto-oncogenes and tumor suppressor genes. In: DM Knowles ed. *Neoplastic hematopathology*. Baltimore: William & Wilkins, 1992: 245–61.
(42) Shibata D, Weiss LM, Hernandez AM, Nathwani BN, Bernstein L, Levine AM. Epstein–Barr virus-associated non-Hodgkin's lymphoma in patients infected with the human immunodeficiency virus. *Blood* 1993; 81, 2102–9.
(43) LevineAM, Meyer PR, Begandy MK et al. Development of B-cell lymphoma in homosexual men: clinical and immunologic findings. *Ann Intern Med* 1984; 100: 7.
(44) Gisselbrecht C, Oksenhendler E, Tirelli U et al. Human immunodeficiency virus-related lymphoma treatment with LNH84 regimen in a 'good risk' population. *Am J Med* 1991; 68: 842–52.
(45) Coiffier B, Gisselbrecht C, Herbrecht R et al. LNH84 regimen: a multicenter

study of intensive chemotherapy in 737 patients with aggressive malignant lymphoma. *J Clin Oncol* 1989; 7: 1018–26.

(46) Tirelli U, Errante D, Oksenhendler E et al. Prospective study with combined low-dose chemotherapy and zidovudine in 37 patients with poor-prognosis AIDS-related non-Hodgkin's lymphoma. *Ann of Oncol* 1992; 3: 843–47.

(47) Kaplan LD, Kahn JO, Crowe S et al. Clinical and virologal effects of recombinant human granulocyte–macrophage colony stimulating factor in patients receiving chemotherapy for human immunodeficiency virus associated non-Hodgkin's lymphoma: results of a randomized trial. *J Clin Oncol* 1991; 9: 929.

(48) Tirelli U. Errante D, Vaccher E et al. Treatment of HIV-related non-Hodgkin's lymphoma (NHL) with chemotherapy (CT) and G-CSF: reduction in the days of hospitalization and toxicity with concomitant overall reduction in the cost. *Proc. ASCO* 1993; 53: 13.

(49) Folks TM, Kessler SW, Orestein JM et al. Infection and replication of HIV-1 in purified progenitor cells of normal human bone marrow. *Science* 1988; 242: 919–22.

(50) Zon LJ, Arkim C, Groopman JE. Hematologic manifestations of the human immune deficiency virus (HIV). *Br J Haematol* 1987; 66: 251–6.

(51) Scadden DT, Zon LJ, Groopman JE. Pathophysiology and management of HIV-associated hematologic disorders. *Blood* 1989; 74: 1455–63.

(52) Berdel WE, Danhauseer–Riedl S, Steinhauser G, Winton EF. Various human hematopoietic growth factors (interleukin-3, GM–CSF, G–CSF) stimulate clonal growth of non hematopoeitic tumor cells. *Blood* 1989; 73: 80–3.

(53) Yoshida T, Nakamura S, Ohtake S et al. Effect of granulocyte colony-stimulating factor or neutropenia due to chemotherapy for non-Hodgkin's lymphoma. *Cancer* 1990; 66: 1904–9.

(54) Kotake T, Miki T, Akaza H et al. Effect of recombinant granulocyte colony-stimulating factor (G-CSF) on chemotherapy-induced neutropenia in patients with urogenital cancer. *Cancer Chemother Pharmacol* 1991; 27: 253–7.

(55) Neidhart J, Mangalik A, Kohler W et al. Granulocyte colony-stimulating factor stimulates recovery of granulocytes in patients receiving dose-intensive chemotherapy without bone marrow transplantation. *J Clin Oncol* 1989; 7: 1685–92.

(56) Herrmann F, Schulz G, Wieser M et al. Effects of granulocyte–macrophage colony-stimulating factor on neutropenia and related morbidity induced by myelotoxic chemotherapy. *Am J Med* 1990; 88: 619–24.

(57) Gianni AM, Bregni M, Siena S et al. Recombinant human granulocyte–macrophage colony-stimulating factor reduces hematologic toxicity and widens clinical applicability of high-dose cyclophosphamide treatment in breast cancer and non-Hodgkin's lymphoma. *J Clin Oncol* 1990; 8: 768–78.

(58) Sheridan WP, Morstyn G, Wolf M et al. Granulocyte colony-stimulating factor and neutrophil recovery after high-dose chemotherapy and autologous bone marrow tranplantation. *Lancet* 1989; 2: 891–5.

(59) Nemunaitis J, Singer JW, Buckner CD et al. Use of recombinant hyuman granulocyte–macrophage colony-stimulating factor in autologous marrow transplantation for lymphoid malignancies. *Blood* 1988; 72: 834–6.

(60) Freund MRF, Luft S, Schober C et al. Differential effect of GM–CSF and G–CSF in cyclic neutropenia. *Lancet* 1990; 336: 313.
(61) Crawford J, Ozzer H, Stoller R et al. Reduction by granulocyte colony-stimulating factor of fever and neutropenia induced by chemotherapy in patients with small-cell lung cancer. *NEJM* 1991; 325: 164–170.
(62) Trillet–Lenoir V, Green J, Manegold J et al. Recombinant granulocyte colony stimulating factor reduces the infections complications of cytotoxic chemotherapy. *Eur J Cancer* 1993; 29A(3): 319–24.
(63) Miles SA, Mitsuyasu RT, Lee K et al. Recombinant human granulocyte colony-stimulating factor increases circulating burst forming unit-erythron and red blood cell production in patients with severe human immunodeficiency virus infection. *Blood* 1990; 75: 2137–42.
(64) Groopman JE, Mitsuyasu RT, DeLeo MJ, Oette DH, Golde DW. Effect of recombinant human granulocyt–macrophage colony-stimulating factor on myelopoiesis in the acquired immunodeficiency syndrome. *N Engl J Med* 1987; 317: 593–8.
(65) Pluda JM, Yarchoan R, Smith PD et al. Subcutaneous recombinant granulocyt–macrophage colony-stimulating factor used as a single agent and in an alternating regimen with azidothymidine in leukopenic patients with severe human immunodeficiency virus infection. *Blood* 1990; 76: 463–72.
(66) Miles SA, Mitsuyasu RT, Moreno J et al. Combined therapy with recombinant granulocyte colony-stimulating factor and erythropoietin decreases hematologic toxicity from zidovudine. *Blood* 1991; 77: 2109–17.
(67) Levine AM, Acquired immunodeficiency syndrome-related lymphoma. *Blood* 1992; 80 (1): 8–20.
(68) Perno CF, Cooney DA, Gao WY et al. Effects of bone marrow granulocyte cytokines on human immunodeficiency virus replication and the antiviral activity of dideoxynucleosides in cultures of microcyte/macrophage. *Blood* 1992, 80(4): 995–1003.
(69) Boyle MJ, Swanson CE, Turner JJ et al: Definition of two distinct types of AIDS-associated non-Hodgkin lymphoma. *Br J of Haematol* 1990; 76: 506–12.
(70) Bermudez MA, Grant KM, Rodvien R et al. Non-Hodgkin's lymphoma in a population with or at risk for acquired immunodeficiency syndrome: indications for intensive chemotherapy. *Am J Med* 1989; 86: 71–6.
(71) Sawka CA, Shepherd FA, Brandwein J et al. Treatment of AIDS-related non-Hodgkin's lymphoma with a twelve week chemotherapy program. *Leukemia and Lymphoma* 1992; 8: 213–20.
(72) Sparano AJ, Wiernik PH, Strack M et al. Infusional cyclophosphamide, doxorubicin, and etoposide in human immunodeficiency virus-and human T-cell leukemia virus type I-related non-Hodgkin's lymphoma: a highly active regimen. *Blood* 1993; 81: 2810–15.
(73) Remick SC, McSharry JJ, Wolf BC et al: Novel oral combination chemotherapy on the treatment of intermediate-grade and high-grade AIDS-related non-Hodgkin's lymphoma. *J Clin Oncol* 1993; 11: 1691–702.

Lymphoma of mucosa-associated lymphoid tissue

W C CHAN and J H CASEY

Introduction

The definitive diagnosis of extranodal lymphoid infiltrates is frequently challenging for pathologists. There are a number of reasons for the difficulties encountered in evaluating these lesions. One of the major criteria for the diagnosis of nodal lymphomas is the effacement of normal nodal architecture which cannot be applied in extranodal sites. On the other hand, the pattern of tissue infiltration in a specific organ may be of diagnostic significance, but lymphoid infiltrates in each specific extranodal site are relatively uncommon and not many pathologists have extensive experience in evaluating them. Frequently, the diagnosis of lymphoma is not anticipated by the clinician and the biopsies are taken without making provisions, such as submission of fresh tissues, for further investigations which are often necessary for the characterization of haematopoietic malignancies. Biopsies of visceral organs tend to be small and may not provide sufficient or representative tissue for diagnosis. Sometimes, this difficulty is compounded by crush artefact induced by the biopsy procedure.

A long list of morphological diagnostic criteria have been proposed in numerous publications attempting to provide useful guidelines for the differential diagnosis between benign and neoplastic lymphoid proliferations consisting of mostly small lymphoid cells.[1–5] None of these criteria is absolute and these 'diagnostic criteria' are often of little assistance in difficult cases where useful guidelines would be most helpful. It is clear that even the absence of clinical progression for an extended period does not prove that a lesion is reactive rather than neoplastic.

All correspondence to: Dr WC Chan, Department of Pathology, University of Nebraska Medical Center, 600 South 42nd Street, Omaha, NE 68198, USA.

Cambridge Medical Reviews: Haematological Oncology Volume 4

With the advent of immunophenotyping, it is possible to obtain additional objective data from tissue biopsies, especially in B-cell lymphoproliferations where restriction of light chain expression is a good indicator of a clonal proliferation.[6] A correlation between morphological findings and clonality is now feasible. The availability of molecular diagnostic assays further enhances our ability to determine T- and B-cell clonality as well as the detection of translocations often observed in specific types of non-Hodgkin's lymphomas.[7–9] These technical advances, together with the increased understanding of lymphoproliferative disorders and the normal immune system, permit a much more meaningful study of extranodal lymphoid proliferations.

The concept of a unique group of lymphomas arising in mucosal sites has been promoted in recent studies based on current techniques and knowledge.[10] This concept has already had a strong impact on diagnostic pathology and will probably influence the management of patients with such lymphomas.

Overview of the mucosa-associated lymphoid system

The lymphoid tissue associated with mucosal surfaces is specialized to respond to the unique situation in mucous membranes which have frequent or continuous exposure to large amounts of foreign antigens. This system needs to respond to pathogens promptly and effectively while at the same time not produce inappropriate or excessive reactions that may cause tissue damage.

The mucosa-associated lymphoid tissue (MALT) contains a significant proportion of the total lymphoid tissue of the body. It has been estimated that the human small intestine contains 10^{10} Ig producing immunocytes per metre.[11] MALT is prominent in the upper aerodigestive tract and the distal ileum while some mucosal surfaces do not normally contain organized lymphoid tissue. There is substantial species variation in the distribution of MALT; for example, bronchial-associated lymphoid tissue is well developed in rodents but appears to be absent in normal human lungs.[12]

In the gastrointestinal tract, MALT is organized into Payer's patches in the distal ileum with scattered lymphoid nodules present elsewhere in the intestine. The gastric mucosa is normally devoid of organized lymphoid tissue. Well-developed MALT contains several components: 1) specialized epithelial cells; 2) intraepithelial lymphocytes; 3) a diffuse lymphoplasmacytic component in the lamina propria; 4) lymphoid aggregates with B-cell follicles and T cells; and 5) regional lymph nodes. In the intestinal epithelium overlying the domes of the lymphoid follicles are interspersed cells specialized in antigen transport from the gut lumen to the intestinal wall, called M-cells,[13] so named because of abundant microfolds seen on the luminal surface of these cells by scanning electron microscopy. Aside from macromolecules, certain microorganisms could enter the intestine through the M-cells. It is obvious that M-cells serve an important function in antigen transport but factors that govern this transport function are not known. Since secretory IgA is an essential component of mucosal immunity,[14] crypt epithelial cells associated with MALT produce and express a transport protein, the secretory component (SC), for polymeric IgA and IgM. SC belongs to the immunoglobulin superfamily and binds polymeric Ig in the presence of the joining (J) chain which connects the monomeric Ig subunits.[15] The SC-polymeric Ig complex is then transported across the epithelial cell and the Ig secreted into the luminal aspect of the mucous membrane.

Scattered lymphocytes are seen between intestinal epithelial cells near the basement membrane. Most of these intraepithelial lymphocytes (IEL) are T cells expressing the T-cell antigen receptor (TCAR) in association with the molecular complex CD3. The majority of them express CD8 rather than CD4 molecules.[16] While in the chicken and some other species, a high proportion of IEL express the $\gamma\delta$-TCAR.[17] human IEL are predominantly $\alpha\beta$ TCAR bearing cells. In addition, there is a small subset of IEL that is CD7−CD3$^-$. About half of these cells contain cytoplasmic granules but they do not express natural killer cell markers.[18] The nature of these cells is still not determined. Intraepithelial lymphocytes increase substantially after birth and they are further expanded in patients with coeliac disease.

The Payer's patches in the gut are similar to the lymph node in their organization and are well defined by the 19th week of gestation.[19] There are primary B-lymphoid follicles containing B cells associated with follicular dendritic cells and surrounded by T lymphocytes. Antigenic stimulation induces the formation of germinal centers with a well-defined mantle zone. Isaacson and co-workers[10] observed the presence of an ill-defined zone outside of the mantle zone probably corresponding to the marginal zone most clearly delineated in splenic follicles. Lymphocytes in the MALT marginal zone have been observed to infiltrate the dome epithelium overlying the lymphoid follicle. The interfollicular cells are mostly T cells expressing CD4 with interspersed dendritic cells. It is believed that these T lymphocytes interact directly with B cells or indirectly via secreted cytokines to facilitate isotype switch of IgM$^+$ B cells into IgA$^+$ cells.[20] These switched B cells then migrate to the lamina propria, probably mainly through the recirculation pathway as described below. In the lamina propria, under the influence of T cells which are mainly of the CD4$^+$ subset, through direct cell contact and/or secreted products, the switched B cells undergo terminal differentiation into IgA secreting plasma cells.[20] Thus, an IgA-dominated humoral immune system is generated.

The phenomenon of lymphocyte recirculation, as described by Gowan and Knight,[21] is well established. In MALT, recirculating lymphocytes migrate into efferent lymphatics draining into regional lymph nodes and eventually enter the blood stream via the thoracic duct. From the bloodstream, these lymphocytes reenter lymphoid tissue via specialized venules. There is evidence that lymphoid cells from MALT tend to recirculate and migrate back to MALT at the same or different locations.[22] This preferential migration suggests that MALT-lymphocytes and vascular endothelium bear complementary adhesion molecules directing the migration to MALT sites rather than to peripheral lymph nodes.[23] Local microenvironmental conditions may alter the antigenic profile of the endothelium, thus influencing the migratory pattern of lymphocytes and hence the immunological activity in different sites.[23]

The concept of MALT-associated lymphoma

The concept of a relationship between mucosa-associated lymphoid tissue (MALT) and non-Hodgkin's lymphoma arising in such sites (MALT-lymphoma) has been popularized chiefly by Isaacson and coworkers.[10,24–26] MALT occurs normally in some sites such as small bowel, especially terminal ileum or it may be 'acquired' as in the stomach, lungs, thyroid and salivary glands where, according to Isaacson, native MALT does not occur. It has been proposed that 'acquired MALT' may be induced by an autoimmune phenomenon or may represent an immune response initiated by a foreign antigen, such as *Helicobacter pylori* in the case of gastric lesions. *H. pylori* has been shown to induce follicular lymphoid hyperplasia in the gastric mucosa which Isaacson suggests may be a non-obligate precursor lesion of low grade MALT-lymphoma. Autoimmunity is almost certainly involved in the development of acquired MALT in the thyroid and salivary glands in association with lymphocytic thyroiditis and Sjogren's syndrome. Paradoxically, low grade MALT-lymphoma only rarely arises at the site where native MALT is most abundant, namely, the terminal ileum and most commonly develops at sites normally lacking MALT, that is, the stomach, lung, salivary glands and thyroid. It thus appears that these lymphomas of MALT type tend to arise in 'acquired' rather than 'native' MALT.

Isaacson believes that these lymphomas arising in MALT deserve special recognition since they share certain features:

1. The pure low grade type has an indolent clinical course, and tends to remain localized to the initial site of origin for a long period. It rarely involves the bone marrow at presentation.
2. The indolent nature of the low-grade lesions lends local control measures, such as surgical resection, more feasible than other non-Hodgkin's lymphomas.
3. The histomorphological appearance of the low grade MALT-

lymphomas tends to recapitulate that of normal MALT and does not fit easily into the currently utilized classifications of malignant lymphomas. With the exception of the node-based monocytoid B-cell lymphoma, it does not have nodal counterparts.

Morphology

The prototypic MALT-lymphoma is a low grade B-cell lymphoma of the gastrointestinal (GI) tract, most commonly the stomach. The lesion is typically polymorphic consisting of a heterogeneous mixture of cell types with both neoplastic and reactive elements.[10] The characteristic neoplastic cell is a small-to-medium-sized lymphocyte with irregular nuclear contours resembling a small cleaved follicular centre cell (centrocyte) but with a moderate amount of pale staining cytoplasm (Fig. 1a). The morphology of this cell, termed centrocyte-like (CCL) cell by Isaacson, is somewhat variable. The CCL cell may also resemble a small lymphocyte with a more uniform nuclear contour. However, there is a distinct rim of pale-to-clear cytoplasm around the nucleus (Fig. 1b). Plasma cells are also present and tend to be more prominent in the superficial (luminal) aspect of the infiltrate. Germinal centers, which may be large and prominent, are a constant feature of the lesion (Fig. 2). The CCL cells surround follicles in aggregates or sheets. They also invade the glandular epithelium and form structures called lymphoepithelial lesions (LEL). The epithelium of a mucosal gland may contain only a few ‘Pautrier's abscess’-like infiltrate of CCL-cells (Fig 3(*A*)) or the epithelial involvement may be so extensive that the epithelium is difficult to recognize without an immunostain for cytokeratin (Fig. 3(*B*)). Large transformed lymphocytes are found scattered among the CCL cells, but they are not prominent in a low-grade lesion. Due to the polymorphic cellular infiltrate and the presence of prominent follicles in the low grade MALT-lymphomas, many of these lesions have been considered ‘pseudolymphomas’ in the past. A major contribution of Isaacson and coworkers is the identification of the constellation of morphological features that make up this form of low grade lymphomas, thereby facilitating the distinction between neoplastic and reactive lesions.

Some morphological features of low grade MALT lymphoma may cause diagnostic confusion. Reactive follicles may be invaded by CCL cells.[27] (Fig. 4). When the follicle infiltration is extensive, the tumour may resemble a follicular center cell lymphoma. The morphological features outside of the follicles should lead one to suspect that the case is in fact a MALT-lymphoma with follicular colonization. While a variable plasma cell infiltrate is a frequent component of a MALT-lymphoma, some cases display a predominance of plasma cells raising the question of a plasmacytoma. Again, the presence of groups and clusters of CCL cells, as well as LELs, would indicate that the lesion is, in fact, a MALT-lymphoma with

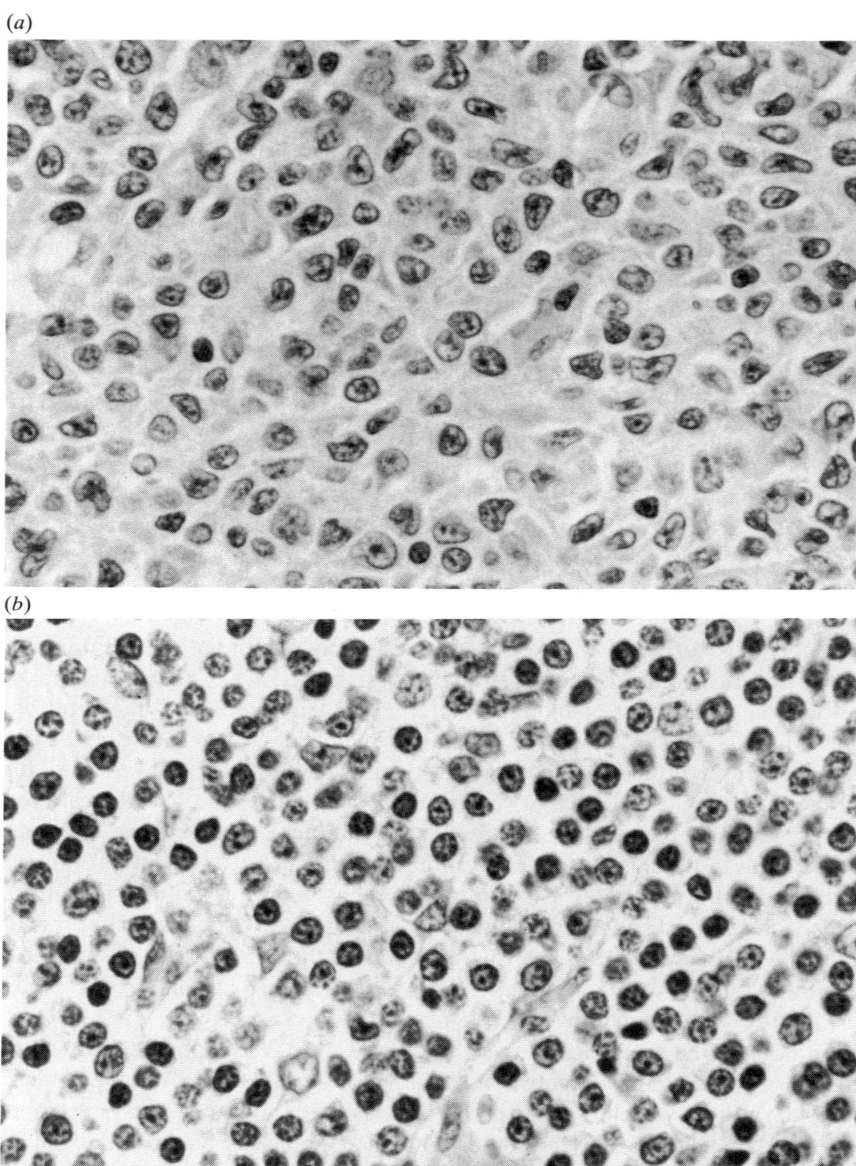

Fig. 1(*a*) Typical centrocyte-like (CCL) cells seen in a low grade MALT-lymphoma. The cells are small to medium sized with irregular nuclear outlines resembling a small follicular centre cell but there is also a moderate amount of pale cytoplasm (H&E × 400). (*b*) The morphological spectrum of the CCL-cells. In some low grade MALT-lymphomas, the neoplastic cells are smaller than the typical CCL cells and with a more regular nuclear outline. A moderate amount of pale to clear cytoplasm is observed (H&E × 400).

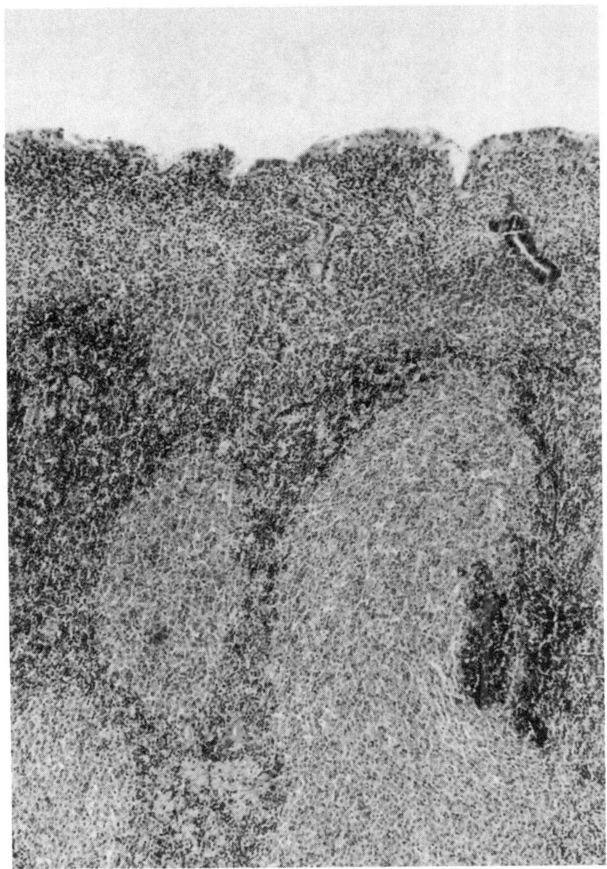

Fig. 2. Germinal centres are present in low grade MALT-lymphomas. In this case, an extensive infiltrate of CCL-cells is seen in the lamina propria. In the submucosa, numerous large germinal centres are observed. (H&E × 40)

plasmacytic differentiation. While scattered large transformed cells are observed in low grade tumours, in some tumours they occur in solid groups and sheets (Fig. 5). Such cases are considered high grade lymphoma evolving from a low grade lesion.[28] Some investigators would consider cases with over 20% large cells as high grade lesions, but the validity of this somewhat arbitrary limit has not been proven.[29,30] Many gastrointestinal lymphomas contain predominantly large cells. The relationship of such lesions to low grade MALT-lymphomas is not as clear as in those lesions in which large areas of the tumour clearly fulfils criteria for low grade MALT-lymphoma. In cases where a low-grade component is detected, it

(*a*)

(*b*)

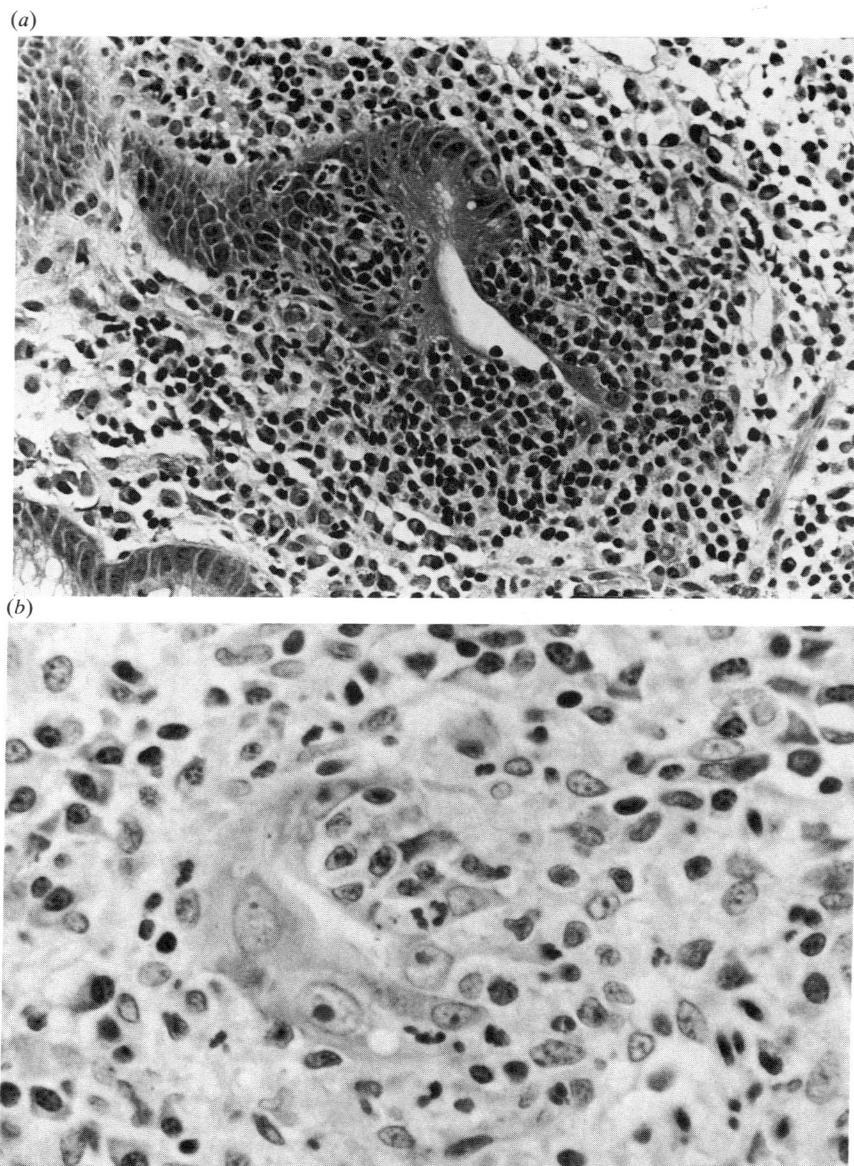

Fig. 3. Lymphoepithelial lesions (LEL) observed in low grade MALT-lymphoma. (*a*) In less involved mucosal glands, the tumour cells infiltrate the epithelium, forming aggregates somewhat resembling the Pautrier's abscess of mycosis fungoides. A few neutrophils are also seen in the epithelium in this case (H&E × 200). (*b*) In some LEL, the glandular structure is largely obliterated by the lymphoid infiltrate. Immunostaining with cytokeratin may be helpful in identifying LEL that are difficult to appreciate with a routine H&E stain. (H&E × 400).

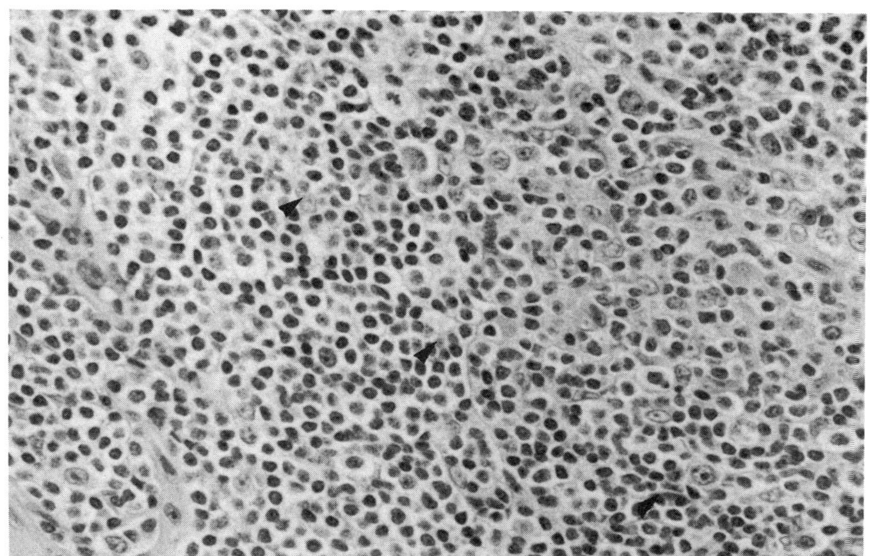

Fig. 4. Follicular colonization observed in a low grade MALT-lymphoma. The CCL-cells outside of a follicle can be seen invading the follicular structure with strands and groups of tumour cells between typical follicular centre cells. The arrowheads indicate the approximate boundary of the follicle which is on the right-hand side of the Figure. (H&E × 200).

has been assumed that the high grade lesion arose from a pre-existing low grade lymphoma. When a low grade MALT-lymphoma is not detectable, such an inference cannot be made.

Low grade lymphomas with the morphological features described above have been observed in other extranodal sites including the salivary glands, thyroid, orbital adnexa, lung, skin, breast, and other rare sites.[31–38] As mentioned previously, many of these sites, including the stomach, where low grade MALT-lymphoma is the most frequent, do not normally contain native MALT. Recognition of MALT-lymphoma in non-gastrointestinal sites is based on the same morphological criteria described for a prototypical gastric MALT-lymphoma.

While low grade MALT-lymphomas do not tend to disseminate to distant sites, involvement of regional lymph nodes is not infrequent. The histological appearance of involved nodes is very similar to, or indistinguishable from, that of monocytoid B-cell lymphoma.[39–41] Both the cytological spectrum and the pattern of infiltration of the two entities overlap. The neoplastic cells in MALT-lymphoma show a peri-follicular, interfollicular and/or sinusoidal or parasinusoidal pattern of infiltration (Fig. 6). Variable

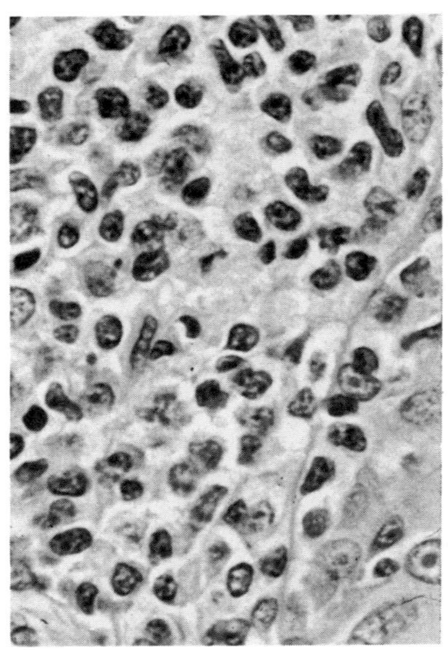

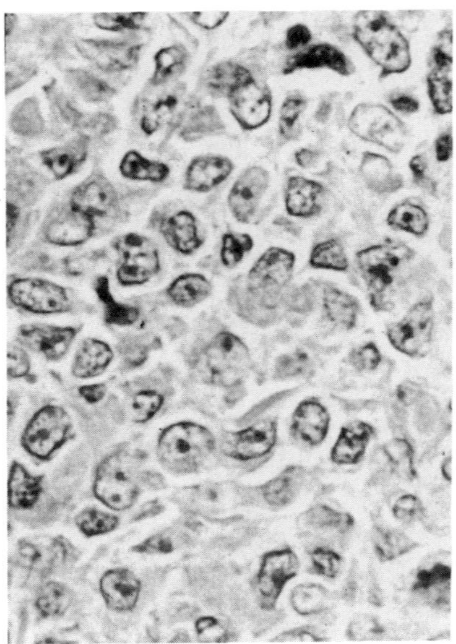

Fig. 5. A MALT-lymphoma of the lung showing a low grade component on the left and a co-existing high grade component on the right with sheets of large tumour cells (H&E × 500).

proportions of large transformed lymphocyte and plasma cells are present. Plasma cells may be numerous forming sheets and aggregates. The phenomenon of follicular colonization by neoplastic cells, as described in extranodal sites, may also be observed in involved lymph nodes.

Immunophenotype

The type of MALT-lymphomas discussed previously are B-cell tumours which express B-cell markers such as CD19, 20, and 22. They are monoclonal proliferations expressing either kappa or lambda light chains. Some immunological markers are useful in distinguishing them from other types of low grade B-cell lymphomas as summarized in Table 1.[10,42–44] The lack of CD10 expression is useful for distinguishing a MALT-lymphoma from a follicular centre cell lymphoma while the absence of CD5 and IgD is helpful in excluding small lymphocytic and mantle cell lymphomas. Paradoxical expression of CD43 is also uncommonly observed in MALT-lymphomas. Plasma cells in the lesions may or may not show light chain restriction (Fig. 7). When they are monoclonal, they express the same light chain as the neoplastic lymphoid cells indicating that they are derived from the same clone.

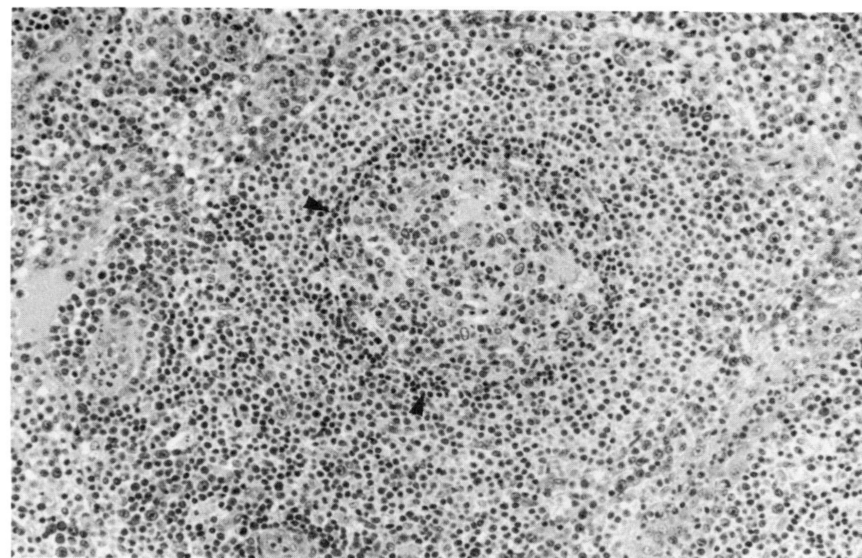

Fig. 6. Lymph node involvement by MALT-lymphoma. Note that the CCL-cells surround a benign germinal centre. A thin interrupted mantle zone is still present (arrow head). (H&E × 100).

Table 1. *Immunophenotypes of low grade lymphomas*

Lymphoma	IgD	CD5	CD10	CD23	CD43
Small lymphocytic	+	+	−	+	+/−
Mantle cell	+	+	−	−	+/−
Follicular centre cell	−	−	+	−	−
Monocytoid-B cell	−	−	−	−	−
MALT	−	−	−	−	−

+: Expressed by the majority of cases; +/−: expressed by a significant proportion of cases; and −: most of the cases do not express the markers.

Cytogenetic and molecular genetic analysis

There is a paucity of reports on cytogenetic findings on MALT-lymphomas. A case of MALT-lymphoma[45] and two additional cases of low grade extranodal lymphomas[46] with t(11;18) (q21;q21) have been reported. Other numerical (Trisomy 3 and 7) and structural (t(1;14)) abnormalities have also been described.[47] More studies are necessary to confirm the specific association of the reported cytogenetic abnormalities with MALT-

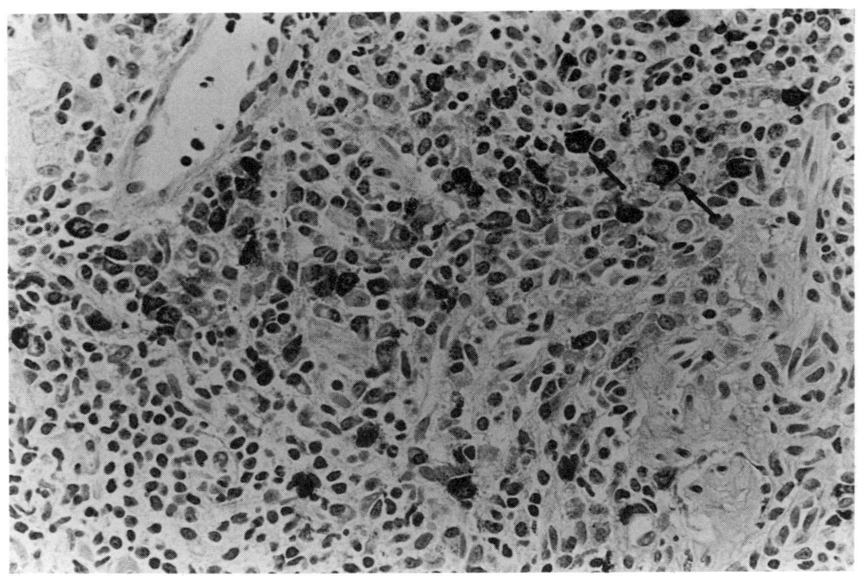

Fig. 7. The plasma cell infiltrate associated with a low grade MALT-lymphoma may be polyclonal or monoclonal. In this particular case, kappa light chain is demonstrated with anti-kappa using an immunoperoxidase technique. Only a fraction of the plasma cells are stained (arrow), suggestive of a polyclonal infiltrate. (Haematoxylin × 200).

lymphomas. Several studies for translocations involving the bcl-2 oncogenes have reported negative findings.[48,49] This has been taken as evidence against a follicular centre cell origin of the neoplastic cells and supports the contention that cases with an apparent follicular pattern are due to follicular colonization by CCL cells and not a concomitant follicular centre cell lymphoma. There is an interesting report of an increased incidence of *c-myc* rearrangement in high grade primary gastric lymphomas compared with nodal high grade lymphomas[50] implicating some basic differences between these two groups of lymphomas. The validity of the latter observation requires confirmation.

Southern blot analysis for immunoglobulin gene rearrangement in MALT-lymphomas shows clonal rearrangements as expected. In difficult cases with only paraffin-embedded tissue, demonstration of clonal IgH rearrangement by the polymerase chain reaction may be attempted.[51–53] A positive result in the presence of compatible histological and clinical findings lends strong support to the diagnosis. The latter technique has also been used in a recent study to demonstrate the clonal identity of two MALT-lymphomas involving distant sites.[54]

Histogenesis of B-low grade MALT-lymphomas

The work of Isaacson and coworkers has demonstrated certain similarities of low grade lymphomas of MALT to the native MALT of the terminal ileum:[10] the Peyer's patch and the overlying 'dome' epithelium. The germinal centre of the Peyer's patch is surrounded by mantle zone lymphocytes which, in turn, are surrounded by a thin rim of 'centrocyte-like cells' referred to as the 'marginal zone'. This architectural and cytological pattern is recapitulated in the usual low grade lymphoma of MALT. The CCL cells of MALT-lymphoma tend to surround follicles in the pattern of marginal zone cells. The tendency of these cells to colonize reactive follicles is also interesting and suggests a close functional relationship with B-lymphoid follicles. The analogy is further strengthened by the presence of marginal zone lymphocytes in the 'dome' epithelium overlying the normal Peyer's patch and the corresponding 'lymphoepithelial lesion' almost invariably found in the low grade lymphomas of MALT.

Immunohistochemical studies demonstrate significant concordance of marker expression between normal marginal zone cells and neoplastic CCL cells (Table 2).[55–57] Low grade MALT-lymphomas are distinct immunophenotypically from follicular centre cell lymphoma and mantle cell lymphoma, tumours that correspond to the follicular centre and mantle zone of normal follicles. In this regard, molecular genetic studies also support the uniqueness of MALT-lymphomas by demonstrating the lack of bcl-2 rearrangements in MALT-lymphomas. bcl-1 rearrangement has not been investigated in sufficient detail for any meaningful discussion.

When a low grade MALT-lymphoma spreads to regional lymph nodes, the pattern of infiltration and the cytological appearance are very similar to that of monocytoid B-cell lymphoma.[39,40] There is also a primary splenic lymphoma with a marginal zone pattern of white pulp involvement and cytological similarity to monocytoid B cells. This lymphoma is considered to originate from splenic marginal zone cells.[57] What then is the relationship between monocytoid B-cell lymphoma, splenic marginal zone lymphoma and low grade MALT-lymphoma? These are closely related entities with striking morphological and immunophenotypical similarity. They may all be related to marginal zone cells, but some degree of heterogeneity may be present.[40,41,57,58] There seems to be a difference in presentation and clinical behaviour that warrants their classification into separate entities. It is possible that neoplastic marginal zone cells arising in different locations express different sets of adhesion molecules that affect cellular localization and trafficking, thus accounting at least partly for the different clinical behaviours.

The pathogenesis of low grade MALT-lymphomas

The aetiology of a malignant neoplasm is generally a multistep process with accumulation of genetic alterations which eventually endow the tumour

Table 2. *Comparison of the immunophenotype of marginal zone cells and MALT-lymphoma cells*

	IgD	CD5	CD10	CD20	CD21	CD22	CD23	CD35	KiB3
Marginal zone cells	–	–	–	+	+	+	–	+	–
MALT-lymphoma cells	–	–	–	+	+	+	–	+	+/–

with all its malignant characteristics.[59] Lymphoid tissue subjected to prolonged, intense antigenic stimulation results in a tremendous expansion of its lymphoid cells. If the antigens involved are very restricted, the immune response may also be restricted and it is possible that a limited number of immunocytes are selected to respond and these cells account for the bulk of the proliferative activity. Cellular proliferation presents an opportunity for genetic errors to occur.[59] If proliferative activity continues for a prolonged period in a clone of cells, there may be sufficient genetic alterations to give rise to a neoplasm.

The fact that the majority of MALT-lymphomas occur in acquired MALT suggests that an abnormal immunological stimulation is taking place at that site. In Hashimoto's thyroiditis and Sjogren's syndrome, an autoimmune process is believed to be the cause of the lymphoid reaction, and the antigenic stimulation could well be restricted under such circumstances. Moreover, one may speculate that, in acquired MALT, as distinct from native MALT, immunoregulation may not be that well established, allowing for a less controlled immune response/proliferation. This scenario probably forms the basis for the evolution from lymphoid hyperplasia to MALT-lymphoma.

There is a close association between *Helicobacter pylori* infection and gastric low grade MALT-lymphoma.[60,61] In six patients with such an association, after eradication of *H. pylori* with antibiotics, histological evidence for a lymphoma was no longer observed in five.[62] These studies suggest that *H. pylori* may be important in the pathogenesis of acquired MALT in the stomach and its subsequent progression to a low grade MALT-lymphoma, some of which may regress on removal of the antigenic stimulus. These results are very preliminary, but if confirmed, will have a significant impact on the management of patients with *H. pylori* gastritis and patients with low grade gastric MALT-lymphoma. This association also provides a very important model for the study of lymphomagenesis.

Uncommon variants of MALT-lymphoma

Mediterranean lymphoma is rare in Western countries and common in certain geographical locations.[63,64] It involves the duodenal and jejunal region of the small bowel although other sites may occasionally be affected as well. Typically, the patient is a young adult who presents with malabsorption syndrome and widespread involvement of the proximal small intestine. In early lesions, the mucosa is infiltrated extensively by plasma cells which usually synthesize and secrete IgA heavy chain of the AI subclass. Features including aggregates of CCL cells, lymphoepithelial lesions and follicular colonization that are typical of the usual type of Western low grade MALT-lymphoma are also observed.[65]

In early disease, administration of broad spectrum antibiotic therapy may induce long-term remission and perhaps cure in some patients. This observation suggests that the lymphoproliferation is dependent on some type of antigenic stimulation and is not completely autonomous in the early stage. There is, however, evidence from the immunohistochemical study of rare cases expressing Ig-light chains and from molecular studies of clonal Ig gene rearrangement that the disease is a clonal proliferation even at presentation.[66,67] The lesion can evolve with time eventuating in a high grade neoplasm with the morphology of an immunoblastic lymphoma. Regional lymph nodes may be involved early in the course of the disease, but wide system dissemination is not observed until late. There is, indeed, an interesting parallel in the pathogenesis and evolution of Mediterranean lymphoma and low grade gastric MALT-lymphoma in Western countries, including the recent observation of regression of gastric MALT-lymphomas with eradication of *H. pylori* infection.

If the category of MALT-lymphoma is broadened to include tumours arising from mucosal sites having features unique and different from their nodal counterparts, the entity termed multiple lymphomatous polyposis (MLP) should be included in our discussion.[68–70] While the usual low grade MALT-lymphoma is probably a marginal-cell lymphoma of MALT, MLP is a mantle cell lymphoma of MALT. There is extensive involvement of the colon, terminal ileum and sometimes other parts of the intestines with numerous lymphomatous polyps and tumourous masses. Morphologically, MLP exhibits the same features as nodal mantle cell lymphoma. The neoplastic mantle cells may surround reactive follicles or appear as nodules without any recognizable central follicles which have probably been invaded and obliterated by the neoplastic cells. Lymphoepithelial lesions are not a feature of MLP. In a biopsy, the morphological distinction of a lesion with many neoplastic nodules composed of small irregular lymphocytes from a true follicular centre cell lymphoma may be very difficult. The paucity of large transformed lymphocytes is a hallmark of mantle cell lymphoma, but in tumour nodules containing germinal centres largely replaced by neoplastic mantle cells, scattered normal small and large follicular centre cells are present and may be mistaken for part of the neoplastic population. Immunohistochemical and molecular studies can be very helpful in the differential diagnosis. Mantle cell lymphoma is usually

$CD5^+$, IgD^+ and $CD10^-$ while the opposite is true for follicular centre cell lymphomas. Bcl-2 protein is absent in normal follicular centre cells but demonstrable in neoplastic follicular and mantle cells. Bcl-1 is often rearranged in mantle cell lymphoma, while bcl-2 rearrangement is frequently detected in follicular centre cell lymphoma. In sharp contrast to the usual low grade MALT-lymphoma, MLP is clinically more aggressive with early dissemination to extragastrointestinal sites and poorer survival.

T-cell lymphomas are rare among MALT-lymphomas but there is a unique type of T-cell lymphoma, often associated with evidence of gluten-sensitive enteropathy,[71–73] which accounts for a substantial proportion of MALT lymphomas of the small intestine and has poor prognosis. Some of the patients have a previous history of coeliac disease, while others have villous atrophy and crypt hyperplasia suggestive of the existence of gluten-sensitive enteropathy.[72–74] A gluten-free diet also appears to reduce the risk of lymphoma in patients with coeliac disease.[75] This lymphoma most often arises in the jejunum and is frequently multifocal. Its morphology is quite variable but typically contains markedly pleomorphic tumour cells. A prominent reactive component with many eosinophils and histiocytes may be present. Necrosis may be prominent. Mesenteric lymph nodes are often involved with the involvement described as predominantly sinusoidal.[74] Much of this sinusoidal infiltrate may consist of reactive histiocytes as the infiltrate 'often shows little pleomorphism but prominent erythrophagocytosis'.[74] Most reported cases have expressed the following phenotype: $CD3^{+/-}$, $CD7^+$, $CD4^-$, $CD8^-$, $HML1^+$, $TCR\gamma\delta^-$. Molecular studies have demonstrated a clonal Tβ gene rearrangement.[76] HML-1, a monoclonal antibody that reacts with intraepithelial T cells and a proportion of mucosal T cells but few peripheral T cells,[77] may be a useful marker for T-cell lymphomas arising from MALT.[78]

There are other types of non-Hodgkin's lymphoma arising in extranodal sites that correspond morphologically and immunohistochemically to nodal lymphomas other than those discussed above. For example, there are authentic cases of follicular centre cell lymphomas, small lymphocytic lymphomas, Burkitt's lymphomas, lymphoblastic lymphomas, and so on, arising in sites usually associated with lymphomas of MALT type. Data are insufficient to determine whether these lymphomas are significantly different in any way from their nodal counterparts. For the present, they should be classified in the same manner as nodal lymphomas.

The diagnosis of MALT-lymphomas

Low grade MALT-lymphoma in various extranodal organs has the same basic components: groups of CCL cells, lymphoepithelial lesions, a plasmacytic infiltrate and reactive follicles with or without tumour colonization.

In an excisional or large biopsy, all these components are usually observed and the diagnosis can be made with a fair degree of certainty. In a small biopsy, however, such as an endoscopic biopsy of the stomach, a definitive diagnosis may be very difficult. The small size of the biopsy may not include tissue showing all the characteristic findings of MALT-lymphoma. Often, crush artefact due to the biopsy procedure obscures diagnostic features. It is essential that technically excellent tissue processing, cutting and staining be maintained, since these biopsies are difficult to interpret at best. For unsatisfactory specimens, repeat biopsies for routine morphologic assessment, as well as fresh tissue for immunophenotyping and molecular studies, should be obtained. For paraffin-embedded specimens that are suspicious for, but not diagnostic of, lymphoma, some ancillary studies may be helpful. When most of the extrafollicular lymphocytes phenotype as B cells, the possibility of a B-cell lymphoma is increased. Immunostaining for kappa and lambda light chains, especially if plasma cells or plasmacytoid lymphocytes are present, may be useful in demonstrating the clonal nature of the lesion. The recently described methods of antigen retrieval[79,80] should make a higher percentage of cases with paraffin-embedded tissue amenable to such studies. Immunohistochemical demonstration of immunoglobulin in frozen tissue is sometimes difficult and flow cytometric analysis may be preferred. When sufficient tissue is available, Southern blot analysis can be performed to demonstrate clonal Ig or TCAR gene rearrangement. For small biopsies, a PCR assay may be used instead. Clonal IgH rearrangements have been detected in over 60% of B-cell non-Hodgkin's lymphomas.[51–53] The PCR assay can also be performed on DNA extracted from formalin-fixed paraffin-embedded tissue.

Some cases of MALT-lymphoma are difficult to differentiate from other types of lymphoma. An immunohistochemical panel as outlined in Table 1 is useful in the differential diagnosis. Certain clinical data, such as the presence of multiple polyps as seen in MLP, the geographical origin of the patient, the clinical stage of the disease, and the presence or absence of a previous biopsy/diagnosis and relevant laboratory studies such as serum and urine immunoglobulin determination, cytogenetics and molecular analysis may be useful in separating MALT-lymphoma from other types of non-Hodgkin's lymphoma.

Clinical considerations

The low grade MALT-lymphoma was initially described in the gastrointestinal tract. Isaacson and coworkers[10] observed that low grade MALT-lymphomas tend to remain localized to the gastrointestinal tract for long periods of time and have an indolent clinical course resulting in prolonged survival. Surgical resection may be curative in lesions limited to the GI mucosa and submucosa. Although gastric MALT-lymphomas have been shown to be multifocal in some cases, extensive involvement of the GI tract is uncommon in Western cases suggesting that the tumour cells do not tend to recirculate and home to other MALT sites. However, a recent case with identical tumours involving two distinct MALT sites indicates that this may occasionally occur.[54]

Since the MALT-lymphoma concept is relatively new, only a limited number of studies have utilized this concept in the classification of extranodal lymphomas. Most of the larger series are studies of gastrointestinal lymphomas. In the stomach, the ratio of combined low and high grade MALT-lymphoma to high grade lymphoma without evidence of a low grade lesion is about 1:1, whereas in the small intestine, the ratio is around 1:2.[30,73,81–87] Although lymphomas of the large intestine are rare, according to the series of Shepherd et al,[29] a large percentage appear to be MALT-lymphomas. In other extranodal sites, such as the salivary glands, thyroid, and orbital adnexa, it appears that many low grade lymphomas are MALT-lymphomas which have indolent behaviour and the tendency to remain localized for prolonged periods of time similar to gastric MALT-lymphomas. This indolent behaviour may account partly for the previous findings that many salivary gland lesions diagnosed as 'Sjogren's syndrome' show a clonal immunoglobulin rearrangement[88] and the rather unexpected findings that in orbital adnexal tumors, clonal or non-clonal lymphoid infiltrates do not seem to have significantly different survival.[89]

In the study by Cogliotti et al,[83] low grade MALT-lymphoma of the stomach has a significantly better survival than high grade lymphomas including high grade MALT-lymphoma. Radaskiewicz et al[30] also demonstrated that gastric low grade MALT-lymphomas have a better survival than high grade lesions while van Kricken and coworkers[81] failed to confirm the superior survival of gastric low grade MALT-lymphoma. Additional studies are needed to confirm the survival advantages of low grade MALT-lymphoma suggested by a number of these studies. Low grade MALT-lymphomas in non-gastric sites are less frequent. Large multi-institutional studies are necessary to address questions properly regarding the clinical behaviour of these lesions.

One of the major difficulties in evaluating the clinical studies of extranodal lymphomas is the highly variable treatments administered to the patients.[90] In future prospective studies, treatment protocols must be standardized in order for the data to be meaningfully analysed. Since low grade MALT-lymphoma may have a prolonged clinical course, evaluation of treatment and survival requires long-term follow-up.

Summary

A unique category of low grade B-cell lymphoma in extranodal sites associated with mucosa or other types of epithelial structures has been recently described. This type of lymphoma is characterized by a polymorphic cellular infiltrate with neoplastic centrocyte-like cells, lymphoepithelial lesions, reactive and/or neoplastic plasma cells and germinal centres. Many of these tumours have previously been misdiagnosed as 'pseudolymphoma' because of their 'reactive' histological appearance and their indolent clinical course. These low grade mucosa-associated lymphoid tissue (MALT)-lymphomas appear to be indolent clonal lymphoid proliferations with a tendency to remain localized to the initial site of presentation for long periods of time. This lymphoma shows morphological and immunophenotypical similarity to monocytoid B-cell lymphoma of lymph nodes and marginal zone lymphoma of the spleen. It is postulated that the cells of these tumors are histogenetically related to marginal zone lymphocytes. A low grade MALT-lymphoma may resemble a follicular lymphoma owing to the phenomenon of follicular colonization. Immunophenotyping and molecular genetic studies, as an adjunct to an adequate morphological study, can be quite helpful in the differential diagnosis. Mediterranean lymphoma is a geographically restricted lymphoma with similarity to, but also with some unique features which differ from the usual Western low grade MALT-lymphoma. Both forms of low grade MALT-lymphoma may undergo transformation to a high grade lesion. It is uncertain what proportion of high grade lesions arise from a pre-existing low grade lymphoma when the latter is not observed at diagnosis. Multiple lymphomatous polyposis is an unusual variant of mantle cell lymphoma which presents with widespread involvement of the intestines. It may perhaps be considered as a lymphoma arising from MALT-mantle cells as distinct from the usual MALT-lymphomas that arise from MALT-marginal zone cells. A high grade T-cell lymphoma of the GI tract has been identified as a special type of MALT-lymphoma which arises as a complication of gluten sensitive enteropathy.

Low grade and high grade lymphomas analogous to their respective nodal counterparts may also be seen as a primary tumour in MALT. Whether they have any unique characteristics compared with the corresponding nodal tumours requires further investigation.

The relative frequency and clinical behaviour of MALT-lymphomas, especially when they arise outside of the gastrointestinal site, have yet to be fully delineated. Since it is unlikely that any single institution will register a sufficient number of cases to answer these questions, large multi-institutional studies should be conducted.

Factors contributing to the pathogenesis of low grade MALT-lymphomas are of great interest. A large proportion of cases arises in acquired MALT suggesting prior and continual stimulation by foreign or autoantigens may be important in the pathogenesis of these lesions. The association of *Helicobacter pylori* with gastric MALT-lymphoma is intriguing and is currently under investigation.

Note added in proof A recent study found trisomy 3 in $\frac{27}{48}$ (56%) cases of MALT-lymphoma suggesting that trisomy 3 may be specifically involved in this type of lymphoma.[91]

References

(1) Salzstein SL. Extranodal malignant lymphomas and pseudolymphomas. *Pathol Annual* 1969; 4: 159–84.
(2) Brooks JJ, Enterline HT. Gastric pseudolymphoma. Its three subtypes and relation to lymphoma. *Cancer* 1983; 51: 476–86.
(3) Colby TV, and Carrington CB. Lymphoreticular tumours and infiltrates of the lung. *Pathol Annu* 1983; 18: 27–70.
(4) Marchevsky A, Padilla M, Kaneko M, Kleinerman J. Localized lymphoid nodules of lung. *Cancer* 1983; 51: 2070–7.
(5) Burke JS. Histologic criteria for distinguishing between benign and malignant extranodal lymphoid infiltrates. *Semin Diag Pathol* 1985; 2: 152–62.
(6) Picker LJ, Weiss LM, Medeiros LJ, Wood GS, Warnke RA. Immunophenotypic criteria for the diagnosis of non-Hodgkin's lymphoma. *Am J Pathol* 1987; 128: 181–201.
(7) Waldmann TA. The arrangement of immunoglobulin and T cell receptor genes in human lymphoproliferative disorders. *Advances in Immunol*, 1987; 40: 247–321.
(8) Weisenburger DD, Chan WC. Lymphomas of follicles: Mantle cell and follicle center cell lymphomas. *Am J Clin Path* 1993; 99: 409–20.
(9) Rowley JD, Aster JC, Sklar J. The clinical applications of new DNA diagnostic technology on the management of cancer patients. *JAMA* 1993; 270: 2331–7.
(10) Isaacson PG, Spencer J. Malignant lymphoma of mucosa-associated lymphoid tissue. *Histopathology* 1987; 11: 445–62.
(11) Brandtzaeg P, Halstensen TS, Kett K et al. Immunobiology and immunopathology of human gut mucosa: humoral immunity and intraepithelial lymphocytes. *Gastroenterology* 1989; 97: 1562–84.
(12) Pabst R. Is BALT a major component of the human lung immune system? *Immunol Today* 1992; 13: 119–22.
(13) Trier JS. Structure and function of intestinal M cells. In: MacDermott RP, Elson CO, eds. *Mucosal immunology I, basic principles. Gastroenterology Clinics of North America*. Philadelphia: WB Saunders Company, 1991: 20: 531–548.
(14) Mazanec MB, Nedrud JG, Kaetzel CS, Lamm ME. A three-tiered view of the role of IgA in mucosal defense. *Immunol Today* 1993; 14: 430–434.
(15) Brandtzaeg P, Farstad IN, Halstensen TS et al. Immune functions in the normal and diseased human gut. *Frontiers of Mucosal Immunol* 1991: 1: 29–36.
(16) Cerf-Bensussan N, Guy-Grand D. Intestinal intraepithelial lymphocytes. In: MacDermott RP, Elson CO, eds. *Mucosal immunology I, basic principles. Gastroenterology Clinics of North America*, WB Saunders Company, Philadelphia, PA 1991; 20: 549–76.
(17) Bucy RP, Chen CLH, Cihok J, Losch U, Cooper MD. Avian T-cells expressing gamma delta receptors localize in the splenic sinusoids and the intestinal epithelium. *J Immunol* 1988; 141: 2200–5.

(18) Jarry A, Cerf-Bensussan N, Brousse N, Selz F, Guy-Grand D. Subsets of $CD3^+$ (T-cell receptor $\alpha\beta^+$ or $\gamma\delta^+$) and $CD3^-$ lymphocytes isolated from normal human gut epithelium display phenotypical features different from their counterparts in peripheral blood. *Eur J Immunol* 1990; 20: 1097–103.
(19) MacDonald TT, Spencer J. Ontogeny of the mucosal immune response. *Springer Semin Immunopathol* 1990; 12: 129–37.
(20) Strober W, Harriman GR. The regulation of IgA B-cell differentiation. In: MacDermott RP, Elson CO eds. *Mucosal immunology I, basic principles. Gastroenterology Clinics of North America*, WB Saunders Company, Philadelphia, PA 1991; 20: 473–94.
(21) Gowans JL, Knight EL. The route of recirculation of lymphocytes in the rat. *Proc R Soc Lond* 1964; 159: 257–82.
(22) Mestecky J. The Common mucosal immune system and current strategies for induction of immune responses in external secretions. *J Clin Immunol* 1987; 7: 265–76.
(23) Salmi M, Jalkanen S. Regulation of lymphocyte traffic to mucosa-assocated lymphatic tissues. In: MacDermott RP, Elson CO, eds. *Mucosal immunology I basic principles. Gastroenterology Clinics of North America*, Philadelphia: WB Saunders Company, 1991: 495–510.
(24) Isaacson P, Wright DH. Malignant lymphoma of mucosa-associated lymphoid tissue. *Cancer* 1983; 52: 1410–16.
(25) Isaacson PT, Wright DH. Extranodal malignant lymphoma arising from mucosa associated lymphoid tissue. *Cancer* 1984; 53: 2515–24.
(26) Isaacson PG. Pathogenesis and early lesions in extranodal lymphoma. *Toxicol Lett* 1993; 67: 237–47.
(27) Isaacson PG, Wotherspoon AC, Diss T, Pan L. Follicular colonization in B-cell lymphoma of mucosa-associated lymphoid tissue. *Am J Surg Pathol* 1991; 15: 819–28.
(28) Chan JKC, Ng CS, Isaacson PG. Relationship between high-grade lymphoma and low-grade B-cell mucosa-associated lymphoid tissue lymphoma (MALToma) of the stomach. *Am J Pathol* 1990; 136: 1153–64.
(29) Shepherd NA, Hall PA, Coates PJ, Levison DA. Primary malignant lymhoma of the colon and rectum. A histopathological and immunohistochemical analysis of 45 cases with clinicopathological correlations. *Histopathology* 1988; 12: 235–52.
(30) Radaszkiewicz T, Dragosics B, Bauer P. Gastrointestinal malignant lymphomas of the mucosa-associated lymphoid tissue: factors relevant to prognosis. *Gastroenterology* 1992; 102: 1628–38.
(31) Addis BJ, Jyjek E, Isaacson PG. Primary pulmonay lymphoma. A re-appraisal of its histiogenesis and its relationship to pseudolymphoma and interstitial pneumonia. *Histopathology* 1988; 13: 1–17.
(32) Hyjek E, Smith WJ, Isaacson PG. Primary B cell lymphoma of salivary gland and its relationship to epithelial sailadenitis. *Hum Pathol* 1988; 19: 766–76.
(33) Hyjek E, and Isaacson PG. Primary B cell lymphoma of the thyroid and its relationship to Hashimoto's thyroiditis. *Hum Pathol* 1988; 19: 1315–26.
(34) Pelstring RJ, Essell JH, Kurtin PJ, Cohen AR, Banks PM. Diversity of organ site involvement among malignant lymphomas of mucosa-associated tissues. *Am J Clin Pathol* 1991; 96: 738–45.

(35) Takahashi H, Cheng J, Fujita S et al. Primary malignant lymphoma of the salivary gland: a tumor of mucosa-associated lymphoid tissue. *J Oral Pathol Med* 1992; 21: 318–25.
(36) Giannotti B, Santucci M. Skin-associated lymphoid tissue (SALT)-related B-cell lymphoma (primary cutaneous B-cell lymphoma). *Arch Dermatol* 1993; 129: 353–5.
(37) Liesegang TJ. Ocular adnexal lymphoproliferative lesions. *Mayo Clin Proc* 1993; 68: 1003–10.
(38) Pawade J, Banerjee SS, Harris M, Isaacson P, Wright D. Lymphomas of mucosa-associated lymphoid tissue arising in the urinary bladder. *Histopathology* 1993; 23: 147–51.
(39) Sheibani K, Burke JS, Swartz WG, Nadamanee A, Winberg CD. Monocytoid B-cell lymphoma: clinicopathologic study of 21 cases of a unique type of low-grade lymphoma. *Cancer* 1988; 62: 1531–8.
(40) Nathwani BN, Mohrmann RL, Brynes RK, Taylor CR, Hansmann ML, Sheibani K. Monocytoid B-cell lymphomas: an assessment of diagnostic criteria and a perspective on histogenesis. *Hum Pathol* 1992; 23: 1061–71.
(41) Nizze H, Cogliatti SB, Von Schilling C, Feller AC, Lennert K. Monocytoid B-cell lymphoma: morphological variants and relationship to low-grade B-cell lymphoma of the mucosa-associated lymphoid tissue. *Histopathology* 1991; 18: 403–14.
(42) Pallesen G. The distribution of CD23 in normal human tissues and in malignant lymphomas. In: McMichael AJ, ed. *Leukocyte typing III: white cell differentiation Antigens*. Oxford: Oxford University Press, 1987: 383–6.
(43) Ngan BY, Pickler LJ, Medeiros LJ, Warnke RA. Immunophenotypic diagnosis of non-Hodgkin's lymphoma in paraffin sections: expression of L60 (Leu-22) and L26 antigens correlates with malignant findings. *Am J Clin Pathol* 1989; 91: 579–83.
(44) Zukerberg LR, Medeiros JL, Ferry JA, Harris NL. Diffuse low-grade B-cell lymphomas: four clinically distinct subtypes defined by a combination of morphologic and immunophenotypc features. *Am J Clin Pathol* 1993; 100: 373–85.
(45) Horsman D, Gascoyne R, Klasa R, Coupland R. t(11; 18)(q21; q21.1): A recurring translocation in lymphomas of mucosa-associated lymphoid tissue (MALT). *Genes Chrom Cancer* 1992; 4: 183–7.
(46) Levine EG, Arthur KJ, Machnicki J et al. Four new recurring translocations in non-Hodgkin's lymphoma. *Blood* 1989 74: 1796–800.
(47) Wotherspoon AC, Pan LX, Diss TC, Isaacson PG. Cytogenetic study of B-cell lymphoma of mucosa-associated lymphoid tissue. *Cancer Genet Cytogent* 1992; 58: 35–8.
(48) Pan L, Diss TC, Cunningham D, Isaacson PG. The *bcl-2* gene in primary B cell lymphoma of mucosa-associated lymphoid tissue (MALT). *Am J Pathol* 1989; 135: 7–11.
(49) Isaacson PG, Androulakis-Papachristou A, Diss TC, Pan L, Wright DH. Follicular colonization in thyroid lymphoma. *Am J Pathol* 1992; 141: 43–52.
(50) van Krieken JHJM, Raffeld M, Raghoebier S, Jaffe ES, van Ommen GJB,

Kluin Ph M. Molecular genetics of gastrointestinal non-Hodgkin's lymphomas: Unusual prevalence and pattern of *c-myc* rearrangements in aggressive lymphomas. *Blood* 1990; 76: 797–800.

(51) Wan JH, Trainor KJ, Brisco MJ, Morley AA. Monoclonality in B cell lymphoma detected in paraffin wax embedded sections using the polymerase chain reaction. *J Clin Pathol* 1990; 43: 888–90.

(52) Davis TH, Yockey CE, Balk SP. Detection of clonal immunoglobulin gene rearrangements by polymerase chain reaction amplification and single-strand conformational polymorphism analysis. *Am J Pathol* 1993; 142: 1841–7.

(53) Inghirami G, Szabolcs MJ, Yee HT, Corradini P, Cesarman E, Knowles DM. Detection of immunoglobulin gene rearrangement of B cell non-Hodgkin's lymphomas and leukemias in fresh, unfixed and formalin-fixed, paraffin-embedded tissue by polymerase chain reaction. *Lab Invest* 1993; 68: 746–57.

(54) Diss TC, Peng H, Wotherspoon AC, Pan L, Speight PM, Isaacson PG. Brief report: a single neoplastic clone in sequential biopsy specimens from a patient with primary gastric-mucosa-associated lymphoid-tissue lymphoma and Sjögren's syndrome. *New Engl J Med* 1993; 329: 172–75.

(55) van Krieken JHJM, von Schilling C, Kluin Ph M, Lennert K. Splenic marginal zone lymphocytes and related cells in the lymph node: a morphologic and immunohistochemical study. *Hum Pathol* 1989; 20: 320–5.

(56) Morente M, Piris MA, Orradre JL, Rivas C, Villuendas R. Human tonsil intraepithelial B cells: a marginal zone-related subpopulation. *J Clin Pathol* 1992; 45: 668–72.

(57) Schmid C, Kirkham N, Diss T, Isaacson PG. Splenic marginal zone cell lymphoma. *Am J Surg Pathol* 1992; 16: 455–66.

(58) Piris MA, Rivas C, Morente M, Cruz MA, Rubio C, Oliva H. Monocytoid B-cell lymphoma, a tumour related to the marginal zone. *Histopathology* 1988; 12: 383–92.

(59) Cohen SM, Purtilo DT, Ellwein LB. Pivotal role of increased cell proliferation in human carcinogenesis. *Mod Pathol* 1991; 4: 371–82.

(60) Wotherspoon AC, Ortiz-Hidalgo C, Falzon MF, Isaacson PG. *Helicobacter pylori*-associated gastritis and primary B-cell gastric lymphoma. *Lancet* 1991; 338: 1175–1176.

(61) Stolte, M. *Helicobacter pylori*-gastritis and gastric MALT-lymphoma. Lancet 1992; 339: 745–6.

(62) Wotherspoon AC, Doglioni C, Diss TC et al. Regression of primary low-grade B-cell gastric lymphoma of mucosa-associated lymphoid tissue type after eradication of *Helicobacter pylori*. *Lancet* 1993; 342: 575–7.

(63) Salem PA, Nassar VH, Shahid MJ et al. Mediterranean abdominal lymphoma: or immunoproliferative small intestinal disease. Part I: Clinical aspects. *Cancer* 1977; 40: 2941–7.

(64) Khojasteh A, Haghshenass M, Haghighi P. Immunoproliferative small intestinal disease. A 'third-world lesion'. *New Engl J Med* 1983; 308: 1401–5.

(65) Isaacson PG, Dogan A, Price SK, Spencer J. Immunoproliferative small intestinal disease: an immunohistochemical study. *Am J Surg Pathol* 1989; 13: 1023–33.

(66) Isaacson PG, and Price SK. Light chains in Medeterranean lymphoma. *J Clin Pathol* 1985; 38: 601–7.
(67) Smith W, Price SK, Isaacson PG. Immunoglobulin gene rearrangement in immunoproliferative small intestinal disease (IPSID). *J Clin Pathol* 1987; 40: 1291–7.
(68) Cornes JS. Multiple lymphomatous polyposis of the gastrointestinal tract. *Cancer* 1961; 14: 249–57.
(69) Isaacson PG, Maclennan KA, Subbuswamy SG. Multiple lymphomatous polyposis of the gastrointestinal tract. *Histopathology* 1984; 8: 641–56.
(70) Triozzi PL, Borowitz MJ, Gockerman JP. Gastrointestinal involvement and multiple lymphomatous polyposis in mantle-zone lymphoma. *J Clin Oncol* 1986; 4: 866–73.
(71) Isaacson PG, Spencer J, Connolly CE et al. Malignant histiocytosis of the intestine: A T-cell lymphoma. *Lancet* 1985; ii: 668–91.
(72) Mead GM, Whitehouse M, Thompson J, Sweetenham JW, Williams CJ, Wright DH. Clinical features and management of malignant histiocytosis of the intestine. *Cancer* 1987; 60: 2791–6.
(73) Domizio P, Owen RA, Shepherd NA, Talbot IC, Norton AJ. Primary lymphoma of the small intestine: a clinicopathological study of 119 cases. *Am J Surg Pathol* 1993; 17: 429–42.
(74) Isaacson P, and Wright DH. Intestinal lymphoma associated with malabsorption. *Lancet* 1978; i: 67–70.
(75) Holmes GKT, Prior P, Lane MR, Pope D, Alan RN. Malignancy in coeliac disease-effect of a gluten free diet. *Gut* 1989; 30: 333–8.
(76) Isaacson PG. Gastrointestinal lymphomas and lymphoid hyperplasias. In Knowles DM, ed. *Neoplastic hematopathology*. Baltimore: Williams & Wilkins, 1992: 953–78.
(77) Cerf–Bensussan N, Jarry A, Brousse N, Lisowska–Grospierre B, Guy–Grand D, Griscelli C. A monoclonal antibody (HML-1) defining a novel membrane molecule present on human intestinal lymphocytes. *Eur J Immunol* 1987; 17: 1279–85.
(78) Stein H, Sperling M, Dienemann, Zeitz M, Riecken E-O. Identification of a T cell lymphoma category derived from intestinal-mucosa-associated T cells. *Lancet* 1988; 2: 1053–4.
(79) Chiu KY. Use of microwaves for rapid immunoperoxidase staining of paraffin sections. *Med Lab Sci* 1987; 44: 3–5.
(80) Shi SR, Key ME, Kalra KL. Antigen retrieval in formalin-fixed, paraffin-embedded tissues: an enhancement method for immunohistochemical staining based on microwave oven heating of tissue sections. *J Histochem Cytochem* 1991; 39: 741–8.
(81) van Krieken JHJM, Otter R, Hermans J et al. Malignant lymphoma of the gastrointestinal tract and mesentery. A clinico-pathologic study of the significance of histologic classification. *Am J Pathol* 1989; 135: 281–9.
(82) Azab MB, Henry–Amar M, Rougier P et al. Prognostic factors in primary gastrointestinal non-Hodgkin's lymphoma. *Cancer* 1989; 64: 1208–17.
(83) Cogliatti SB, Schmid U, Schumacher U, et al. Primary B-cell gastric lymphoma: A clinicopathological study of 145 patients. *Gastroenterology* 1991; 101: 1159–70.

(84) Lim FE, Hartman AS, Tan EGC, Cady B, Meissner WA. Factors in the prognosis of gastric lymphoma. *Cancer* 1977; 39: 1715–20.

(85) Filippa DA, Lieberman PH, Weingrad DN, Decosse JJ, Bretsky SS. Primary lymphomas of the gastrointestinal tract. Analysis of prognostic factors with emphasis on histological type. *Am J Surg Pathol* 1983; 7: 363–72.

(86) Brooks JJ, Enterline HT. Primary gastric lymphomas. A clinicopathologic study of 58 cases with long-term follow-up and literature review. *Cancer* 1983; 51: 701–11.

(87) Gobbi PG, Dionigi P, Barbieri F et al. The role of surgery in the multimodal treatment of primary gastric non-Hodgkin's lymphomas. A report of 76 cases and review of the literature. *Cancer* 1990; 65: 2528–36.

(88) Fishleder A, Tubbs R, Hesse B, Levine H. Uniform detection of immunoglobulin-gene rearrangement in benign lymphoepithelial lesions. *New Engl J Med* 1987; 316: 1118–21.

(89) Knowles DM, Jakobiec FA, McNally FA, Burke JS. Lymphoid hyperplasia and malignant lymphoma occurring in the ocular adnexa (orbit, conjunctiva and eyelids): a prospective multiparametric analysis of 108 cases during 1977–1987. *Hum Pathol* 1990; 21: 959–73.

(90) Haber DA, Mayer RJ. Primary gastrointestinal lymphoma. *Sem Oncol* 1988; 15: 154–69.

(91) Wotherspoon AC, Finn T and Isaacson PG. Numerical abnormalities of chromosome 3 and 7 in lymphomas of mucosa-associated lymphoid tissue and the splenic marginal zone. *Lab Invest* 1994; 70: 124A.

Ki-1 positive anaplastic large cell lymphoma – a useful concept?

J P GREER, J A WHITLOCK and M C KINNEY

Anaplastic large cell Ki-1+ lymphoma (ALCL) is a recently described entity; it is defined by characteristic histological features, reactivity with a monoclonal antibody Ki-1 (CD30), and frequent association with a unique chromosomal marker, t(2;5) (p23;q35). Controversies about ALCL's validity as a distinct entity evolve from defining it by a non-specific marker (CD30); a variable immunophenotype, albeit predominantly a peripheral T-cell; a variable clinical course, and overlap with other diseases, particularly Hodgkin's disease (HD) and cutaneous lymphoproliferations. Distinguishing primary ALCL from secondary Ki-1 lymphoma is important because the de novo primary ALCL appears to have a higher cure rate. Secondary Ki-1+ lymphomas with anaplastic morphology may follow preexisting lymphoproliferative disorders, including Hodgkin's disease, lymphomatoid papulosis, and cutaneous T cell lymphoma, and probably represent evolution to a higher grade process that is distinct from de novo ALCL. In addressing the issue of whether ALCL is a useful concept, we review the historical background, the significance of the CD30 antigen, histopathology, clinical features, and therapy of primary Ki-1 lymphoma.

Historical background

In 1982, Schwab et al reported the production of a monoclonal antibody Ki-1 raised against the Reed–Sternberg (RS) cell line L428 which reacted with RS cells and some normal cells in the parafollicular regions of normal or reactive lymphoid tissue.[1] In 1985, Stein et al reported that Ki-1 strongly marked tumour cells in 45 cases of non-Hodgkin's large cell lymphomas that had a pleomorphic appearance with a sinusoidal growth pattern and were frequently misdiagnosed as carcinoma or malignant histiocytosis.[2] In

All correspondence to: Dr JP Greer, Hematology Division, Vanderbilt University Medical Center, C-3119 MCN, Nashville, TN 37232, USA.

Cambridge Medical Reviews: Haematological Oncology Volume 4

1986, Kadin et al recognized this lymphoma was present in children and showed a predilection for skin and regional lymph nodes.[3] Several groups in 1988 and 1989 identified a recurring chromosomal abnormality, t(2;5) (p23; q35), in patients with primary Ki-1 lymphoma.[4–7] Morris et al recently cloned the genes altered by the t(2;5) and reported the rearrangement involves the NPM nucleolar phosphoprotein gene on chromosome 5q35 and a protein tyrosine kinase gene on chromosome 2p23, referred to as ALK.[8]

Molecular cloning studies have characterized the CD30 antigen and its ligand. In 1992, Durkop et al cloned the cDNA encoding the CD30 antigen and reported that the CD30 protein is a transmembrane receptor whose extracellular domain is homologous to the nerve growth factor receptor (NGFR) superfamily which includes tumour necrosis factor (TNF) receptors (I and II), T-cell activation antigens (OX-40 and CD27); 4-1BB, an inducible T-cell antigen of uncertain function; B cell antigen CD40; and Fas, a cell surface antigen that affects apoptosis.[9]

Using a chimeric probe consisting of the extracellular domain of CD30 fused to truncated immunoglobulin heavy chains, Smith et al cloned the cDNA cognate of CD30 from a murine T cell clone 7B9.[10] The encoded protein is a 239 amino acid type II membrane protein whose C-terminal domain has homology to TNF-alpha, TNF-beta, and CD40 ligand. They suggested that all members of the TNF/NGF family may be receptors whose cognate ligands are cytokines. Further evidence of the probable role of cytokines and their receptors in CD30+ lymphomas is the recognition of a restricted expression of the c-kit receptor in both HD and ALCL and its absence in other NHL.[11]

Fonatsch et al localized the CD30 gene to chromosome 1p36, a similar site for the gene for type II TNF receptor and near the site (1p35) for Epstein–Barr virus (EBV) insertion; they hypothesized that expression of CD30 could be secondary to either genomic instability due to viral integration or to control by a viral promotor or activator.[12] Viral components, particularly EBV and less commonly HTLV-1, have been identified in tissue from both anaplastic large cell lymphoma (ALCL) and HD, and may participate in the pathogenesis of these disorders.[13,14]

Ki-1, or CD30 antigen, is a non-specific marker and its role in the pathogenesis of de novo ALCL is uncertain; it is an activation antigen that can be induced on normal lymphocytes after exposure to mitogens (phytohaemagglutinin, staphylococcal protein A) and viruses (HTLV-1 and 2, EBV).[2] CD30 expression appears late in T-cell activation[15] and is found in a variety of disorders (Fig. 1). CD30 is uniformly found in tumour cells of virtually all cases defined as ALCL, but is also found in some cases of other peripheral T-cell lymphomas, particularly immunoblastic and pleomorphic T-cell lymphomas.[2,16] CD30 antigen may be identified in

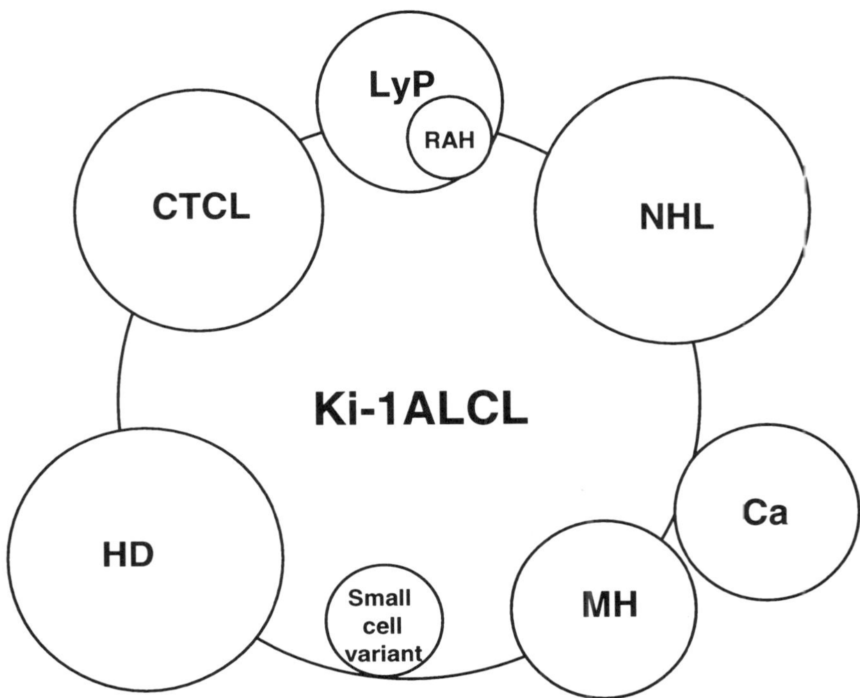

Fig. 1. Venn diagram of Ki-1 lymphomas: CD30 (Ki-1) expression is uniformly found in Ki-1 ALCL (anaplastic large cell lymphoma); but can also be found in other disorders: HD (Hodgkin's disease), CTCL (cutaneous T-cell lymphoma), LyP (lymphomatoid papulosis), RAH (regressing atypical histiocytosis), NHL (non-Hodgkin's lymphoma), Ca (carcinoma), and MH (malignant histiocytosis).

a minority of transformed cells in some low grade peripheral T cell lymphomas and is absent in lymphoblastic lymphoma.[16] Lymphomatoid papulosis and regressing atypical histiocytosis (RAH) have large cells that express CD30. RAH may be particularly difficult to distinguish from cutaneous ALCL;[16,17] recent publications, moreover, suggest RAH is a form of ALCL.[18] Most cases previously diagnosed as malignant histiocytosis express CD30 antigen and have been recognized as Ki-1+ ALCL.[19] CD30 antigen expression is common in Hodgkin's disease and can be found in embryonal cell carcinoma,[20] pancreatic carcinoma,[21] and some B cell lymphomas.[22] Other histological and immunophenotypical data are required to separate these Ki-1 (CD30)+ disorders (see Diagnosis).

Biochemical studies indicate that CD30 antigen exists in multiple molecular weight forms (57, 90, 105, and 120 kD) that are cytoplasmic, membrane associated, or released into the extracellular environment.[23,24] The smaller 57 kD molecule has protein kinase activity while the larger membrane form does not.[25] Soluble CD30 antigen can be detected in serum of patients with Hodgkin's disease and ALCL using an ELISA assay and may be a useful clinical marker to follow disease activity.[26]

The clinical significance of CD30 expression in malignant lymphoid cells is controversial, but, in general, its presence appears to be associated with a more favourable prognosis in primary lymphomas. The favourable impact of CD30 may be most pronounced in cutaneous lymphomas.[27,28] Beljaards et al reported a series of 47 patients with primary cutaneous CD30-positive large cell lymphoma: 42 had localized lesions, 15 had frequent relapses, 11 had complete spontaneous remissions, and 12 patients developed extracutaneous disease. Thirty-five (74%) of 47 patients with CD30+ tumour were alive compared to less than 15% survival at 3 years in 21 patients with CD30-negative cutaneous lymphomas.[28] Offit et al similarly reported a better survival in ten patients with CD-30 positive non-B cell diffuse large cell lymphoma compared to eight patients who were CD30 negative ($p<.001$); however, they did report a continued trend for relapse.[29] Conversely, Kadin et al reported no impact on prognosis of CD30 positivity in 24 (53%) of 45 paediatric patients with disseminated diffuse large cell lymphoma.[30]

Diagnosis and pathology

As previously discussed, Ki-1 antigen expression may be seen in several reactive and malignant lymphoproliferative processes including infectious mononucleosis, lymphomatoid papulosis, angio-immunoblastic lymphadenopathy, non-Hodgkin's lymphomas (particularly peripheral T cell type), and Hodgkin's disease.[2,3,22,31,32] This widespread expression of CD30 makes the term Ki-1 lymphoma imprecise, and its use should be discouraged.[16] Based on morphological and immunological features, anaplastic large cell lymphoma is a specific entity that has been added as a high grade lymphoma to the Kiel classification of T-cell lymphomas.[33,34] The following discussion of pathology will be limited to ALCL and its morphological variants. Other 'Ki-1+ lymphomas' will be mentioned in the differential diagnosis of this more specific entity.

Histology

The presence of a pleomorphic large cell infiltrate with a predilection for nodal sinuses is characteristic of ALCL (Fig. 2). The large cells extend from the subcapsular sinus into the paracortical region of the node often sparing follicles. The tumour cells are large with folded or indented, U-shaped nuclei with vesicular chromatin, prominent nucleoli, and abundant, pyroninophilic cytoplasm. Tumour giant cells, sometimes resembling

(*a*)

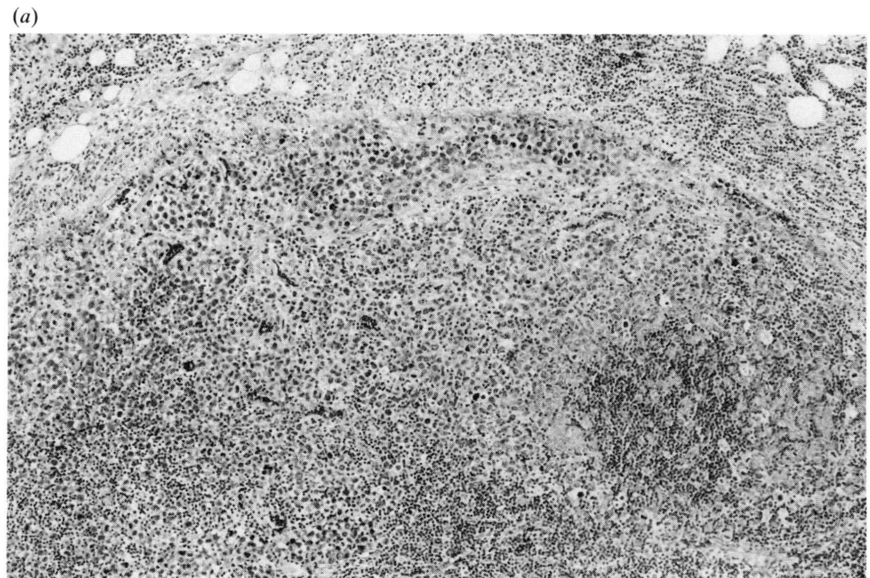

Fig. 2(*a*). ALCL showing paracortical and subcapsular sinus infiltration of node (H+E × 75).

Reed–Sternberg cells, are usually present. Mitotic figures are numerous. Large numbers of plasma cells often surround the tumour cells. The histological appearance varies somewhat according to tumour cell size, the degree of nuclear pleomorphism, cytoplasmic features, number of giant cells, type and number of reactive cells, and fibrous tissue deposition. Histological variants of ALCL include: pale cell or basophilic cell,[35] monomorphic,[36] sarcomatous,[37] histiocyte-rich,[38] Hodgkin's like.[39] Kinney et al described a small cell predominant primary Ki-1+ lymphoma with a similar pattern of nodal involvement as ALCL but with a large number of small, irregular lymphocytes and only a minor population of large cells (Fig. 3).[40] Several of these cases had a t(2;5) (p23;q35) (Fig. 4) and progressed to monomorphic ALCL. These findings suggest that some ALCLs have a histological spectrum that may initially be composed of small cells.

Extranodal involvement, particularly the skin, is common in ALCL and the cytological features of the tumour cells are identical to those in the node.[41,42] The skin infiltrate is primarily dermal and often extends to the subcutaneous tissue. Epidermotropism by small lymphocytes is minimal. Epidermal hyperplasia may be present as well as ulceration. Reactive inflammatory cells as described in the node are often present. Bone marrow

(*b*)

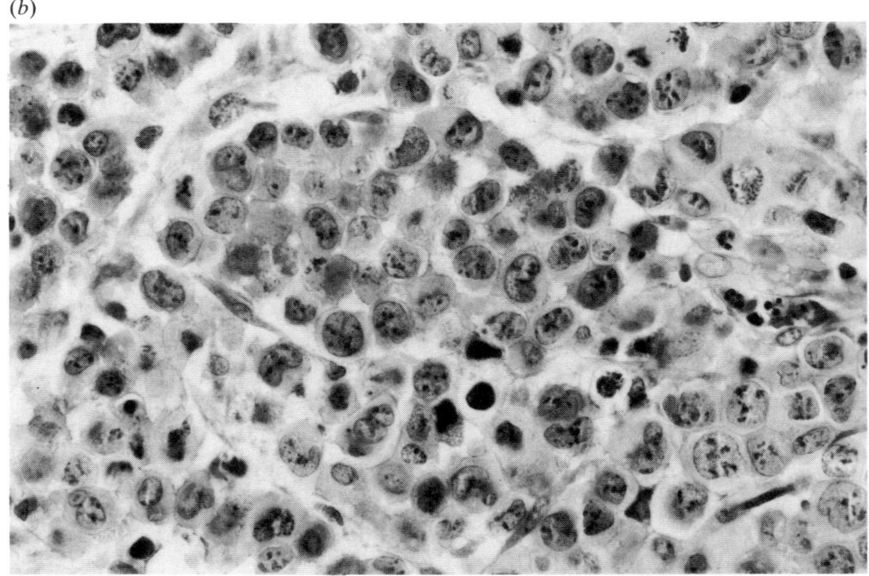

Fig. 2(*b*). Tumour cells are large, pleomorphic, and have irregular, indented nuclei with vesicular chromatin and prominent nucleoli (H+E × 450).

involvement is infrequent except in the small cell variant.[40,43] Bone marrow involvement tends to be subtle with single or very small clusters of large tumour cells that may be recognized only after immunoperoxidase staining with Ber-H2 (CD30). Large basophilic, finely vacuolated tumor cells may be seen circulating in the peripheral blood, particularly in the small cell variant or monomorphic variant of ALCL. Other sites of involvement include gastrointestinal tract,[44,45] lung and pleural fluid, bone,[46] and rarely central nervous system.[47]

Immunopathology

The majority of ALCLs are T-cell lymphomas although B and very rarely B + T cell phenotypes occur.[2,36,48,49] Approximately 10–20% of ALCLs remain unclassified as to immunophenotype. B-cell ALCLs may be a form of transformation of follicular centre cell lymphoma.[50] Most ALCLs are leukocyte common antigen (LCA, CD45) and epithelial membrane antigen (EMA) positive. Cases which lack LCA but are EMA positive can be confused with carcinoma if a limited immunological marker panel is performed. Activation antigens, interleukin 2 receptor (CD25), and HLA–DR are frequently expressed.[51] ALCLs also express blood group H and Y

(c)

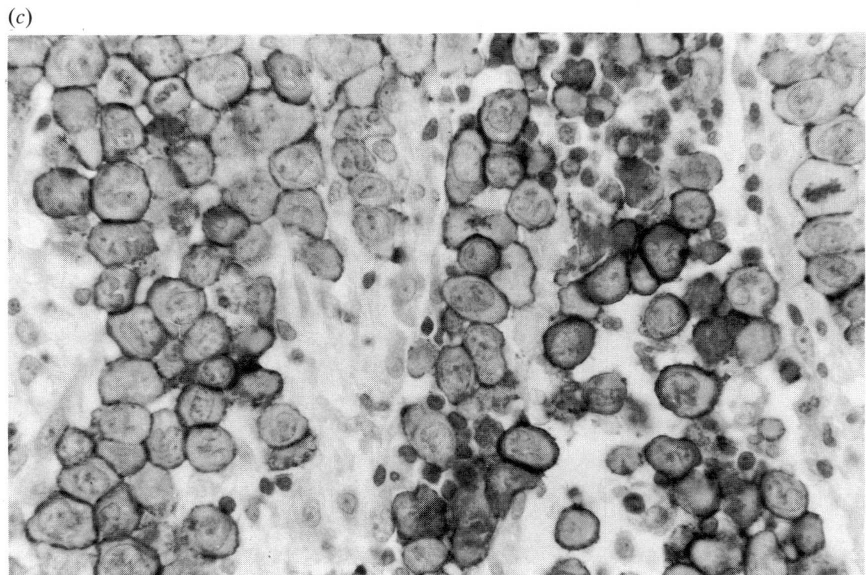

Fig. 2(*c*). Tumour cells show strong immunoperoxidase membrane reactivity with anti-CD30 antibody Ber-H2 (Paraffin immunoperoxidase × 450).

determinants recognized by antibody BNH9[52,53] and sialosylated Lewis X antigen (SLEX), a ligand for endothelial leukocyte adhesion molecule 1.[54] Only 15–25% of ALCLs express CD15 (LeuM1), and this can be used in many cases to distinguish ALCL and HD.

Molecular genetics In most cases, molecular genetic analyses have confirmed the T or B cell nature of ALCL. Some cases that are unclassified (null immunologically) do not show evidence of immunoglobulin or T-cell receptor rearrangements.[55,56] Discrepant results between the immunophenotype and the genotype may be seen.[55,56] The significance of this finding is unclear since T-cell receptor beta chain rearrangements have been reported in 5–10% of B-cell neoplasms.[57–59] The presence of activation antigens without the production of functional immunoglobulin molecules or T-cell antigen receptors led Stein's group to propose ALCLs may be derived from a transformation process that superimposes characteristics of mature activated lymphocytes on immature lymphocytes.[55]

Differential diagnosis ALCLs share some histological features with other large cell neoplasms including Hodgkin's disease, metastatic carcinoma or

(*a*)

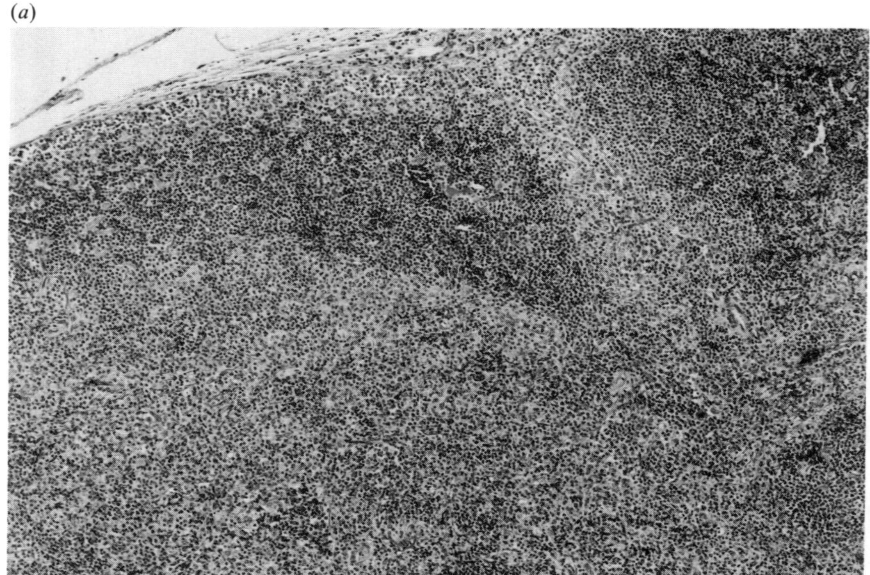

Fig. 3(*a*). Small cell predominant variant showing a similar sinus and paracortical distribution as seen in ALCL (Fig. 1(*a*) (PAS × 75).

melanoma, malignant histiocytosis and microvillous lymphoma.[48,49,51] For the most part, ALCL can be distinguished from these other malignancies using a panel of paraffin immunoperoxidase markers (see Table 1). Many cases previously diagnosed as malignant histiocytosis have proven to be T-cell lymphomas, primarily ALCLs.[19,48] Due to the lack of 'specific' histiocyte markers, some large cell Ki-1+ cases remain difficult to classify.[60] Overlap cases between Hodgkin's disease with large numbers of Reed–Sternberg cells and ALCL also present diagnostic difficulties.[61–63] More sophisticated studies are required to distinguish these entities. The recent cloning of the t(2;5)(p23;q35) has provided a molecular probe that may be useful in resolving these difficult cases and more precisely defining ALCL.[8] Other CD30+ B or T cell lymphomas (B cell immunoblastic lymphomas, cutaneous T cell lymphoma, AILD-like peripheral T cell lymphomas, and pleomorphic T cell lymphoma) can be distinguished from ALCL by clinical features, morphology, and cytogenetic data.

Clinical features

Distinctive clinical features of ALCL are being recognized along with the histopathological, immunological, and molecular genetic characteristics.[64,65] Subsets of ALCL are being proposed and include childhood, adult

(*b*)

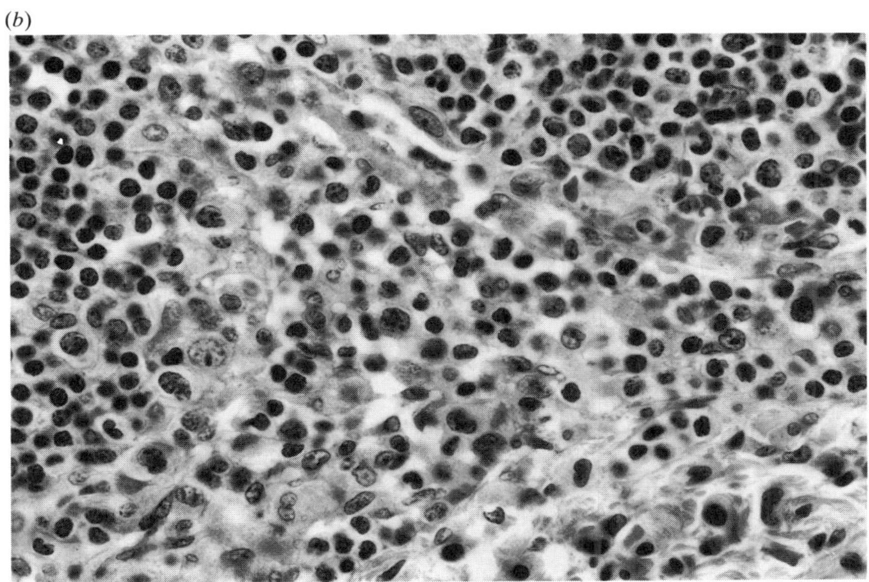

Fig. 3(*b*). The infiltrate is composed predominantly of small irregular lymphocytes with scattered large tumour cells (PAS × 450).

cutaneous, adult nodal and HIV associated.[66] Table 2 outlines series of ALCL previously reported.[2,3,27,28,35,36,64,65,67–80]

Vanderbilt series

In order to describe the clinical features of de novo ALCL the series previously reported was extended to 58 cases diagnosed at Vanderbilt from September 1986 until December 1991; no patient had a preexisting condition or lymphoproliferative disorder that has been associated with secondary Ki-1 lymphomas. Fifty-two cases represented the prototypic ALCL while six cases were the recently recognized small cell predominant variant.[40] Immunophenotyping studies revealed 44 cases had a peripheral T immunophenotype, six were B cell; and eight remained unclassified as to immunological type.

The present series suggests there is a bimodal presentation with the largest peak in childhood (second decade) and a smaller peak in older adults (Fig. 5); a similar bimodal presentation has been previously reported.[81] The median age of the patients was 33 years with a range from 0.4 to 78 years; the male : female ratio was 1.9 : 1.

Table 3 summarizes the presenting features in primary ALCL. A common problem is an erroneous diagnosis; the initial diagnosis was incorrect in

(c)

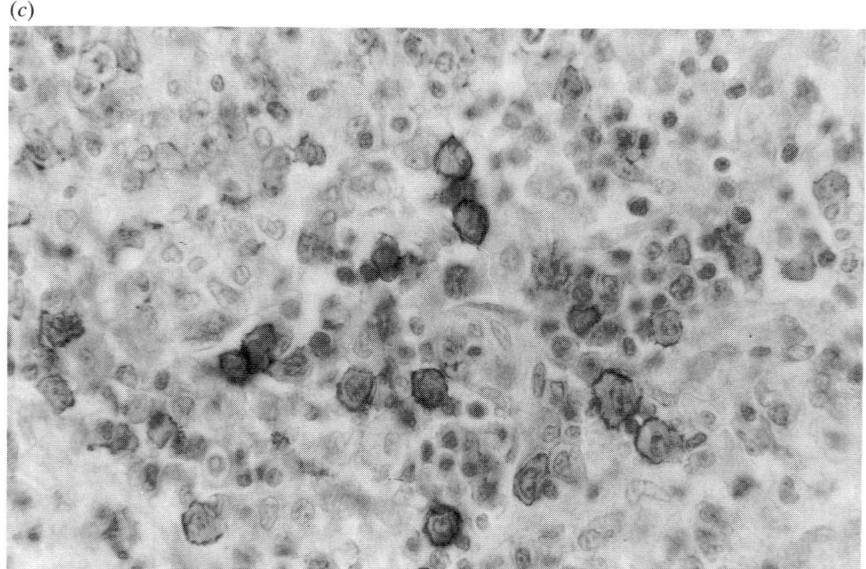

Fig. 3(*c*). The large cells are Ber-H2 positive and are more readily apparent after immunoperoxidase staining (paraffin immunoperoxidase × 450).

18 (31%) patients and included carcinoma (seven patients), Hodgkin's disease (four), infections (four), malignant histiocytosis (two), and regressing atypical histiocytosis (one). Peripheral adenopathy was frequent, occurring in 46 (79%) patients, and there was relative sparing of the mediastinum with involvement in only seven (12%) patients. Extranodal disease occurred in 28 (48%) patients with skin being the most common extranodal site (28% of patients). The skin lesions varied from papular rashes to small nodules to the more common ulcerated tumourous masses; an inflammatory component with erythema and tenderness was occasionally noted on the skin lesions or over sites of nodal involvement. Adequate cytogenetic data was available on only eight patients, but six had the characteristic t(2;5). HIV or HTLV-1 serology was negative but only limited numbers of patients were tested.

Initial therapy was heterogeneous and is outlined in Table 4. Of the five patients who did not receive initial therapy, three died rapidly with fulminant disease; one had progressive nodal involvement at 14 months but now has responded to CHOP chemotherapy; the remaining patient had surgical biopsy with spontaneous regression of a localized skin mass and remains free of disease over four years from biopsy. One of three

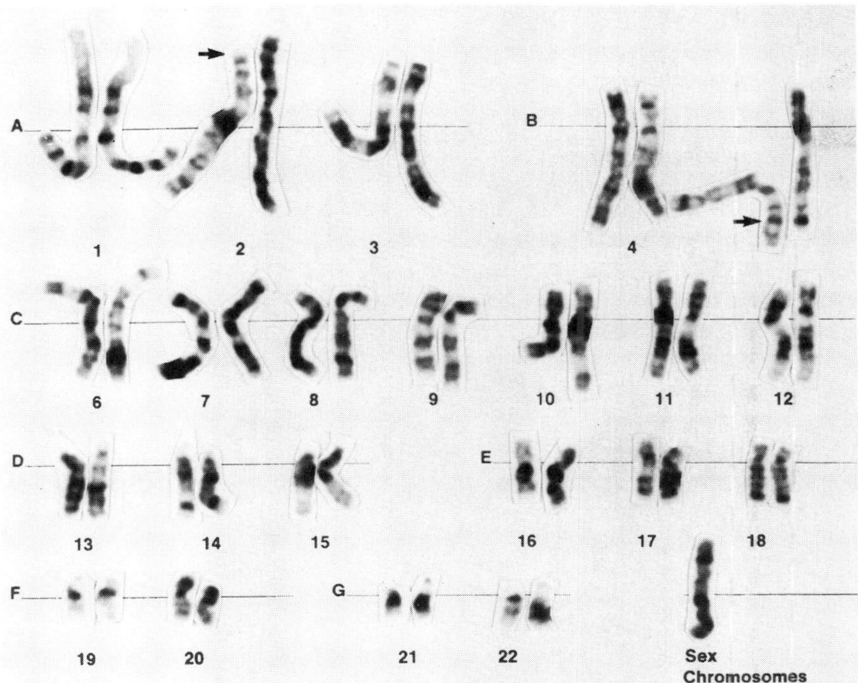

Fig. 4. Cytogenetics: a reciprocal translocation involving the short arm of chromosome 2 (band p23) and the long arm of chromosome 5 (band q35), t(2;5) (p23;q35) is characteristic of ALCL.

patients who received local radiation therapy has had prolonged survival and one of three patients had a prolonged response to single agent therapy, but died of another malignancy 25 years after the initial diagnosis.[82]

Initial combination chemotherapy included conventional chemotherapy for NHL in 36 patients, mega therapy[83] in 7 patients, and other therapy in 4 patients, including two who received platinum-based regimens and two patients who received therapy for Hodgkin's disease. The complete remission rate was 89% with 62% of patients remaining in continuous complete remission. The overall survival was 67% at 3 years while the disease-free survival (DFS) was 57% (Fig. 6). One reason for the discrepancy between overall survival and disease-free survival is that patients who have relapsed have had prolonged responses to additional therapy. This includes three of six patients who underwent bone marrow transplantation (BMT) with survival at 20, 50, and 70 months. Several other groups have utilized bone marrow transplantation as salvage therapy in relapsed ALCL.[62,84,85]

Table 1. *Differential antigen expression in nodal large cell malignancies with a sinus and diffuse growth pattern*

	Antigen[a]								
	CD45	EMA	Keratin	CD20	CD45RO	CD30	CD15	Lysozyme	CD68
ALCL Hodgkin's disease	+	+	−	±	+	+	±	−	±
Hodgkin's disease (other than lymphocyte predominant)	−	±	−	−	−	+	+	−	−
Microvillous malignant lymphoma	+	−	−	+	−	−	−	−	−
Malignant histiocytosis	±	±	−	−	±	−	±	+	+
Metastatic carcinoma	−	+	+	−	−	−*	±	−	−

+ = >50% of cases positive based on paraffin immunoperoxidase studies.

± = <25% positive.

− = Negative or rare (<1%) cases positive.

[a]CD45 (LCA = leukocyte common antigen, usually expressed in non-Hodgkin's lymphoma), CD20 (L26 = B-cell), CD45RD (UCHL-1 = T-cell), CD30 (Ber-H2), CD15 (LeuM-1 = Reed–Sternberg cell), CD68 (KP-1 = histiocyte).

* Embryonal carcinoma and pancreatic carcinoma may be positive for CD30.

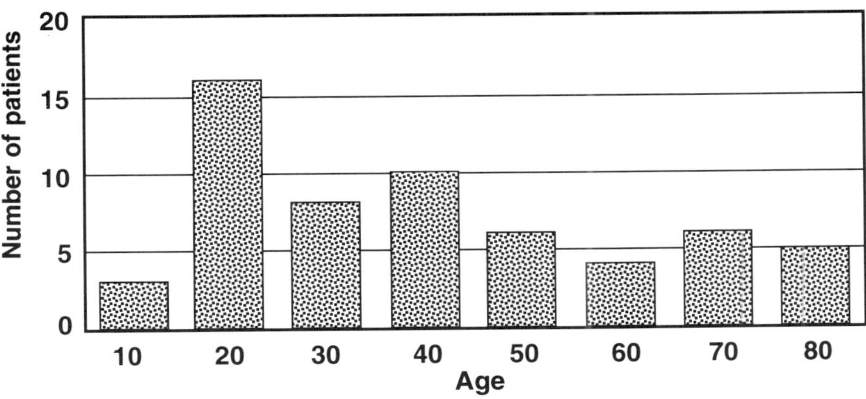

Fig. 5. Age distribution in primary Ki-1 lymphoma.

There were significant differences in overall survival and disease-free survival between limited stage I and II and advanced stage III and IV disease (Fig. 7). Univariate analysis of prognostic factors on survival (Table 5) indicated that extranodal disease, B symptoms, bulk disease, and Stage IV disease were significant factors; however, only Stage IV disease remained statistically significant in disease-free survival for patients receiving combination chemotherapy.

Childhood Ki-1+ ALCL is probably a more uniform disease than that reported in adults in part due to the predominant T immunophenotype, the frequent skin involvement, and the relative infrequency of secondary Ki-1 lymphomas.[3,67–72] In the initial description by Stein et al, eight (18%) of the 45 patients with Ki-1+ ALCL were 19 years or less in age.[2] In Kadin's initial report of six children with Ki-1+ ALCL, four marked as T cells, all six had cutaneous involvement and peripheral adenopathy, and two patients treated with chemotherapy early in the course of disease had sustained clinical remissions.[3] In a large series of 31 children with ALCL, Heitger et al reported 8 (26%) patients with skin involvement and 24 (77%) patients with advanced stage disease; 30 (97%) patients achieved a complete remission after chemotherapy with 23 (74%) patients remaining in first remission with a median follow-up of 35 months.[68]

In the Vanderbilt series, 17 patients were less than 20 years of age; 14 (82%) patients had peripheral adenopathy while 12 (71%) patients had extranodal involvement, including 9 (53%) with skin involvement.[70] Twelve cases had histological features of prototypic ALCL while five had the small cell predominant variant.[40] Fifteen (88%) tumours were of the peripheral T cell immunophenotype. Fourteen (82%) patients attained a complete remission, but six patients subsequently relapsed. The overall survival was

Table 2. *Series of Ki-1 anaplastic large cell lymphoma*

Series	No. Pts	Median age (Range)	M:F	Involved sites Nodes (%)	Involved sites Skin (%)	Stage III/IV (%)	Immunophenotype[b] T	B	Null	B/T	Response[a] CR (%)	Response[a] CCR (%)	Comments
Stein[2]	45	41 (3–72)	29:16	89	7	–	26	7	3	9	–	–	Initial series
Paediatric													
Kadin[3]	6	12 (8–19)	4:2	83	100	67	4	–	2	–	100	33	CCR in 2 pts treated promptly
Schnitzer[67]	3	11 (8–14)	3:0	100	0	33	3	–	–	–	67	67	Germline by DNA analysis
Wollman[68]	9	12 (1–19)	3:6	77	67	–	51	–	–	–	88	67	6 had monocytosis, 3 eosinophilia, 1 CNS
Fabretti[69]	11	9 (2–16)	6:5	100	27	80	–	–	–	–	82	55	Most were T cell
Whitlock[70]	17	14 (3–19)	12:5	82	53	41	15	–	–	2	82	50	Small cell variant had worse survival
Heitger[71]	31	13 (4–19)	17:14	90	26	77	–	–	–	–	97	74	Early large series
Vecchi[72]	13	9 (3–12)	7:6	62	23	38	11	2	–	–	100	75	LSA_2L_2 in 12 patients; two late relapses
Sandlund[86]	18	13 (2–20)	13:5	88	28	78	9	–	9	–	–	61	CD30+ cases with advanced disease had better overall survival compared to CD30– cases
Reiter[87]	62	10 (0.8–18)	41:21	90	14	58	32	3	15	–	93	81	Largest series; skin involvement associated with risk of tx failure
Adult													
Chan[35]	16	40 (8–82)	11:5	56	31	75	9	3	3	1	75[b]	75	60% overall survival; including 3 pts with recurrent regressing skin lesions
Tashiro[73]	12	54 (13–77)	8:4	75	42	58	6	2	4	–	–	58	5/10 HTLV-1+ (Japan)
Chott[36]	41	50 (5–91)	23:18	56	15	41	28	4	9	–	–	61[c]	>40 yo inferior survival (68% dead)

Romaguera[74]	18	38	–	–	47	–	8	2	7	–	76	73	Possible EBV association
Bitter[75]	5	20 8–48)	1:4	100	40	80	3	–	2	–	80	80	t (2;5) (p23;q35) in 2 pts
Penny[76]	24	57 (19–73)	17:7	92	21	54	16	6	2	–	55	30	Includes 7 secondary Ki-1 lymphomas
Greer[64]	31	35 (0.3–78)	18:13	84	23	55	24	4	3	–	91[d]	52	Extended to 58 pts in text
Marosi[77]	9	37 (24–67)	6:3	100	33	88	9	–	–	–	55	44	All received MACOP-B (2 relapsed, 6 stage IV)
Shulman[65]	31	44 (16–86)	18:13	–	32	71	13	8	6	–	81	48	3 of 7 patients salvaged with BMT
Nakamura[78]	30	18 (2–81)	13:17	80	30	–	24	–	6	–	77	52	Japanese series; 9/13 TCR gene rearranged, 2 HTLV-1+
De Bruin[79]	18	24 (14–72)	6:12	100	–	56	12	–	6	–	83	44	Inferior survival compared to cutaneous
Cutaneous													
Beljaards[27]	10	68 (27–89)	5:5	–	100	30	10	–	–	–	90	90	CD30 (Ki-1)+ good prognosis compared to CD30−
Beljaards[28]	47	60 (2–95)	28:19	–	100	–	45	–	2	–	98[e]	38	36 (76%) alive w/o disease; 12 (25%) developed extra-cutaneous disease
Krishnan[80]	27	67 (19–83)	23:4	–	100	–	21	3	–	3	–	80[f]	20/25 alive w/o disease; 2 (5%) died with disseminated disease
De Bruin[79]	19	61 (29–89)	14:5	–	100	–	16	–	3	–	100	42	11 recurrences (4 extra-cutaneous); 15/19 alive w/o disease

[a] Response percentages are determined if curative therapy given which was usually combination chemotherapy; CR=complete remission. CCR=continuous complete remission.
[b] Response was in 6/8 patients who received combination chemotherapy as initial therapy; overall 40% of series is in CCR.
[c] Response was in 8/13 patients <40 yo.
[d] Response was in 23 patients who received combination chemotherapy as their initial therapy.
[e] Initial therapy: chemotherapy (6), radiation (9), surgical excision (23), excision and radiation (4).
[f] CR occurred in 13/15 receiving chemotherapy, 5/9 surgical excision, 1/1 radiation.

Table 3. *Presenting features in Ki-1 lymphoma*

Erroneous diagnoses	18 (31%)	Extranodal disease	28 (48%)
B symptoms	20 (34%)	Skin	16 (28%)
Lymphadenopathy		Bone marrow	6 (11%)
Peripheral	46 (79%)	Bone	5 (8%)
Mediastinal	7 (12%)	Liver	4 (7%)
Retroperitoneal	24 (41%)	Bulk disease	10 (17%)
Stage: I (16), II (12), III (12), IV (18)			

Table 4. *Initial therapy/response in Ki-1 NHL*

	No.		CR		Relapse	CCR	
None	5		–		–	–	
Radiation	3		2		1	1	
Single agents	3		2		1	0	
Combination chemotherapy							
Conventional	36	47	33	42 (89%)	10	23	29 (62%)
Mega	7		5		2	3	
Other	4		4		1	3	

65% and the two year DFS was 53%. Preliminary data indicated an inferior prognosis for the small cell variant.[70]

In a report of 22 children with peripheral T-cell lymphoma, Gordon et al questioned the specificity of the CD30 antigen, as well as the t(2;5) marker.[84] Twenty (95%) of 21 patients tested expressed CD30 on the large tumours cells, but only five patients had morphology characteristic of ALCL, and only one of four patients with t (2;5) had this histology. The remaining histologies included diffuse large cell[10] and mixed cell[7] and it is likely the majority of these cases fit into the histologic spectrum described for primary ALCL. Nine patients initially seen at diagnosis had a 61% 2 year relapse-free survival while 13 patients who were referred after relapse underwent salvage therapy, predominantly with bone marrow transplantation.[84, 85]

Two recent series have added information to the distinguishing features, prognosis, and therapy of childhood Ki−1+ ALCL. Sandland et al reported a series of 18 CD30+ patients from St Jude's Research Hospital and compared them to 27 CD30− patients with large cell lymphoma.[86] Skin involvement was significantly more frequent in CD30+ cases (p=.007), and all CD30+ cases had either a T-cell or null-cell phenotype while the

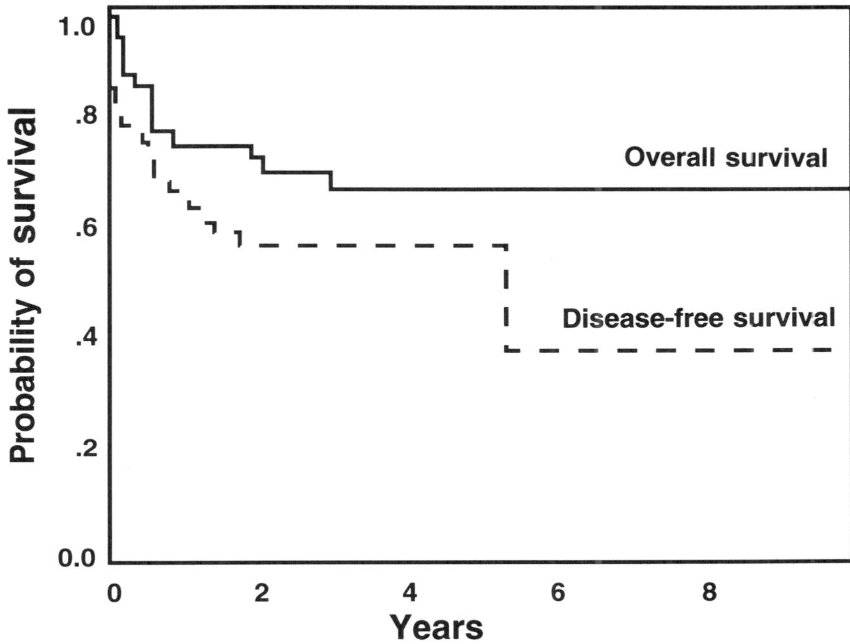

Fig. 6. Survival of primary Ki-1 lymphoma: The 3-year overall survival was 67% and the 3-year disease-free survival was 57%.

majority of CD30− cases were of B-cell origin (p<.001). For patients with advanced stage disease, CD30+ expression was associated with a better 5-year overall survival than CD30− (84% ± 12% vs 27% ± 16%, p= .0016).[86] Reiter et al reported a series of 62 patients treated prospectively in three consecutive Berlin–Frankfurt–Munster Group studies.[87] Ki−1+ ALCL was distinguished by predominantly a T immunophenotype, more frequent bone, soft tissue and skin involvement, and the relative lack of bone marrow and CNS disease. The therapy was primarily short-pulse chemotherapy over 2 to 5 months without local radiation or CNS radiation with a CR rate of 93% and a 9 year event-free survival of 81% ± 5%.[87]

Cutaneous presentation

The diagnosis and management of Ki−1 ALCL with disease limited to the skin are controversial areas.[38, 39] Patients with cutaneous ALCL tend to be older than patients with nodal ALCL.[79] The skin lesions usually are over 1 cm and often have ulcerations. De Bruin et al reported absence of expression of the epithelial membrane antigen in cutaneous ALCL in contrast to nodal disease and the presence of a cutaneous lymphocyte

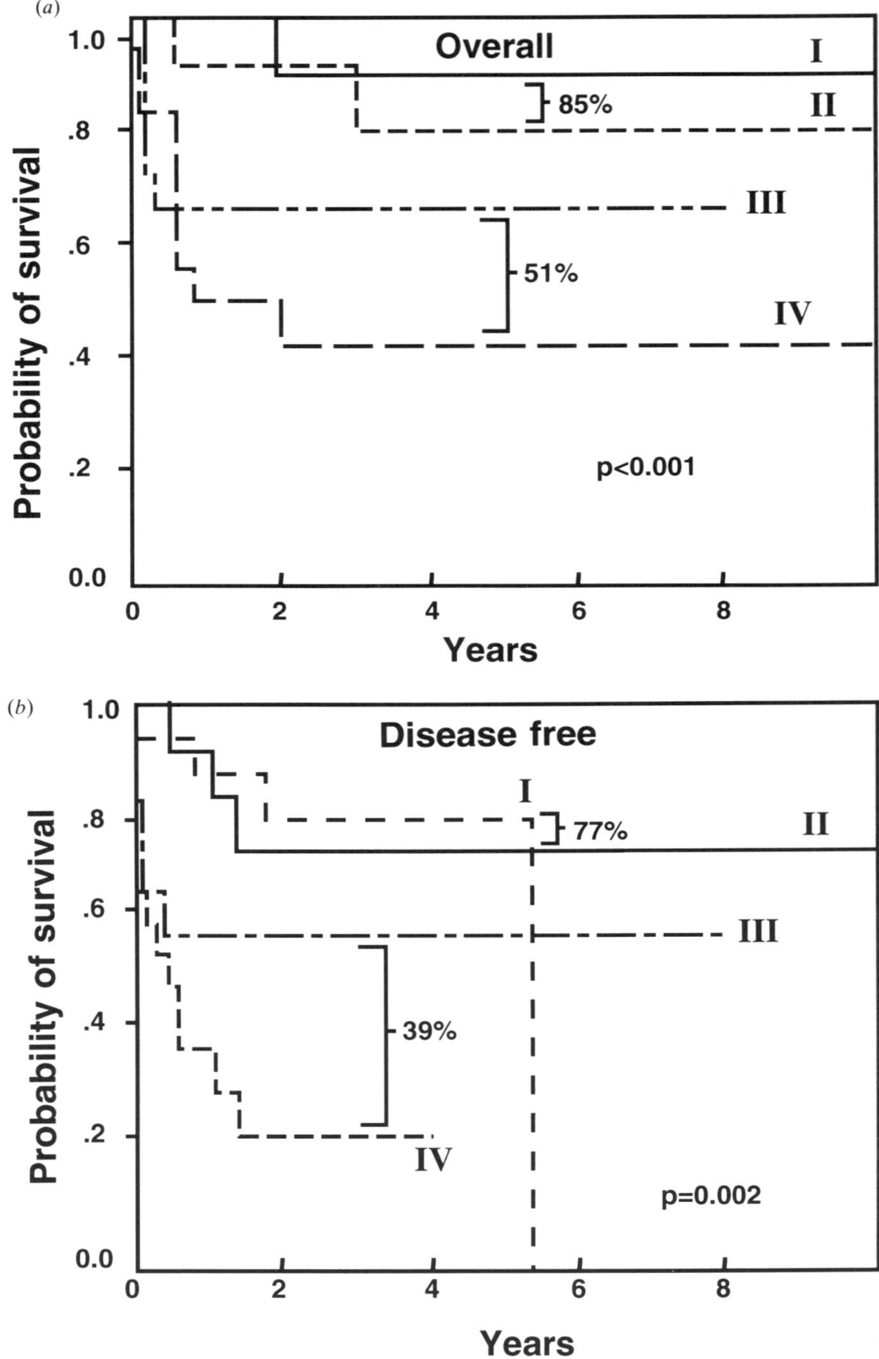

Fig. 7. Survival of primary Ki-1 lymphoma (*a*) overall and (*b*) disease-free survival for limited Stage (I/II) vs advanced Stage (III/IV).

Table 5. *Univariate analysis of prognostic factors on survival*

	Overall survival	Disease-free survival (DFS)	DFS after chemotherapy
Extranodal disease	0.043	0.131	0.056
B symptoms	0.003	0.034	0.136
Bulk disease	0.001	0.027	0.136
Stage IV disease	<0.001	0.001	0.001

antigen (HECA-452).[79] Distinguishing cutaneous ALCL from benign dermatoses and lymphomatoid papulosis may be difficult.[88] Lymphomatoid papulosis contains CD30+ large cells and may have T cell gene rearrangements; additionally, 5–20% of lymphomatoid papulosis patients develop overt lymphoma.[42]

The optimal therapy for cutaneous ALCL is uncertain owing to regressions and spontaneous remissions, particularly with localized lesions. Because there is an overall good prognosis, Beljaards et al have recommended local radiation therapy for patients with localized cutaneous lesions or even simple excision for small solitary lesions; with this approach, however, there is a high relapse rate.[28] Krishnan et al reported 13 of 15 patients had a sustained remission with combination chemotherapy in a series of 25 patients with cutaneous ALCL; five of nine patients who underwent surgical excision were without disease along with one patient who received radiation therapy.[80] Therapy in cutaneous ALCL should be based on the age of the patient, performance status, size and extent of lesions and may include observation, surgical excision, radiation, and/or chemotherapy; extracorporeal photophoresis, *cis*-retinoic acid, and other cutaneous directed therapies have achieved responses in some patients.[64,89]

Unique extranodal presentation

In addition to cutaneous disease, presentations at unusual sites may add to the difficulty in diagnosing ALCL. Bone pain may be the initial symptom and involvement may be either monostotic or polyostotic; radiologically, the lesions are lytic with ill-defined borders and bone scans may reveal more extensive involvement.[46] Although bony involvement usually represents Stage IV disease, chemotherapy with or without radiation often achieves sustained remissions.[43] ALCL developing in the gastrointestinal tract, lung, and muscle may present with clinical features suggestive of carcinomas.[44,45]

HIV and ALCL

Recent series of AIDS lymphomas have shown ALCL represents 2 to 15% of cases. HIV-related ALCLs have predominantly been B cell or unclassified immunophenotypes in contrast to the predominant T cell phenotype seen in immunocompetent patients. There is disagreement about the prognostic significance of histology in AIDS lymphomas and their relationship to EBV, but recent studies indicate emerging trends. In a series of 49 patients, Pederson et al reported that immunoblastic B lymphomas occurred later in the course of AIDS and were more commonly associated with EBV than Burkitt's lymphoma; two patients (4%) had ALCL, one of one tumour tested was positive for EBV, and both patients had a prolonged survival.[90]

Chadburn et al reported a series of eight AIDS patients with ALCL; four were T, one was B, and three were indeterminate for cell of origin.[91] EBV was present in two of three patients tested. Seven patients were Stage IE, including four with cutaneous disease, and one patient was Stage IV. These patients primarily had aggressive disease with a median survival of only three months, but two patients had localized, regressing cutaneous lesions. Although histology varies, the prognosis in AIDS lymphomas appears principally to be related to the immune status of the patient.[91]

Viral studies indicate a role for EBV in the pathogenesis of AIDS lymphomas including ALCL. Carbone et al reported 12 (14%) ALCL in a series of 87 patients and separated all the lymphomas into two groups, one which was positive for EBV-DNA and latent membrane protein-1 (LMP-1), including the majority of ALCL and a proportion of immunoblastic lymphoma, and another which was positive for EBV-DNA but negative for LMP-1 and included small noncleaved cell lymphomas.[92] Hamilton-Dutoit et al reported only one (2%) T-ALCL in 49 AIDS lymphomas, but also reported a correlation of CD30 expression with immunoblastic/large cell lymphoma, EBV positivity, and LMP-1 expression.[93] They reported three patterns of EBV latency in AIDS lymphomas based on EBV encoded small RNA-2 (EBER-1), EBV nuclear antigen-2(EBNA-2), and LMP-1: broad (EBER+/EBNA-2+/LMP-1+), restricted (EBER+/EBNA-2-/LMP-1-), and intermediate (EBER+/EBNA-2-/LMP-1+). The one ALCL had an intermediate pattern, the immunoblastic/large cell lymphomas expressed all three patterns, and the small non-cleaved (Burkitt-type) lymphomas predominantly had a restricted pattern.[93] The role of EBV in AIDS lymphomas remains to be determined but appears to be significant in ALCL, immunoblastic lymphomas, and in the advanced stage of AIDS.

Viral studies

Viral interactions, particularly EBV, appear to be important in the pathogenesis of ALCL and may account for some of the heterogeneity seen in ALCL. Expression of EBV from tumor tissue has been variable at least in part due to the sensitivity of the methods employed to identify the virus.[94,95] By Southern blotting, Anagostopoulos et al identified EBV-DNA in one of 22 (4.5%) patients with ALCL[13] while by polymerase chain reaction, Herbst et al detected EBV-DNA in 15 of 47 (32%) patients.[96] EBER transcripts were detected in tumour cells by in situ hybridization (ISH) in 9 of 11 EBV-DNA-positive cases; LMP positivity was present in tumour cells in 5 of 28 (18%) cases and two B-cell cases also expressed EBNA-2.[96] Kanavaros et al reported similar findings: eight of 17 (47%) cases were PCR-positive, three of seven ISH-positive, and two of 15 (13%) LMP-positive.[97] Lytic cycle antigens, BZLF1 protein and gp 250/350, have not been detected. Latent infection by EBV, with variable expression of latent gene products, appears to be significant in the pathogenesis of some primary ALCL. A combination of Southern blotting and PCR has detected HTLV-1 proviral sequences in cutaneous T-cell ALCL in patients from Germany and suggests HTLV-1 may be involved in some cutaneous ALCL.[14]

Cytokines have an integral role in the pathogenesis of malignant lymphoma.[98] Clinical, pathological, and molecular genetic data support involvement of cytokines in ALCL. CD30 and its ligand have homology to members of the TNFR/NGFR family[9], TNFα and β, and CD40 ligand,[10] suggesting a cytokine network. Kadin et al have demonstrated that the progression of lymphomatoid papulosis to a Ki-1+ lymphoma is due to the loss of receptors for transforming growth factor beta (TGFβ) which normally inhibits the clonal expansion of T cells.[42] Newcom et al supported the theory by showing a marked in vitro increase in DNA synthesis by Ki-1 lymphoma cells after exposure to neutralizing antibodies to TGFβ.[99]

Clinical and pathological features such as leukocytosis, monocytosis, eosinophilia and a marked inflammatory response in some skin and nodal lesions suggest involvement of cytokines in ALCL. Increased G-CSF production in tumor cell culture supernates has been demonstrated in a patient with ALCL and neutrophilia.[100] Other cytokine studies in ALCL include increased IL-6 in a patient with extensive bone involvement[101] and IL-9 expression in ALCL and Hodgkin's disease.[102]

Conclusions

Primary Ki-1+ ALCL is a unique clinicopathologic entity which should be distinguished from secondary ALCL, other Ki-1+ non-Hodgkin's lymphomas, Hodgkin's disease, malignant histiocytosis, carcinomas, and cutaneous lymphoproliferative disorders. Morphology and immunology, possibly in conjunction with the cytogenetic marker t(2;5), can usually confirm the diagnosis. Morphological variants, variable immunophenotype and the inability to detect t(2;5) in all cases indicate some heterogeneity within primary ALCL.

Distinguishing clinical features include a bimodal age distribution with the largest peak in the second decade, frequent peripheral adenopathy with sparing of the mediastinum, and extranodal disease with skin the most common site of involvement. Primary Ki-1+ ALCL probably represents the most common subtype of peripheral T-cell lymphoma of childhood and unlike other childhood lymphomas has infrequent marrow and central nervous system involvement.

The management of primary ALCL is controversial particularly if localized cutaneous involvement is the only site of disease. Because there may be spontaneous remissions with cutaneous disease and there is an overall good prognosis, simple excision and/or local radiation have been advocated by some investigators; however, relapse rates appear to be less with combination chemotherapy. For most patients, combination chemotherapy for large cell lymphoma is warranted with cure rates approaching two-thirds of all patients. Marrow transplantation has been used as salvage therapy in some relapsed patients.

The recent identification of the genes involved in the (2;5) translocation associated with ALCL provides a tumour-specific marker for this disorder which will permit advances in the understanding of its pathogenesis, diagnosis and classification. The availability of a tumour-specific marker will facilitate clinical studies looking at detection of minimal residual disease, and may provide a basis for novel therapeutic approaches.

Continued investigations of cytokines, specifically IL-9 and TGF-B, and viruses, particularly EBV, may define additional pathogenetic mechanisms in ALCL.

Acknowledgement

The authors wish to thank Mrs Willa Bean for preparation of the manuscript.

References

(1) Schwab U, Stein H, Gerdes J et al. Production of a monoclonal antibody specific for Hodgkin and Sternberg–Reed cells of Hodgkin's disease and a subset of normal lymphoid cells. *Nature* 1982; 299: 65–7.

(2) Stein H, Mason J, Gerdes N et al. The expression of the Hodgkin's disease associated antigen Ki-1 in reactive and neoplastic lymphoid tissue: evidence that Reed–Sternberg cells and histiocytic malignancies are derived from activated lymphoid cells. *Blood* 1985; 66: 848–58.

(3) Kadin ME, Sako DY, Berliner J et al. Childhood Ki-1 lymphoma presenting with skin lesions and peripheral lymphadenopathy. *Blood* 1986; 68: 1042–9.

(4) Fischer P, Nacheva E, Mason DY et al. A Ki-1 (CD30) positive human cell

line (karpas 299) established from a high grade non-hodgkin's lymphoma, showing a 2;5 translocation and rearrangement of the T-cell receptor B-chain gene. *Blood* 1988; 72: 234–40.

(5) Rimokh R, Magaud J-P, Berger F et al. A translocation involving a specific breakpoint (q35) on chromosome 5 is characteristic of anaplastic large cell lymphoma ('Ki-1 lymphoma'). *Br J Haematol* 1989; 71: 31–6.

(6) Kaneko Y, Frizzera G, Edamura S et al. A novel translocation, t(2;5) (p23;q35), in childhood phagocytic large T-cell lymphoma mimicking malignant histiocytosis. *Blood* 1989; 73: 806–13.

(7) LeBeau MM, Bitter MA, Larson RA et al. The t(2; 5) (p23; q35): A recurring chromosomal abnormality in Ki-1-positive anaplastic large cell lymphoma. *Leukemia* 1989; 3: 866–70.

(8) Morris SW, Kirstein MN, Valentine MB et al. Fusion of the tyrosine kinase gene ALK to the nucleolar phosphoprotein gene NPM in human t(2; 5)-positive lymphomas. *Science* 1994; 263: 1281–4.

(9) Dürkop H, Latza U, Hummel M, Eitelbach F, Seed B, Stein H. Molecular cloning and expression of a new member of the nerve growth factor receptor family that is characteristic for Hodgkin's disease. *Cell* 1992; 68: 421–7.

(10) Smith C, Grus H-J, Davis T et al. CD30 antigen, a marker for Hodgkin's lymphoma, is a receptor whose ligand defines an emerging family of cytokines with homology to TNF. *Cell* 1993; 73: 1349–60.

(11) Pinto A, Gloghini A, Gattei V, Aldinucci D, Zagonel V, Carbone A. Expression of the *c-kit* receptor in human lymphomas is restricted to Hodgkin's disease and CD30+ anaplastic large cell lymphomas. *Blood* 1994; 83: 785–92.

(12) Fonatsch C, Latza U, Dürkop H, Rieder H, Stein H. Assignment of the human CD30 (Ki-1) gene to 1p36. *Genomics* 1992; 14: 825–6.

(13) Anagnostopoulos I, Herbst H, Niedobitek G, Stein H. Demonstration of monoclonal EBV genomes in Hodgkin's disease and Ki-1-positive anaplastic large cell lymphoma by combined Southern blot and in situ hybridization. *Blood* 1989; 74: 810–16.

(14) Anagnostopoulos I, Hummel M, Kaudewitz P, Herbst H, Braun–Falco O, Stein H. Detection of HTLV-1 proviral sequences in CD30-positive large cell cutaneous T-cell lymphomas. *Am J Pathol* 1990; 137: 1317–22.

(15) Chadburn A, Inghirami G, Knowles DM. The kinetics and temporal expression of T-cell activation-associated antigens CD15 (LeuM1), CD30 (Ki-1), EMA, and CD11c (LeuM5) by benign activated T cells. *Hematol Pathol* 1992; 6: 193–202.

(16) Pallesen G. The diagnostic significance of the CD30 (Ki-1) antigen. *Histopathol* 1990, 16: 409–13.

(17) Jaworsky C, Cirillo–Hyland V, Petrozzi JW, Lessin SR, Murphy GF. Regressing atypical histiocytosis: aberrant prothymocyte differentiation, T-cell receptor gene rearrangements, and nodal involvement. *Arch Dermatol* 1990; 126: 1609–16.

(18) Motley RJ, Jasani B, Path MMRC. Regressing atypical histiocytosis, a

regressing cutaneous phase of Ki-1-positive anaplastic large cell lymphoma. *Cancer* 1992; 70: 476–83.

(19) Wilson MS, Weiss LM, Gatter KC, Mason DY, Dorfman RF, Warnke RA. Malignant histiocytosis: a reassessment of cases previously reported in 1975 based on paraffin section immunophenotyping studies. *Cancer* 1990; 66: 530–36.

(20) Pallesen G, Hamilton–Dutoit SJ. Ki-1 (CD30) antigen is regularly expressed by tumor cells of embryonal carcinoma. *Am J Pathol* 1988; 133: 446–50.

(21) Schwarting R, Gerdes J, Durkop H, Falini B, Pileri S, Stein H: Ber-H2: a new anti-Ki-1 (CD30) monoclonal antibody directed at a formol-resistant epitope. *Blood* 1989; 74: 1678–89.

(22) Piris M, Brown DC, Gatter KC, Mason DY. CD30 expression in non-Hodgkin's lymphoma. *Histopathology* 1990; 17: 211–18.

(23) Hansen H, Lemke H, Bredfeldt G, Konnecke I, Havsteen B. The Hodgkin-associated Ki-1 antigen exists in an intracellular and a membrane-bound form. *Biol Chem Hoppe-Seyler* 1990; 141: 13–31.

(24) Froese P, Lemke H, Gerdes J et al. Biochemical characterization and biosynthesis of the Ki-1 antigen in Hodgkin-derived and virus-transformed human B and T-cell lymphoid cell lines. *J Immunol* 1987; 139: 2081–7.

(25) Hansen H, Bredfeldt G, Havsteen B, Lemke H. Protein kinase activity of the intracellular but not of the membrane-associated form of the Ki-1 antigen (CD30). *Res Immunol* 1990, 141: 13–31.

(26) Josimovic-Alasevic O, Dürkop H, Schwarting R, Backe E, Stein H, Diamanstein T. Ki-1 (CD30) antigen is released by Ki-1-positive tumor cells in vitro and in vivo. I. Partial characterization of soluble Ki-1 antigen and detection of the antigen in cell culture supernatants and in serum by an enzyme-linked immunosorbent assay. *Eur J Immunol* 1989; 19: 157–62.

(27) Beljaards RC, Meijer CJL, Scheffer E et al. Prognostic significance of CD30 (Ki-1/Ber-H2) expression in primary cutaneous large-cell lymphomas of T-cell origin. *Am J Pathol* 1989; 135: 1169–78.

(28) Beljaards RC, Kaudewitz P, Berti E et al. Primary cutaneous CD30-positive large cell lymphoma: definition of a new type of cutaneous lymphoma with a favorable prognosis. A European multicenter study of 47 patients. *Cancer* 1993; 71: 2097–104.

(29) Offit K, Ladanyi M, Gangi MD, Ebrahim SAD, Filippa D, Chaganti RSK. Ki-1 antigen expression defines a favorable clinical subset of non-B cell non-Hodgkin's lymphoma. *Leukemia* 1990; 4: 625–30.

(30) Kadin ME, Anderson JR, Chilcote et al. Lack of prognostic significance of Ki-1 (CD30) positivity in disseminated pediatric large cell lymphoma. *Blood* 1991; 78: 121a.

(31) Abbondanzo SL, Sato N, Straus SE, Jaffe ES. Acute infectious mononucleosis: CD30 (Ki-1) antigen expression and histologic correlations. *Am J Clin Pathol* 1990; 93: 698–702.

(32) Hall PA, d'Ardenne AJ, Stansfeld AG. Paraffin section immunohistochemistry. I: non-Hodgkin's lymphoma. *Histopathology* 1988; 13: 149–60.

(33) Suchi J, Lennert K, Tu L–Y et al. Histopathology and immunohistochemistry

of peripheral T cell lymphomas: a proposal for their classification. *J Clin Pathol* 1987; 40: 995–1015.
(34) Stansfeld AG, Diebold J, Kapanci Y et al. Updated Kiel classifications for lymphomas. *Lancet* 1988; 1: 292–3.
(35) Chan JKC, Ng CS, Hui PK et al. Anaplastic large cell Ki-1 lymphoma. Delineation of two morphological types. *Histopathology* 1989; 15: 11–34.
(36) Chott A, Kaserer K, Augustin I et al. Ki-1-positive large cell lymphoma: a clinicopathologic study of 41 cases. *Am J Surg Pathol* 1990; 14: 439–48.
(37) Chan JKC, Buchanan R, Fletcher CDM. Sarcomatoid variant of anaplastic large-cell Ki-1 lymphoma. *Am J Surg Pathol* 1990; 14: 983–88.
(38) Pileri S, Falini B, Delsol G et al. Lymphohistiocytic T-cell lymphoma (anaplastic large cell lymphoma CD30+/Ki-1+ with a high content of reactive histiocytes). *Histopathology* 1990; 16: 383–91.
(39) Rosso R, Paulli M, Magrini U et al. Anaplastic large cell lymphoma, CD30/Ki-1 positive, expressing the CD15/Leu-M1 antigen. Immunohistochemical and morphological relationships to Hodgkin's disease. *Virchows Archiv A Pathol Anat* 1990; 416: 229–35.
(40) Kinney MC, Collins RD, Greer JP, Whitlock JA, Sioutos N, Kadin ME. A small-cell-predominant variant of primary Ki-1 (CD30)+ T-cell lymphoma. *Am J Surg Pathol* 1993; 17: 859–68.
(41) Kadin ME. Cutaneous Ki-1 lymphoma: pathology, immunology and clinical characteristics. *Int Symp Princess Taka-Matsu Cancer Res Fund* 1988; 18: 187–95.
(42) Kadin ME. The spectrum of Ki-1+ cutaneous lymphomas. *Curr Probl Dermatol* 1990; 19: 132–43.
(43) Wong KF, Chan JKC, Ng CS et al. Anaplastic large cell Ki-1 lymphoma involving bone marrow: marrow findings and association with reactive hemophagocytosis. *Am Med J* 1991; 37: 112–9.
(44) Ross CW, Hanson CA, Schnitzer B. CD30 (Ki-1)-positive, anaplastic large cell lymphoma mimicking gastrointestinal carcinoma. *Cancer* 1992; 70: 2517–23.
(45) Paulli M, Rosso R, Kindl S et al. Primary gastric CD30 (Ki-1)-positive large cell non-Hodgkin's lymphoma. *Cancer* 1994; 73: 541–9.
(46) Chan JKC, Chi-Sing N, Pak-Kwan P et al. Anaplastic large cell Ki-1 lymphoma of bone. *Cancer* 1991; 68: 2186–91.
(47) Feldges A, Gerhard L, Reinhardt V, Budach V. Primary cerebral anaplastic T-cell lymphoma (Type Ki-1): review and case report. *Clin Neuropathol* 1991; 11: 55–9.
(48) Kinney MC, Greer JP, Glick AD, Salhany KE, Collins RD. Anaplastic large-cell Ki-1 malignant lymphomas: recognition, biological and clinical implications. *Pathol Annu* 1991; 26: 1–24.
(49) Kinney MC, Glick AD, Stein H, Collins RD. Comparison of anaplastic large cell Ki-1 lymphomas and microvillous lymphomas in their immunologic and ultrastructural features. *Am J Surg Pathol* 1990; 14: 1047–60.
(50) Hugh J, Poppema S. Ki-1 (CD30) expression on transformed follicular lymphomas. *Lab Invest* 1990; 62: 46A (abstract).
(51) Delsol G, Al Saati T, Gatter KC. Coexpression of epithelial membrane

antigen (EMA), Ki-1, and interleukin-2 receptor by anaplastic large cell lymphomas. Diagnostic value in so-called malignant histiocytosis. *Am J Pathol* 1988; 130: 59–70.
(52) Delsol G, Blancher A, Al Saati T et al. Antibody BNH9 detects red blood cell related antigens on anaplastic large cell (CD30+) lymphomas. *Br J Cancer* 1991; 64: 321–6.
(53) Carbone A, Gloghini A, Volpe R. Immunohistochemistry of Hodgkin and non-Hodgkin lymphomas with emphasis on the diagnostic significance of the BNH9 antibody reactivity with anaplastic large cell (CD30 positive) lymphomas. *Cancer* 1992; 70: 2691–8.
(54) Kasai K, Sato Y, Kuwao S, Kawakubo Y, Inoue H, Kameya T. Sialosylated Lewis X expression in CD30 positive anaplastic large cell lymphomas. *J Cancer Res Clin Oncol* 1992; 119: 87–90.
(55) Herbst H, Tippelmann G, Anagnostopoulos I et al. Immunoglobulin and T-cell receptor gene rearrangements in Hodgkin's disease and Ki-1 positive anaplastic large cell lymphoma: Dissociation between phenotype and genotype. *Leuk Res* 1989; 13: 103–16.
(56) O'Connor NTJ, Stein H, Gatter KC et al. Genotypic analysis of large cell lymphomas which express the Ki-1 antigen. *Histopathology* 1987; 11: 733–40.
(57) O'Connor NTJ, Wainscoat JS, Weatherall DJ et al. Rearrangement of the T-cell receptor B-chain gene in the diagnosis of lymphoproliferative disorders. *Lancet* 1985; 1: 1295–97.
(58) Tawa A, Hozumi N, Minden M, Mak TW, Gelfand EW. Rearrangement of the T-cell receptor B-chain gene in non-T-cell, non-B-cell acute lymphoblastic leukemia of childhood. *N Engl J Med* 1985; 313: 1033–7.
(59) Waldmann TA, Davis MM, Bongiovanni KF, Korsmeyer SJ. Rearrangements of genes for the antigen receptor on T cells as markers of lineage and clonality in human lymphoid neoplasms. *N Engl J Med* 1985; 313: 776–83.
(60) Carbone A, Gloghini A, Volpe R, Pinto A. KP-1(CD68)-positive large cell lymphomas: a histopathologic and immunophenotypic characterization of 12 cases. *Hum Pathol* 1993; 24: 886–96.
(61) Frizzera G. The distinction of Hodgkin's disease from anaplastic large cell lymphoma. *Semin Diagnostic Pathol* 1992; 9: 291–6.
(62) Kadin ME: Primary Ki-1-positive anaplastic large-cell lymphoma: a distinct clinicopathologic entity. *Ann Oncol* 1994; 5: S25–30.
(63) Leoncini L, Del Vecchio MT, Kraft R et al. Hodgkin's disease and CD30 – positive anaplastic large cell lymphomas – a continuous spectrum of malignant disorders. A quantitative morphometric and immunohistologic study. *Am J Pathol* 1990; 137: 1047–57.
(64) Greer JP, Kinney MC, Collins RD et al. Clinical features of 31 patients with Ki-1 anaplastic large-cell lymphoma. *J Clin Oncol* 1991; 9: 539–47.
(65) Shulman LN, Frisard B, Antin JH et al. Primary Ki-1 anaplastic large-cell lymphoma in adults: clinical characteristics and therapeutic outcome. *J Clin Oncol* 1993; 11: 937–42.
(66) Stein H. Ki-1-anaplastic large cell lymphoma: is it a discrete entity? *Leukemia Lymphoma* 1993; 10: 81–4.

(67) Schnitzer B, Roth MS, Hyder DM, Ginsburg D. Ki-1 lymphomas in children. *Cancer* 1988; 61: 1213–21.
(68) Wollman M, Blatt J, Nelson K et al. Ki-1 lymphomas in childhood: a report of 9 cases from a single institution. *ASCO Proc* 1992; 11: 342 (abstract).
(69) Fabretti G, Comelli A, Piombo M, et al. Ki-1 large cell lymphoma in children. *Med Pediatr Oncol* 1991; 19: 369 (abstract).
(70) Whitlock JA, Kinney MC, Greer JP: Childhood Ki1+ lymphoma: Effect of small cell predominant histology on outcome. *Blood* 1992; 80: 43a.
(71) Heitger A, Gadner H, Bucksy P, Feller AC, Ritter J, Riehm H. Das grosszellige anaplastische Lymphom im Kindesalter – klinische Erfahrungen bei einer histologisch neu definierten Entität. *Klin Padiatr* 1989; 201: 237–41.
(72) Vecchi V, Burnelli R, Pileri S, et al. Anaplastic large cell lymphoma (Ki-1+/CD30+) in childhood. *Med and Pediatr Oncol* 1993; 21: 402–10.
(73) Tashiro K, Kikuchi M, Takeshita T, Yoshida T, Ohshima K. Clinicopathological study of Ki-1-positive lymphomas. *Path Res Pract* 1989; 185: 461–7.
(74) Romaguera J, Hagemeister F, McLaughlin P, et al. Adult Ki-1 diffuse large cell lymphoma (DLCL): a distinct clinicopathologicaal (CPC) entity with a favorable prognosis. *J Clin Oncol* 1990; 9: 266 (abstract).
(75) Bitter MA, Franklin WA, Larson RA. Morphology in Ki-1 (CD30)-positive non-Hodgkin's lymphoma is correlated with clinical features and the presence of a unique chromosomal abnormality, t(2; 5) (p23; q35). *Am J Surg Pathol* 1990; 14: 305–16.
(76) Penny RJ, Blaustein JC, Longtine JA, Pinkus GS. Ki-1-positive large cell lymphomas, a heterogenous group of neoplasms. Morphologic, immunophenotypic and clinical features of 24 cases. *Cancer* 1991; 68: 362–73.
(77) Marosi Ch, Heinz R, Steger G et al. MACOP-B treatment in patients with Ki-1-positive large-cell anaplastic lymphoma. *J Cancer Res Clin Oncol* 1992; 118: 314–17.
(78) Nakamura S, Takagi N, Kojima M et al. Clinicopathologic study of large cell anaplastic lymphoma (Ki-1-positive large cell lymphoma) among the Japanese. *Cancer* 1991; 68: 118–29.
(79) De Bruin PC, Beljaards RC, Van Heerde P, et al. Differences in clinical behaviour and immunophenotype between primary cutaneous and primary nodal anaplastic large cell lymphoma of T-cell or null cell phenotype. *Histopathology* 1993; 23: 127–35.
(80) Krishnan J, Tomaszewski M-M, Kao GF. Primary cutaneous CD30-positive anaplastic large cell lymphoma. Report of 27 cases. *J Cutan Pathol* 1993; 20: 193–202.
(81) Lennert K, Feller AC. *Histopathology of non-Hodgkin's lymphomas*. 2nd ed. New York: Springer-Verlag, 1992: 203.
(82) Salhany KE, Collins RD, Greer JP, Kinney MC. Long-term survival in Ki-1 lymphoma. *Cancer* 1991; 67: 516–22.
(83) Waits TM, Greco FA, Greer JP et al. Effective therapy for poor prognosis non-Hodgkin's lymphoma with 8 weeks of high dose intensity combination chemotherapy. *J Clin Oncol* 1993; 11: 943–49.

(84) Gordon BG, Weisenburger DD, Warkentin PI et al. Peripheral T-cell lymphoma in childhood and adolescence. *Cancer* 1993; 71: 257–63.
(85) Chakravarti V, Kamani NR, Bayever E et al. Bone marrow transplantation for childhood Ki-1 lymphoma. *J Clin Oncol* 1990; 8: 657–60.
(86) Sandland JT, Pui C–H, Santana VM et al. Clinical features and treatment outcome for children with CD30+ large-cell non-Hodgkin's lymphoma. *J Clin Oncol* 1994; 12: 895–8.
(87) Reiter A, Schrappe M, Tiemann M et al. Successful treatment strategy for Ki-1 anaplastic large-cell lymphoma of childhood: a prospective analysis of 62 patients enrolled in three consecutive Berlin–Frankfurt–Munster Group studies. *J Clin Oncol* 1994; 12: 899–908.
(88) Camisa C, Helm TN, Sexton C, Tuthill R. Ki-1-positive anaplastic large-cell lymphoma can mimic benign dermatoses. *J Am Acad Dermatol* 1993; 29: 696–700.
(89) Chow J–M, Cheng A–L, Su I–J, Wang C–H. 13-*cis*-retinoic acid induces cellular differentiation and durable remission in refractory cutaneous Ki-1 lymphoma. *Cancer* 1991; 67: 2490–4.
(90) Pedersen C, Gerstoft J, Lundgren JD et al. HIV-associated lymphoma: histopathology and association with Epstein–Barr virus genome related to clinical, immunological and prognostic features. *Eur J Cancer* 1991; 27: 1416–23.
(91) Chadburn A, Cesarman E, Jagirdar J, Subar M, Mir RN, Knowles DM. CD30 (Ki-1) positive anaplastic large cell lymphomas in individuals infected with the human immunodeficiency virus. *Cancer* 1993; 72: 3078–90.
(92) Carbone A, Tirelli U, Gloghini A, Volpe R, Boiocchi M. Human immunodeficiency virus-associated systemic lymphomas may be subdivided into two main groups according to Epstein–Barr viral latent gene expression. *J Clin Oncol* 1993; 11: 1674–81.
(93) Hamilton–Dutoit SJ, Rea D, Raphael M et al. Epstein–Barr virus-latent gene expression and tumor cell phenotype in acquired immunodeficiency syndrome-related non-Hodgkin's lymphoma. Correlation of lymphoma phenotype with three distinct patterns of viral latency. *Am J Pathol* 1993; 143: 1072–85.
(94) Borisch B, Gatter K, Tobler A et al. Epstein–Barr virus-associated anaplastic large cell lymphoma in renal transplant patients. *Am J Clin Pathol* 1992; 98: 312–18.
(95) Hamilton–Dutoit SJ, Pallesen G. A survey of Epstein–Barr virus gene expression in sporadic non-Hodgkin's lymphomas. Detection of Epstein–Barr virus in a subset of peripheral T-cell lymphomas. *Am J Pathol* 1992; 140: 1315–25.
(96) Herbst H, Dallenbach F, Hummel M et al. Epstein–Barr virus DNA and latent gene products in Ki−1 (CD30)-positive anaplastic large cell lymphomas. *Blood* 1991; 78: 2666–73.
(97) Kanavaros P, Jiwa NM, De Bruin PC et al. High incidence of EBV genome in CD30− positive non-Hodgkin's lymphomas. *J Pathol* 1992; 168: 307–15.
(98) Hsu S-M, Waldron JW, Hsu P-L, Hough AJ. Cytokines in malignant lymphomas: review and prospective evaluation. *Hum Pathol* 1993; 24: 1040–57.

(99) Newcom SR, Tagra KK, Kadin ME. Neutralizing antibodies against transforming growth factor B potentiate the proliferation of Ki−1 positive lymphoma cells. Further evidence for negative autocrine regulation by transforming growth factor β. *Am J Pathol* 1992; 140: 709–18.
(100) Nishihira H, Tanaka Y, Kigasawa Y, Sasaki Y, Fujimoto J. Case Reports: Ki−1 lymphoma producing G-CSF. *Br J Haematol* 1991; 80: 556–7.
(101) Agematsu K, Takeuchi S, Ichikawa M et al. Spontaneous production of interleukin-6 by Ki−1-positive large-cell anaplastic lymphoma with extensive bone destruction. *Blood* 1991; 77: 2299–301 (letter).
(102) Merz H, Houssiau FA, Orscheschek K et al. Interleukin-9 expression in human malignant lymphomas: unique association with Hodgkin's disease and large cell anaplastic lymphoma. *Blood* 1991; 78: 1311–17.

What is the best treatment for diffuse large cell lymphoma?

E R GAYNOR and R I FISHER

Introduction

The non-Hodgkin's lymphomas are a diverse group of diseases with varying natural history and varying responses to chemotherapy. The Working Formulation provides a conceptual framework in which the lymphomas are grouped as indolent, intermediate or high grade with respect to their natural history.[1] Ironically those which have an unfavourable course if untreated (the intermediate and high grade histologies) are the same lymphomas which are potentially curable if treated with aggressive combination chemotherapy. Those lymphomas which have an unfavourable, i.e. aggressive natural history are shown in Table 1. In this chapter we will discuss the staging, prognostic features and treatment of diffuse large cell lymphoma which is the most common entity encountered clinically within the intermediate and high grade categories. Treatment approaches to diffuse large

Table 1. *Working formulation nomenclature: intermediate and high grade lymphomas*

Intermediate grade
Malignant lymphoma, follicular predominantly large cell
Malignant lymphoma, diffuse mixed, small and large cell
Malignant lymphoma, diffuse large cell
High grade
Malignant lymphoma, large cell, immunoblastic
Malignant lymphoma, lymphoblastic
Malignant lymphoma, small non-cleaved cell

All correspondence to: Dr RI Fisher, Division of Hematology and Oncology, Loyola University School of Medicine, 2160 South 1st Avenue, Maywood, IL 60153, USA.

Cambridge Medical Reviews: Haematological Oncology Volume 4

cell lymphoma provide a framework for management decisions regarding patients with follicular large cell, diffuse small cleaved cell and diffuse mixed small and large cell. The approach to treatment of diffuse small, non-cleaved cell, non-Burkitt's lymphoma remains to be defined, although many clinicians would approach treatment of this lymphoma in the same way as the treatment of diffuse large cell lymphoma. Because standard therapy is not curative in many cases, the answer to the question of what is the best treatment necessitates a discussion of newer approaches to staging and treatment.

Staging and prognostic factors

The purpose of any staging system for the non-Hodgkin's lymphomas is to identify patients who are more or less likely to respond to a given program of treatment. The most widely used staging system has been the Ann Arbor System (Table 2) which is based on the anatomical extent of the disease as well as the presence or absence of symptoms.[2] Originally devised for use in the staging of Hodgkin's disease (HD), the system has proven inadequate for the staging of NHL because patterns of spread are quite different for HD and NHL. Unlike HD which commonly spreads through contiguous groups of lymph nodes, NHL is infrequently localized at the time of diagnosis, and frequently involves extranodal sites of disease.

Table 2. *The Ann Arbor staging classification*

Stage I
Involvement of a single lymph node region or of a single extranodal organ or site (I_E).

Stage II
Involvement of two or more lymph node regions on the same side of the diaphragm, or localized involvement of an extranodal site or organ (II_E) and of one or more lymph node regions on the same side of the diaphragm.

Stage III
Involvement of lymph node regions on both sides of the diaphragm, which may also be accompanied by localized involvement of an extranodal organ or site (III_E) or spleen (III_S) or both (III_{SE}).

Stage IV
Diffuse or disseminated involvement of one or more distant extranodal organs with or without associated lymph node involvement.

Fever >38°, night sweats, and/or weight loss >10% of body weight in the 6 months preceding diagnosis are defined as sytemic symptoms, and denoted by the suffix B. Asymptomatic patients are denoted by the suffix A.

Because of the shortcomings of the Ann Arbor System as it is applied to staging of NHL, several other prognostic factors have been identified as useful in predicting outcome. These factors include patient age, presence or absence of 'B' symptoms, serum LDH, performance status, the presence or absence of bulky disease, the number of nodal and extranodal sites of disease and the stage of disease, i.e. localized (I and II) vs extensive (III and IV). Most investigators would separate patients into two groups, localized disease (I and II non-bulky) and advanced disease (II bulky, III, IV) when making therapy decisions. There is, however, a growing awareness that, particularly among patients with advanced disease, there is a need to identify patients who are at risk of not being cured with currently available combination chemotherapy regimens.

Standard treatment

Diffuse large cell lymphoma is best viewed as a systemic disease; chemotherapy is therefore the mainstay of treatment. The most commonly used chemotherapy regimens are those outlined in Table 3.

Localized disease

By definition, localized disease includes those patients with stage I or II disease which is non-bulky (i.e. no tumour mass ≥ 10 cm; no mediastinal mass > one-third of the thoracic diameter). Cure is attainable in a very high percentage of patients in this subgroup, and a variety of treatment approaches have been successfully employed.

Studies conducted at the University of Chicago demonstrated that patients with pathologically staged early disease could be cured with a tumouricidal dose of radiation (4000 cGy) delivered to an extended field port. In the most recent update of this series, Vokes et al reported a 70% 10-year survival for patients with pathologic stage I disease.[3] The morbidity associated with the staging laparotomy required to identify patients with early stage disease is not acceptable, and hence these studies are now mainly of historical interest. Furthermore, the results obtained with RT alone in pathologically staged patients is not superior to results obtained in clinically staged patients treated with chemotherapy alone or in combination with RT. Patterns of failure in patients treated with RT suggest that more extensive radiation ports would not prevent relapses since many occur in extranodal sites.[4]

One of the earliest reported studies using an Adriamycin-based chemotherapy regimen either alone or in combination with RT was a non-randomized trial by Jones et al.[5] All patients received CHOP chemotherapy usually for a total of eight cycles. Patients having an inadequate response to chemotherapy or experiencing toxicity requiring significant modification in chemotherapy dosages, were treated with RT to an involved field

Table 3. *Chemotherapeutic regimens*

Regimens	Dose and route	Day	Frequency
CHOP			
C=cyclophosphamide	750 mg/m² IV	1	Repeat every 21 days
H=Adriamycin	50 mg/m² IV	1	
O=Oncovin	1.4 mg/m² IV (max. 2.0 mg)	1	
P=prednisone	100 mg PO	1–5	
M-BACOD			
M=methotrexate*	3000 mg/m² IV	15	Repeat every 21 days
B=bleomycin	4 mg/m² IV	1	
A=Adriamycin	45 mg/m² IV	1	
C=cyclophosphamide	600 mg/m² IV	1	
O=Oncovin	1 mg/m² IV	1	
D=Decadron	6 mg/m² PO	1–5	
m-BACOD			
M=methotrexate*	200 mg/m² IV	8, 15	Repeat every 21 days
B=bleomycin	4 mg/m² IV	1	
A=Adriamycin	45 mg/m² IV	1	
C=cyclophosphamide	600 mg/m² IV	1	
O=Oncovin	1.0 mg/m² IV	1	
D=Decadron	6 mg/m² PO	1–5	
ProMACE-MOPP			
Pro=prednisone	60 mg/m² PO	1–14	Repeat every 28 days
M=methotrexate*	1500 mg/m² IV	15	
A=Adriamycin	25 mg/m² IV	1, 8	
C=cyclophosphamide	650 mg/m²	1, 8	
E=etoposide	120 mg/m² IV	1, 8	
Followed by MOPP after maximal response			
M=mechlorethamine	6 mg/m² IV	1, 8	Repeat every 28 days
O=Oncovin	1.4 mg/m² IV	1, 8	
P=Procarbazine	100 mg/m² PO	1–14	
P=prednisone	40 mg/m² PO	1–14	
ProMACE-CytaBOM			
Pro=prednisone	60 mg/m² PO	1–14	Repeat every 21 days
A=Adriamycin	25 mg/m² IV	1	
C=cyclophosphamide	650 mg/m² IV	1	
E=etoposide	120 mg/m² IV	1	
Cyta=cytarabine	300 mg/m² IV	8	
B=bleomycin	5 mg/m² IV	8	
O=Oncovin	1.4 mg/m² IV	8	
M=methotrexate*	120 mg/m² IV	8	
MACOP-B			
M=methotrexate*	400 mg/m² IV	8, 36, 64	
A=Adriamycin	50 mg/m² IV	1, 15, 29, 43, 57, 71	
C=cyclophosphamide	350 mg/m² IV	1, 15, 29, 43, 57, 71	
O=Oncovin	1.4 mg/m² IV (max. 2.0 mg)	8, 22, 36, 50, 64, 78	
P=prednisone	75 mg/m² PO	1–84	
B=bleomycin	10 mg/m² IV	22, 50, 78	

* Leucovorin rescue is given 24 hours after each methotrexate dose.

(IFRT). When patients treated with chemotherapy alone were compared to those treated with combined modality therapy, there was no significant difference in the relapse rate or survival.

Connors et al employed a short course of chemotherapy (three cycles of CHOP) followed by IFRT in 78 patients with clinical stage I or II disease.[6] None of these patients had poor prognostic features such as bulky disease. In this highly favourable subgroup, 99% achieved a CR with 85% being long-term survivors.

The Southwest Oncology Group (SWOG) is currently conducting a randomized trial comparing CHOP for three cycles followed by IFRT vs CHOP for eight cycles in patients with clinical Stage I and II non-bulky disease. The primary objective of this study is to evaluate differences in survival, time to treatment failure, and toxicity of these two approaches both of which as noted above have been shown to be curative in this subset of patients with diffuse large cell lymphoma.

Whether RT is needed in addition to the CHOP regimen is also being addressed in a randomized trial being conducted by the Eastern Cooperative Oncology Group (ECOG). In this trial, patients are randomized to eight cycles of CHOP alone or eight cycles followed by IFRT. The data from Connors suggest that RT adds to chemotherapy by reducing the cumulative toxicity of chemotherapy which is of particular importance in the treatment of the elderly. The optimal number of chemotherapy cycles given prior to RT is unknown but the available data would suggest that three cycles may be adequate to insure a high cure rate.

There is little data on the use of more aggressive combination therapy regimens either alone or in combination with RT in the treatment of early stage disease. Investigators at the National Cancer Institute (NCI) have treated 49 patients with Stage I or IE disease with four cycles of the $ProMACE_1/MOPP_8$ regimen followed by IFRT.[7] Myelotoxic drugs were given at 75% of full dose to this subgroup of patients. 47 of 49 patients achieved a CR and with a median follow up of four years, 94% are alive. Hence this is a very active treatment programme for patients with very early stage disease, although it is unlikely that such an aggressive approach is needed.

The best approach for treatment of patients with localized disease is participation in a clinical trial. If this is not possible, available data would suggest that a full course of eight cycles of CHOP alone or an abbreviated course of three to four cycles of combination chemotherapy followed by a tumouricidal dose of RT to an involved field are appropriate choices of therapy.

Advanced disease (II Bulky, III, IV)

Investigators at the NCI were among the first to demonstrate the curability of these advanced stage lymphomas using combination chemotherapy regimens.[8,9] CR was achieved in 45% of treated patients with 80% of these remissions being durable. In these early trials the vast majority of relapses and deaths occurred in the first two years after therapy was completed, and hence a disease-free survival of two years was considered to be equivalent to cure. Long-term follow-up of these patients verified that late relapses were unusual. Based on these observations, investigators sought to devise treatment strategies which would result in increased numbers of complete remissions with the expectation that this would ultimately translate into improved survival.

CHOP was one of the first combination therapies to employ the drug Adriamycin. This regimen has subsequently been studied extensively in the setting of co-operative group trials and it remains today as the standard against which newer therapies must be compared.[10–12] As had been hoped, CHOP did result in an increased number of complete responses. However, in contrast to earlier studies, relapses and deaths were not limited to the first two years. In fact, relapses continued to be seen 6–7 years after the completion of therapy. Hence, despite a higher percentage of complete responses, the percentage of patients cured was very similar to those seen in the early NCI studies.

Recognizing the need to improve on the results obtained with CHOP, new and more complex chemotherapy protocols were tried and reported from single institutions in the 1980s. These are often referred to in the literature as the second and third generation regimens to distinguish them from the earlier regimens such as CHOP which might be considered as a first generation treatment. While retaining the most active drugs, Adriamycin and cytoxan, multiple other drugs with less single agent activity such as methotrexate, cytarabine, etoposide and bleomycin were introduced into the newer regimens. Initial reports appeared very promising and suggested that the percentage of patients cured by these regimens might be doubled as compared to earlier regimens which were used as historic controls.

Two of the more widely used second generation regimens are ProMACE/MOPP developed and piloted at the NCI and M-BACOD which was developed and piloted at the Dana Farber Cancer Center.[13,14] ProMACE/MOPP employed etoposide and high dose methotrexate in addition to the standard lymphoma drugs. Of 74 patients with Stage IIE, III and IV diffuse mixed, diffuse large cell and undifferentiated lymphoma treated, 74% achieved a CR, and 65% of all patients were projected to be alive at 4 years. After 9 years of follow-up, however, the projected long-term survival excluding deaths unrelated to therapy has decreased to 50%. It is important to note that the median age of patients in this trial was 44 years compared to a median age of 55 years for patients treated with the CHOP regimen. In addition, it should be noted that the ProMACE/MOPP trial included patients with Stage II disease whereas prior NCI studies and studies utilizing CHOP included only patients with Stage III and IV disease.

M-BACOD utilized high dose methotrexate in addition to standard lymphoma drugs. Patients participating in the study were relatively young with a median age of 48. In addition to patients with advanced stage disease, patients with I, IE, II and IIE were treated. The initial results were very promising with 72% of patients achieving a CR and a projected 5-year survival of 65% for 101 patients treated. Subsequent follow-up has seen a decrease in the 3-year survival to 54%.

Attempting to improve on results obtained with the second generation regimens, several large institutions piloted and reported results with third generation regimens including m-BACOD which utilized a much lower dose of methotrexate than had been used in M-BACOD, ProMACE/CytaBOM which employed cytarabine and bleomycin in addition to the ProMACE drugs, and the MACOP-B regimen which is an intensive 12-week treatment employing conventional drugs given on an unconventional dosing schedule.[15–17] CR rates of 68–86% and projected survival of 58–69% were reported with the newer regimens; these results certainly appeared superior to those achieved with CHOP.

The SWOG conducted confirmatory trials of each of these third-generation regimens.[18–20] Results were, unfortunately, considerably poorer than those reported by the single institutions with percentage CR ranging from 49–65% and survival projected at 50–61%. The results obtained by SWOG were, in fact, very similar to those which had been achieved with CHOP. These results were not surprising, however, because as noted above, many of the patients treated in single institution studies had less advanced stage disease and were younger than patients treated in the co-operative group studies. There is in addition, a selection bias in any single institution study which favours better response rates and outcomes as compared to multi-institutional trials. This occurs in part because the elderly and more debilitated patients are not referred to the larger lymphoma centres.

Because of the increased costs and toxicity of the third-generation regimens, it was felt to be important to compare them in a randomized fashion with CHOP. Increased costs and toxicity are acceptable only if associated with an improved outcome. The results of the Intergroup trial which was a randomized comparison of CHOP vs m-BACOD vs ProMACE/CytaBOM vs MACOP-B in patients with intermediate or high grade lymphoma have recently been published.[21]

1138 previously untreated patients with bulky Stage II, III or IV disease were randomized to one of four treatment arms between 1986 and 1991. Each treatment was administered exactly as had been initially described. There were 239 ineligible patients, and hence the results which have been reported are for the 899 eligible patients.

Treatment arms were well balanced for all patient characteristics. It should be noted that the group as a whole had several poor prognostic characteristics. For example, the median age was 56 years with greater than one-fourth of patients being over 64. In addition, 40% of patients had bulky disease and 45% had an elevated LDH. At the time the results were reported, the median follow up was 49 months with a maximum follow-up of 84 months.

There was no significant difference between treatment arms in overall or complete response rates. Because it is difficult to assess complete response owing to persistent radiographical abnormalities on post treatment CT scans, the time to treatment failure which is a measure of time to progression, relapse or death from any cause, was looked at as a more accurate estimate of the fraction of patients cured by the initial therapy. Of all eligible patients 43% were estimated to be alive and disease free at three years. By treatment arm, 43% on the CHOP arm, 43% on the m-BACOD arm, 44% on ProMACE/CytaBOM and 40% on the MACOP-B arm were estimated to be alive and disease free at 3 years. There was no statistical difference in survival between the treatment arms. 52% of all eligible patients are estimated to be alive at 3 years; the breakdown by specific treatment is 49% MACOP-B, 51% m-BACOD, 53% ProMACE/CytaBOM and 55% CHOP.

The toxicities resulting from treatment were similar to those reported in Phase II studies. The most severe toxicities were those related to granulocytopenic infection. Fatal toxicities occurred in 1% of CHOP treated patients, 5% of m-BACOD treated patients, 3% of ProMACE/CytaBOM and 6% of MACOP-B treated patients.

In a smaller randomized trial done by ECOG, 325 patients with diffuse mixed or diffuse large cell lymphoma were treated with either CHOP or m-BACOD.[22] With a median follow-up of 4 years, there was no difference in complete response rate, time to treatment failure or survival when the two treatment arms were compared.

Experimental approaches to therapy

Based on the available data as well as on the lower cost and less severe toxicity associated with CHOP therapy, it remains the best available standard treatment for patients with advanced stage diffuse large cell lymphoma. With a reported durable CR rate of 43%, CHOP certainly cannot be considered as ideal therapy for patients with this disease and clearly more efficacious therapies are needed. There are several approaches to improving the therapy of this disease including (a) the use of more appropriate prognostic factors models to identify prior to therapy those patients who are unlikely to achieve a durable CR and who thus constitute the target population for more aggressive approaches and (b) the development of more effective therapeutic strategies. Newer therapeutic approaches include: (1) increasing the dose intensity of drugs used in standard regimens (2) the use of strategies to overcome drug resistance and (3) autologous bone marrow transplant and or peripheral stem cell support as rescue from marrow ablative chemotherapy. Each of these approaches will be explored below.

Newer prognostic factor models

As noted above there are several limitations to the use of the Ann Arbor System for the staging of NHL. Recently, Shipp and a large number of collaborators involved in the International Non-Hodgkin's Lymphoma Prognostic Factors Project have proposed a predictive model for aggressive NHL based on the pretreatment characteristics of several thousand patients with aggressive NHL treated with doxorubicin based combination chemotherapy.[23] Five pretreatment characteristics which were found to be independently statistically significant with respect to outcome included age ($\leqslant$ 60 vs $>$ 60), tumour Stage I or II (localized) vs III or IV (advanced), the number of extranodal sites of involvement ($\leqslant$ 1 vs $>$ 1), patient performance status (0 or 1 vs $\geqslant$ 2), and serum LDH (normal vs abnormal).

With these five pretreatment characteristics, patients could be assigned to one of four risk groups based on the number of presenting risk factors, low risk (0–1), low intermediate risk (2), high intermediate risk (3) and high risk (4 or 5). When analysed according to risk groups, patients were found to have remarkably different rates of complete response (CR), relapse-free survival (RFS) and overall survival (OS). Patients in the low risk category had an 87% CR rate and a five-year survival of 73%. This is in contrast to patients identified prior to therapy as being in high risk categories who had a 44% CR rate and five-year survival of 26%.

As noted above, the value of any staging system is its ability to predict the likelihood of a response to a proposed treatment. Because the Ann Arbor System has proven inadequate in this regard, it is hoped that the use of newer staging systems and predictive models will allow clinicians to identify, prior to therapy, the patient's chance of responding to conventional approaches to therapy. Those in whom an adequate response to standard therapy is unlikely would be identified as candidates for a more aggressive experimental approach.

New therapeutic approaches

Dose intensification The concept of dose intensity may be an important determinant of treatment outcome and, simply stated, argues that increasing the drug dose per unit time will increase its effectiveness. It does appear that treatment-related variables such as the dose intensity of drug delivered play a role in determining outcome. What is not clear is the independence of treatment related variables from pretreatment characteristics.

The third generation regimens focused on the delivery of six to eight active drugs given at the highest possible dose intensity. As noted above, in the Intergroup trial, there was no improvement in outcome when three different third-generation regimens were randomly compared to CHOP. With the availability of colony stimulating factors (CSF), the ability to maximize dose intensity has been improved as compared to dosages which can be delivered without CSF support. Hence one very rational approach at maximizing the efficacy of therapy is to dose escalate the drugs given in standard regimens with CSF support. The SWOG is undertaking a randomized Phase II study of dose intensified CHOP and dose-intensified ProMACE/CytaBOM with G–CSF support. In both arms the doses of cytoxan and Adriamycin will be escalated to determine in a pilot study if the results appear better than those seen in prior studies employing these drugs given at conventional doses.

Strategies to overcome drug resistance Multidrug resistance (MDR) is the phenomenon of cross-resistance to a group of natural products which are structurally and functionally distinct that occurs following exposure to one member of this group. MDR is believed to result from reduced intracellular drug concentration which results from active efflux of the drug by P-glycoprotein which is a membrane bound protein. This protein is encoded by the mdr-1 gene. The normal physiological function of this protein is unknown. One proposed function is that of inhibition of absorption and facilitation of excretion of toxic natural products.

There are various patterns of P-glycoprotein expression in tumors in humans. Some tumours, e.g. lymphomas, are derived from normal cell types where P-glycoprotein is not found. As Miller and colleagues have demonstrated, P-glycoprotein is rarely present in untreated lymphomas, but is commonly found in lymphomas which have recurred following exposure to chemotherapy.[24] While this data suggests a role for P-glycoprotein as a determinant of treatment outcome, clinical trials using P-glycoprotein inhibitors such as verapamil and quinine to restore sensitivity provide further evidence that this is the case. When Verapamil was given with cyclophosphamide, Adriamycin, Vincristine and Decadron (CVAD), as shown by Miller et al, responses were observed in patients with relapsed intermediate grade lymphomas.[25]

Based on the data from treatment of patients with relapsed lymphoma, SWOG has recently conducted a trial of verapamil and quinine given concurrently with the CVAD regimen in previously untreated patients with intermediate grade lymphomas. The goal of this approach is to suppress MDR development and/or to overcome any low level P-glycoprotein which may be present but undetected. Results of this trial are pending. Toxicity attributable to verapamil and quinine has been minimal, however.

Autologous bone marrow transplant (ABMT)

High dose chemotherapy with autologous bone marrow support has established itself as effective salvage therapy for selected patients with refractory or relapsed diffuse aggressive lymphoma. In several series, 20–25% of treated patients have achieved prolonged disease-free survival employing this approach.[26–29] While there has been considerable variability in the selection criteria in these studies, several consistent findings have been observed. The patients who are likely to achieve a complete remission and possible cure are those who responded well to initial therapy, who respond well to salvage therapy pretransplant, and who enter transplant with no or minimal residual disease. Patients progressing on salvage therapy as well as those who responded poorly to initial therapy are unlikely to benefit. A variety of regimens have been used and shown to be effective.

Results from single institution trials prompted the initiation of randomized trials comparing conventional salvage therapy vs high dose therapy. In 1986, the PARMA Study proposed randomizing patients with DHAP (dexomethasone, cytarabine, cisplatin) sensitive disease after relapse to further therapy with DHAP or high dose therapy with ABMT.[30] 172 patients were enrolled with 97 of these achieving a CR or PR after two cycles of DHAP. Among these 97 patients, 84 were randomized to four additional courses of DHAP or ABMT. At the time of interim analysis there was no statistical difference in disease-free survival or overall survival between the two treatment arms. An obvious selection bias is present in this study with only patients showing a good response to DHAP proceeding to the randomized portion of the study. Hence the survival of randomized patients is better than expected with a probability of survival at 3 years of 50%. Accrual to this study has unfortunately been very slow.

The role of ABMT as initial therapy for patients judged to be at high risk of treatment failure with conventional therapy remains to be defined. Few randomized studies comparing ABMT with conventional therapy have been completed.

In a trial conducted by Gianni et al, 33 patients with diffuse large cell lymphoma were randomized to MACOP-B or a novel high dose sequential chemoradiotherapy regimen.[31] Three of the first five patients randomized to the transplant arm died of transplant related causes; with modification of the treatment regimen there were no subsequent transplant-related deaths. The overall survival of 21 months was almost identical between the two arms (73% vs 74%) but the event-free survival was higher in the transplant arm (74% vs 48%).

The Groupe d'Etudes des Lymphomes des l'Adulte (GELA) reported on a subset of 727 patients treated with the LNH87 protocol.[32] 370 patients were randomized after achieving a CR with induction therapy to a consolidation phase in which patients were randomized to sequential chemotherapy (188) or ABMT (182). Only one patient died of transplant-related complications. With a median follow-up of 21 months the overall 2 year survival was 62% and disease-free survival was 58%. Overall survival and disease free survival did not differ between the consolidation arms (p = .089).

Finally, the Italian Cooperative group compared DHAP to ABMT following very aggressive initial chemotherapy.[33] Patients identified as partial responders to induction therapy were eligible for randomization. 25 patients were randomized to receive DHAP and 22 to undergo ABMT. A CR was subsequently achieved in four (14%) of the patients in the DHAP arm and in three (13.6%) of the patients on the ABMT arm. Stable clinical status was observed in ten (40%) of the DHAP group and 18(81.8%) of the ABMT group. Progression of disease was ultimately seen in ten (40%) of the DHAP patients but only one (4.5%) of the ABMT patients, Probability of progression-free survival at 40 months was 74% for patients undergoing ABMT vs 22% for patients treated with DHAP.

The recommendations of a Consensus Conference on Intensive Chemotherapy plus Hematopoietic Stem Cell Transplant in Malignancies were recently published.[34] While some regard their recommendations regarding the use of this approach in malignant lymphomas as too conservative, their recommendations include the following. High dose chemotherapy (HDC) should not be considered standard care in malignant lymphomas because no definitive study has established that HDC is either superior to or significantly worse than conventional combination chemotherapy in any stage of NHL. While retrospective studies suggest that HDC improves survival in relapsed aggressive NHL, the panel members believe that randomized trials are needed to confirm these data. Hence they recommend that for high grade or intermediate grade NHL, a randomized trial of conventional therapy vs high dose therapy with bone marrow +/or peripheral stem cell support be developed for those patients defined to be in poor prognostic groups. For those patients with relapsed disease, the panel recommended that the PARMA study be completed.

While there is reason to hope that high dose therapy may represent an advance in the therapy of aggressive lymphomas, there is an obvious need for data from randomized trials to prove that this is the case. It is appropriate to use this modality as first-line therapy in selected poor risk patients, but only in the context of a randomized trial assessing the value of this approach compared to conventional therapy. The cost and toxicity of ABMT can only be justified if, in randomized trials, this approach is shown to result in a significant improvement in survival.

What is the best therapy?

The majority of patients with advanced stage large cell lymphoma are not cured with conventional therapy. Hence each treating physician must recognize the inadequacy of current therapy and urge all eligible patients to participate in well-designed clinical trials. The best therapy remains to be defined and therefore the best approach for the patient is an experimental approach designed to improve our ability to cure the disease. If a patient is not eligible or does not wish to participate in a clinical trial, CHOP as inadequate as it is, remains the gold standard against which all new therapy must be compared.

References

(1) The non-Hodgkin's Lymphoma Pathologic Classification Project. National Cancer Institute sponsored study of classifications of non-Hodgkin's lymphomas. Summary and description of a working formulation for clinical usage. *Cancer* 1982; 49: 2112–35.

(2) Carbone PP, Kaplan HS, Musshoff K, Smithers DW, Tubiana M. Report of the Committee on Hodgkin's Disease Staging Classification. *Cancer Res* 1971; 31: 1860–1.

(3) Vokes EE, Ultmann JE, Golomb HM et al. Long-term survival of patients with localized diffuse histiocytic lymphoma. *J Clin Oncol* 1985; 3:1309–17.

(4) Hallahan DE, Farah R, Vokes EE et al. The patterns of failure in patients with pathological Stage I and II diffuse histiocytic lymphoma treated with radiation therapy alone. *Int J Radiat Oncol Biol Phys* 1989; 17: 767–71.

(5) Jones SE, Miller TP, Connors JM. Long term follow-up and analysis for prognostic factors for patients with limited-stage diffuse large-cell lymphoma treated with initial chemotherapy with or without adjuvant radiotherapy. *J Clin Oncol* 1989; 7: 1186–91.

(6) Connors JM, Klimo P, Fairey RN, Voss N. Brief chemotherapy and involved field radiation therapy for limited-stage histologically aggressive lymphoma. *Ann Intern Med* 1987; 107: 25–30.

(7) Longo DL, Glatstein E, Duffey PL et al. Treatment of localized aggressive lymphomas with combination chemotherapy followed by involved-field radiation therapy. *J Clin Oncol* 1989; 7: 1295–1302.

(8) DeVita VT, Canellos GP, Chabner B, Schein P, Hubbard SP, Young RC. Advanced diffuse histiocytic lymphoma, a potentially curable disease. *Lancet* 1975; 1: 248–50.

(9) Schein PS, DeVita VT, Hubbard S et al. Bleomycin, Adriamycin, Cyclophosphamide, Vincristine, and Prednisone (BACOP) combination chemotherapy in the treatment of advanced diffuse histiocytic lymphoma. *Ann Intern Med* 1976; 85: 417–422.

(10) Jones SE, Grozea PN, Metz EN et al. Superiority of adriamycin-containing combination chemotherapy in the treatment of diffuse lymphoma: a Southwest Oncology Group Study. *Cancer* 1979; 43: 417–25.

(11) Jones SE, Grozea PN, Metz EN et al. Improved complete remission rates and survival for patients with large cell lymphoma treated with

chemoimmunotherapy: a Southwest Oncology Group Study. *Cancer* 1983; 51: 1083–90.

(12) Jones SE, Grozea PN, Miller TP et al. Chemotherapy with cyclophosphamide, Doxorubicin, Vincristine, and Prednisone alone or with Levamisole or with Levamisole plus BCG for malignant lymphoma: a Southwest Oncology Group Study. *J Clin Oncol* 1985; 3: 1318–24.

(13) Fisher RI, DeVita VT, Hubbard SM et al. Diffuse aggressive lymphomas: increased survival after alternating flexible sequences of ProMACE and MOPP chemotherapy. *Ann Intern Med* 1983; 98: 304–9.

(14) Skarin AT, Canellos GP, Rosenthal DS et al. Improved prognosis of diffuse histiocytic and undifferentiated lymphoma by use of high dose methotrexate alternating with standard agents (M-BACOD). *J Clin Oncol* 1983; 1: 91–8.

(15) Shipp MA, Harrington DP, Klatt MM et al. Identification of major prognostic subgroups of patients with large-cell lymphoma treated with m-BACOD or M-BACOD. *Ann Intern Med* 1986; 104: 757–65.

(16) Longo DL, DeVita VT, Duffey PL et al. Superiority of ProMACE-CytaBOM over ProMACE-MOPP in the treatment of advanced diffuse aggressive lymphoma: results of a prospective randomized trial. *J Clin Oncol* 1991; 9: 25–38.

(17) Connors JM, Klimo P: MACOP-B chemotherapy for malignant lymphomas and related conditions. 1987 update and additional observations. *Semin Hematol* 1988; 25: 41–6.

(18) Dana BW, Dahlberg S, Miller TP et al. m-BACOD treatment for intermediate and high-grade malignant lymphomas: a Southwest Oncology Group Phase II Trial. *J Clin Oncol* 1990; 8: 1155–1162.

(19) Miller TP, Dahlberg S, Weick JK et al. Unfavorable histologies of non-Hodgkin's lymphoma treated with ProMACE-CytaBOM. a Groupwide Southwest Oncology Group Study. *J Clin Oncol* 1990; 8: 1951–8.

(20) Weick JK, Dahlberg S, Fisher RI et al. Combination chemotherapy of intermediate-grade and high-grade non-Hodgkin's lymphoma with MACOP-B. a Southwest Oncology Group Study. *J Clin Oncol* 1991; 9: 748–53.

(21) Fisher RI, Gaynor ER, Dahlberg S et al. Comparison of a standard regimen (CHOP) with three intensive chemotherapy regimens for advanced non-Hodgkin's lymphoma. *N Engl J Med* 1993; 328: 1002–6.

(22) Gordon LI, Harrington D, Andersen J et al. Comparison of a second-generation combination chemotherapeutic regimen (m-BACOD) with a standard regimen (CHOP) for advanced diffuse non-Hodgkin's lymphoma. *N Engl J Med* 1992; 327: 1342–9.

(23) The International Non-Hodgkin's Lymphoma Prognostic Factors Project: a predictive model for aggressive non-Hodgkin's lymphoma. *N Engl J Med* 1993; 329: 987–94.

(24) Miller TP, Grogan TM, Spier CM, Salmon SE, Dalton WS. High dose Verapamil infusion added to chemotherapy reverses drug resistance in lymphoma patients in relapse. *Proc Am Soc Clin Oncol* 1989; 8: 252. (Abstract)

(25) Miller TP, Grogan TM, Dalton WS, Spier CM, Scheper RJ, Salmon SE. P-Glycoprotein expression in malignant lymphoma and reversal of clinical

drug resistance with chemotherapy plus high-dose Verapamil. *J Clin Oncol* 1991; 9: 17–24. (Abstract)

(26) Armitage JO. Bone marrow transplantation in the treatment of patients with lymphoma. *Blood* 1989; 73: 1749–58.

(27) Gribben JG, Goldstone AH, Linch DC et al. Effectiveness of high-dose combination chemotherapy and autologous bone marrow transplantation for patients with non-Hodgkin's lymphomas who are still responsive to conventional-dose therapy. *J Clin Oncol* 1989; 7: 1621–1629.

(28) Carey PJ, Proctor SJ, Taylor P, Hamilton PJ. Autologous bone marrow transplantation for high-grade lymphoid malignancy using Melphalan/irradiation conditioning without marrow purging or cryopreservation. *Blood* 1991; 77: 1593–8.

(29) Philip T, Chauvin F, Armitage J et al. Parma International Protocol – pilot study of DHAP followed by involved-field radiotherapy and BEAC with autologous bone marrow transplantation. *Blood* 1991; 77: 1587–92.

(30) Philip T, Guglielmi C, Hagenbeek A et al. The PARMA international randomized prospective study in relapsed non Hodgkin lymphoma: second interim analysis of 172 patients. *Blood* 1992; 80: 67. (Abstract)

(31) Gianni AM, Bregni M, Siena S et al. Prospective randomized comparison of MACOP-B vs. rhGM-CSF-supported high-dose sequential myeloablative chemoradiotherapy in diffuse large cell lymphomas. *Proc Am Soc Clin Oncol* 1991; 10: 274. (Abstract)

(32) Haioun C, Lepage E, Gisselbrecht C et al. Autologous bone marrow transplantation (ABMT) versus sequential chemotherapy in first complete remission aggressive non-Hodgkin's lymphoma (NHL): 1st interim analysis on 370 patients (LNH87 Protocol). *Proc Am Soc Clin Oncol* 1992; 11: 316. (Abstract)

(33) Tura S, Zinzani PL, Mazza P et al. ABMT vs. DHAP in residual disease following third generation regimens for aggressive non-Hodgkin's lymphomas. *Blood* 1992; 80: 157. (Abstract)

(34) Coiffier B, Philip T, Burnett AK, Symann ML. Consensus conference on intensive chemotherapy plus hematopoietic stem-cell transplantation in malignancies: Lyon, France, June 4–6, 1993. *J Clin Oncol* 1994; 12: 226–31.

Clinical and laboratory features of splenic lymphoma with villous lymphocytes

E MATUTES and D CATOVSKY

Introduction

Splenic lymphoma with villous lymphocytes (SLVL) is a recently recognized disorder of mature B cells characterized by distinct clinical and laboratory features.[1,2] In common with other B-cell diseases, its recognition as a distinct entity has resulted from greater attention to the morphology of peripheral blood lymphocytes, a better definition of the histological patterns of the affected tissues and the systematic use of immunological markers and molecular techniques which provide information which is often unique or characteristic of a particular disease.

SLVL is a low grade lymphoma usually evolving with leukaemia which may be considered within the spectrum of lymphoplasmacytic lymphomas because of morphological evidence of plasma cell differentiation and the frequent presence of a small monoclonal band in the serum. SLVL has been confused in the past with other lymphoproliferative disorders, namely chronic lymphocytic leukaemia (CLL), hairy-cell leukaemia (HCL) and HCL-variant, the latter two conditions also characterized as SLVL by circulating 'hairy' lymphocytes.

SLVL has been described in the past under a variety of designations namely malignant lymphoma simulating reticulo-endotheliosis[3,4] or splenomegalic immunocytoma with circulating hairy cells.[5] Neiman et al[3] reported in 1979 ten patients presenting with massive splenomegaly, minimal or no lymphadenopathy, variable degree of cytopenia, circulating lymphoid cells with villous projections and a serum monoclonal band in half of them. They pointed out to the clinical similarities of this lymphoma with HCL but emphasized the major differences in spleen histology from HCL. Spriano et al in 1986[5] described eight cases and referred to the favourable

All correspondence to: Professor D Catovsky, Academic Department of Haematology and Cytogenetics, The Royal Marsden Hospital, Fulham Road, London SW3 6JJ, UK.

Cambridge Medical Reviews: Haematological Oncology Volume 4

course of the disease following splenectomy. SLVL has also been included in series of patients described as primary splenic lymphoma.[6–8] Narang (1985) series included some of the cases originally reported by Neiman et al (1979). More recently, SLVL cases have been probably included disorders of CD11c positive B lymphocytes with intermediate features between CLL and HCL[9] or described as an unusual group of CLL.[10] These various designations reflect the main clinical and cytological features of SLVL, namely splenomegaly without or with minimal lymphadenopathy, circulating villous lymphocytes with some lymphoplasmacytic differentiation and evidence of a monoclonal band in the serum.

In 1987, our group proposed the term splenic lymphoma with villous lymphocytes[11] to account for the likely splenic origin of this lymphoma and described the distinct morphology of the circulating cells. In subsequent years, SLVL has been more fully characterized on clinical, immunological and molecular/genetic grounds.[12–16]

We will outline here the characteristics which allow the distinction between SLVL and other low grade B-cell malignancies and update our experience on its natural history and management.

Etiology and incidence

There is so far no data on etiological factors, e.g. viral, chemical carcinogens, radiation, etc. which might be involved in the development of SLVL. The disease has been described in Western countries and has also been recognised in Africa.[17] Neither is there evidence for familial clustering although two sisters with SLVL have been reported.[18]

The incidence of SLVL among the B-lymphoproliferative disorders is difficult to ascertain at present because SLVL may still be underdiagnosed and has only been recognized in the last seven years. In our experience, the disease accounts for a significant minority of cases referred to our laboratory under the diagnosis of CLL and represents the form of low grade lymphoma which more often involves the peripheral blood. Its frequency is of the order of 5% within the chronic B-cell disorders, and thus similar or slightly higher than HCL and around seven times more common than the HCL variant.

Clinical features

SLVL affects adults, preferentially elderly, and is rarely seen under the age of 50 years. The median age in a series of 100 patients studied by us was 68; only three patients were less than 50 years. In contrast to earlier reports[5] which suggested a higher proportion of females, our data shows a slight male predominance (Table 1).

Presenting symptoms relate to cytopenias such as fatigue, abdominal discomfort due to splenomegaly or the incidental discovery of lymphocytosis

Table 1. *Clinical and laboratory features of SLVL**

Feature		Incidence (%)
Sex (M/F ratio)	1.3	
Age (median, range)	68 years (24–89)	
Splenomegaly		90
Hepatomegaly		50
Lymphadenopathy		15
Hb (<10 g/dl)		30
Platelets (<100×10⁹/l)		25
Lymphocytes (5–10×10⁹/l)		15
(10–50×10⁹/l)		75
(>50×10⁹/l)		10

* Based on a series of 100 cases studied by the authors.

in a routine blood count. 'B' symptoms such as fever, night sweats and weight loss are rare. The main physical sign is a moderate to marked splenomegaly.

Although in a minority of patients, the spleen may not be palpable at diagnosis it often becomes enlarged during the course of the disease. A monoclonal B-cell lymphocytosis with circulating CD11c positive villous lymphocytes without organomegaly has been reported as an early form of SLVL.[19] Hepatomegaly is detected in half of the patients and palpable lymphadenopathy, usually small volume lymph nodes, is rare (Table 1). Other organ involvement such as prominent tonsil enlargement, affection of the gastrointestinal tract, e.g. stomach or bowel is rare and seen in less than 5% of patients.

A consistent finding is an absolute lymphocytosis with distinct morphology (see below). The white blood cell (WBC) count is usually raised ranging from 10 to 40 × 10⁹/l. In our series, as in others,[3,5,8] few patients are leucopenic but have typical villous lymphocytes. A minority have a markedly raised WBC over 100 × 10⁹/l, even reaching 400 × 10⁹/l in one case.

The degree of anaemia and or thrombocytopenia is variable but usually moderate (Table 1). The cytopenia in SLVL is mainly related to hypersplenism rather than bone marrow failure, although the latter may contribute in some patients. Autoimmune haemolytic anaemia (Coombs positive) and/or immune thrombocytopenia are well documented but uncommon.[3,20] We have observed autoimmune complications in a few patients. In SLVL, the monocyte count is within the normal range in contrast to HCL. The most characteristic biochemical abnormality is the presence of a small monoclonal band in the serum, usually not exceeding 30 g/l.[3,5,11,12] The paraprotein is often IgM but in few cases it may be IgG; free light chains can also be detected in the urine (Bence–Jones proteinuria). Both these parameters may be useful to monitor the disease and its response to treatment.

We have documented an acquired deficiency of the complement component 1 (C1) inhibitor with consequent angioedema in two patients. One of them had overt SLVL at presentation whereas in the other, angioedema preceded the onset of SLVL by four years. This abnormality has also been observed in other low grade B-cell disorders, often with a serum paraprotein. In our two cases the monoclonal band was IgM kappa.[21]

Cell morphology

The morphology of SLVL cells is best appreciated on May–Grumwald–Giemsa stained peripheral blood films. The villous lymphocytes are slightly larger than CLL lymphocytes but smaller than hairy cells or HCL-variant cells. The nucleo-cytoplasmic ratio is high but slightly smaller than in CLL. The nucleus is round or oval in shape and has a mature condensed chromatin. The chromatin may be clumped as in CLL lymphocytes or is more dispersed. A small nucleolus is visible in a variable proportion of lymphocytes. The nucleolus is never as prominent and vesicular in SLVL as in the HCL-variant or B-prolymphocytic leukemia (B–PLL). The cytoplasm is moderately basophilic and the most distinct feature is the presence of a variable number of short, rarely long, thin projections or villi, which often appear to be localized in one or the two poles of the cell (Fig. 1 (*a*), (*b*)). Lymphoplasmacytic features including few circulating plasma cells are apparent in c.20% of cases.

The acid phosphatase reaction resistant to tartaric acid (TRAP) has been documented by some workers.[3–5] In our experience, although most cases stain moderately to strong with acid phosphatase, they are, as a rule, TRAP negative.[11]

Ultrastructural analysis show that most SLVL cells have a round nucleus, sometimes slightly indented with abundant heterochromatin and a small or medium size nucleolus. The cytoplasm contains numerous ribosomes and short strands of rough or smooth endoplasmic reticulum which account for the basophilia seen at light microscopy. The cytoplasmic outline is irregular and show multiple short or few long projections which are not broadly based as in hairy cells (Fig. 2). Ribosome–lamella complex, another feature of hairy cells is absent in SLVL.[4, 11]

Histopathology

The histology of the spleen provides an important distinction between SLVL and HCL and its variant form. Because lymph node involvement is infrequent, the histological material regularly available in SLVL are bone marrow trephines as well as spleen sections from splenectomized patients.

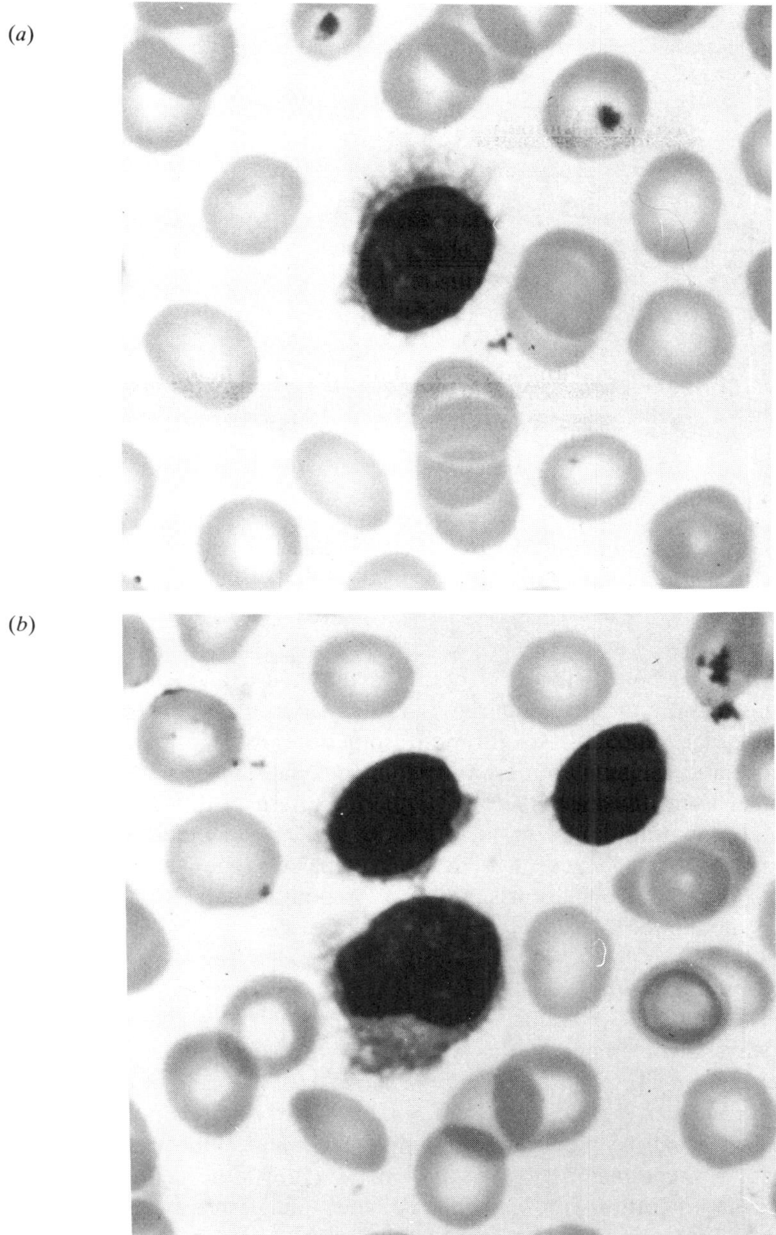

Fig 1 (*a, b*) May–Grumwald–Giemsa stained peripheral blood films from two SLVL cases showing lymphocytes with condensed nuclear chromatin and small cytoplasm with multiple thin projections.

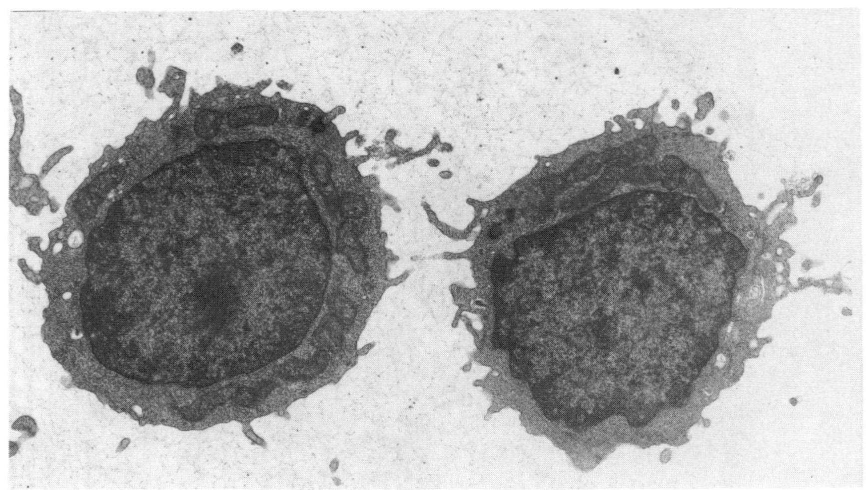

Fig. 2. Electron micrograph of SLVL cells showing a round nucleus with patches of nuclear heterochromatin and a cytoplasm with several villi and multiple ribosomes (uranyl acetate and Reynold's lead citrate stain).

Bone marrow The bone marrow is easily aspirated in SLVL, unlike HCL, and the films show usually moderate lymphocytic infiltration. The sections show a nodular pattern of infiltration, sometimes with a paratrabecular localization, and mild interstitial infiltration by small lymphocytes admixed with normal haemopoietic cells (Fig. 3).[1–11] A pattern of diffuse infiltration is rare. The lymphocytes are arranged in clusters or nodules with no evidence of spacing between them; lymphoplasmacytic cells are easily identified. Bone marrow fibrosis is not a predominant feature and when present is moderate.

Spleen In common with other B-cell lymphomas, the sections of the spleen reveal white nodules of variable size (0.1–1 mm). Microscopic examination shows always involvement of the white pulp with variable degree of red pulp infiltration. This contrasts with findings in HCL and HCL variant which show exclusively red pulp involvement. The white pulp nodules are integrated by small to medium size lymphocytes and some large cells. A characteristic phenomenon of margination with the large cell component located predominantly in the periphery of the nodules has been described (Fig. 4).[8,11] Expansion of the marginal zone without or few remaining reactive germinal centres has been noted in four cases of primary splenic lymphoma reported by Kraemer (1984).[6] Schmid et al (1992)[22] described a splenic lymphoma arising from the B lymphocytes of the splenic marginal

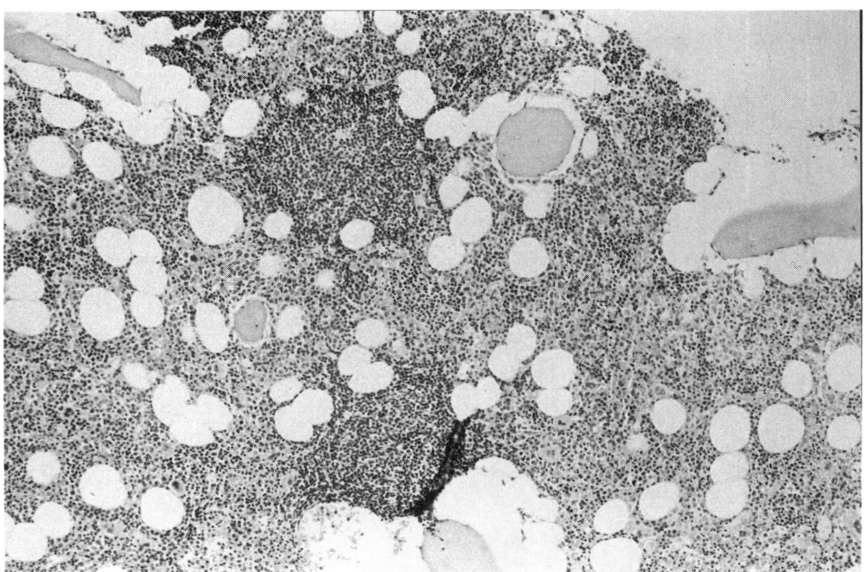

Fig. 3. Bone marrow trephine biopsy from an SLVL showing two nodules composed by small to medium mature lymphocytes (haematoxylin and eosin stain).

zone which may represent the cell of origin in SLVL. We are currently reviewing histological material from 27 cases in collaboration with Professor P.G. Isaacson to confirm this hypothesis.

Lymphoplasmacytic cells admixed with lymphocytes and PAS positive material can be seen in the central nodular areas.[3, 8] Although the red pulp may be infiltrated in SLVL, there is no evidence of blood lakes or the formation of pseudosinuses as in HCL.[3, 4, 11] Non-caseiting sarcoid granulomas may be present in few cases.[3, 8]

Lymph node Lymph nodes show diffuse effacement of the normal architecture by mature small to medium sized lymphocytes involving cortical and paracortical areas, sometimes adopting a vaguely nodular pattern; lymphoplasmacytic differentiation is common.[3+5]

Immunological markers

SLVL is a clonal disorder of mature B lymphocytes with a phenotype distinct from that of CLL and HCL. We have recently reported the immunological profile in 100 SLVL cases.[15] The cells in most cases expressed strong surface immunoglobulin (Smlg) with light chain restriction. The kappa/lambda ratio was 1.5. The most common heavy chain

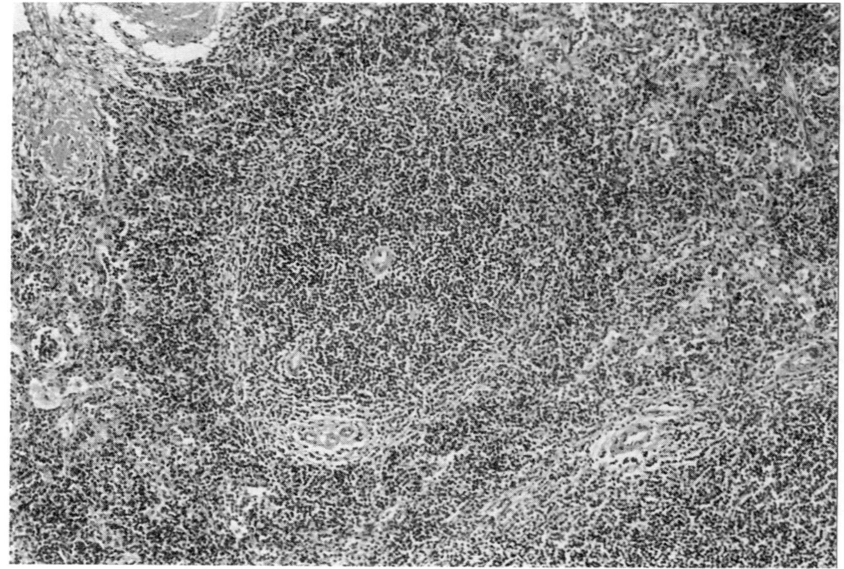

Fig. 4. Spleen section from an SLVL showing nodular infiltration of the white pulp by small mature lymphocytes. Note expansion of the perifollicular area (haematoxylin and eosin stain).

expressed was IgM with or without IgD (50% of cases); in 20% of cases the heavy chain was IgG and in the remaining 30%, IgG and IgM were coexpressed, or only IgD or IgA.

SLVL cases express strongly CD22 and FMC7 in the cell membrane (Table 2, Fig. 5). This profile is similar to findings in other B-cell disorders, B-PLL, HCL and other B-cell lymphomas in leukaemic phase except CLL, which is, as a rule, FMC7 and CD22 negative or express the latter antigen weakly.[23] Reactivity with CD5, a marker characteristic of CLL and mantle-cell lymphoma, is seen in 20% of cases. In none of these CD5 positive cases, however, have we observed the typical phenotypic profile of CLL.[23] CD23 is positive in a third of cases, a feature seen in other B-cell disorders;[24] this marker is positive in 92% of CLL cases.[23]

Considering four markers which can be regarded as characteristic of HCL, namely CD11c, CD25, HC2 and B-ly-7, each of them may be positive in a proportion of SLVL, more often CD11c and CD25. (Table 2). However, we have not observed yet a single case of SLVL positive with more than two of these markers. Over 85% of HCL cases are positive with the above four markers and in the remainder at least three of them

Table 2. *Immunological markers in SLVL**

Membrane marker	% of positive cases
Smig	100
Intensity: moderate/strong	88
weak	12
Light chain: kappa	60
lambda	40
CD22	95
FMC7	89
CD24	89
CD11c	47
CD23	31
CD5	19
CD25	25
B-ly-7	15
HC2	9
CD10	30
CD38	30

* Based on a series of 100 cases (Matutes *et al.*, 1994).

are positive.[25] The differences with these markers are not so apparent between SLVL and HCL variant. Two of the only differences which can be observed are the reactivity with CD24, which is positive in 89% of SLVL and usually negative in HCL variant and CD25 which is negative in HCL variant but may be positive in SLVL (Table 2).[25,26]

Measurement of the proliferative rate with the McAb Ki-67 shows that only a small percentage of circulating cells (mean: 2.9%) are Ki-67 positive. This parallel the findings in CLL.[27]

Cytogenetics

Chromosome abnormalities have been documented in a series of 30 cases.[13] The majority of cases have clonal abnormalities which in half of them are complex. Although there is no unique chromosome translocation associated with SLVL, four recurring abnormalities were demonstrated. These included: deletions or translocations involving the long arm of chromosome seven at bands 7q22 and 7q35 (20% of cases), t(11;14)(q13;q32) identical to that seen in mantle-cell lymphoma (18% of cases), iso17q (18% of cases) and translocations involving 2p11 (18% of cases). Abnormalities frequent in CLL such as trisomy 12 and deletions or rearrangements of 13q14 appear to be very rare and no single case had t(14;18) which is characteristic of follicular lymphoma.

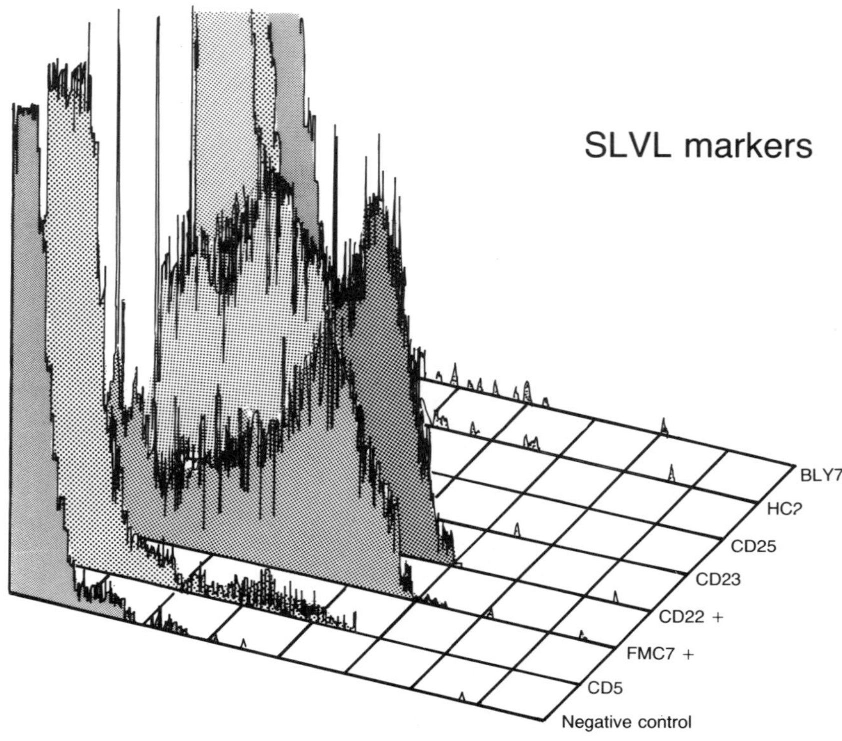

Fig. 5. FACS profile on SLVL cells showing a marker profile different to that of CLL.

Molecular analysis with pulse field electrophoresis and probes specific to the BCL-1/PRAD gene in 16 SLVL cases showed rearrangement of this gene in two cases with t(11;14) and in a third one with a t(11;22)(q23;q11).[16] The chromosome 11 breakpoints mapped within 28kb telomeric to the major translocation cluster where rearrangement occurs in most mantle-cell lymphomas and in the case with t(11;22) the breakpoint was 100 kb centromeric to the major translocation cluster. RNA analysis showed that the three SLVL cases with BCL-1 rearrangement but not the others exhibited low levels of a normal size cyclin D1 transcript.[16]

Differential diagnosis

The differential diagnosis of SLVL often arises with other B-cell disorders which evolve with lymphocytosis and splenomegaly. These include the two other diseases with circulating 'hairy' lymphocytes, HCL and HCL-variant, B-PLL, the splenomegalic form of CLL and other B-cell lymphomas which may evolve with leukaemia. Cell morphology, immunological markers and histology allow to differentiate SLVL from the other disorders (Table 3).

When considering CLL, the lymphocytes lack villi are smaller and display a different phenotypic marker profile.[23] Cell morphology rather than markers is necessary to distinguish SLVL from B-PLL (Table 3). The degree of bone marrow infiltration is greater in B-PLL. Differences in morphology, markers (Table 3) and bone marrow and spleen histology are marked between SLVL and HCL. Therefore, the distinction between these two disorders should only rarely present problems. Difficulties may arise instead with the HCL variant because of the similarities in immunological profile (Table 3); the diagnosis is based largely on cell morphology in well-prepared peripheral blood films. In such difficult cases, the bone marrow trephine and spleen histology may help as the findings in HCL variant are closer to that of HCL.

Prognosis and treatment

SLVL has a chronic clinical course with a minority of patients not requiring treatment for many years. Treatment is indicated to control symptomatic

Table 3. *Differential diagnosis with other B-cell disorders*

Disease	Morphlogy	Membrane immunophenotype*
CLL	small cells, clumped no villi, high N/C ratio	SmIg (weak), FMC7−, CD22 (weak) or −; CD5+
B-PLL	medium size, nucleolus no villi	
HCL	large size, abundant villous cytoplasm, low N/C ratio	CD24−/+, CD25+, HC2+, B-ly-7+
HCL-V	large size, nucleolus villous cytoplasm, low N/C ratoo	CD24−/+, CD25−
FL	small size, cleaved nucleus, very high N/C ratio	CD25−/+, HC2−, B-ly-7−
Mc-NHL	heterogeneous, cleaved nucleus	CD5+, CD25−/+, B-ly-7−

SLVL: splenic lymphoma with villous lymphocytes: CLL: chronic lymphocytic leukaemia; PLL: prolymphocytic leukaemia; HCL: hairy cell leukaemia; HCL-V: HCL-variant; FL: follicular lymphoma; N/C nucleo/cytoplasmic.

* Differences from findings in SLVL (see Table 2).

Number of + in McAb indicates the proportion of positive cases as follows: <20% of cases (−/+); 20–35% of cases (+/−); >50% of cases (+).

splenomegaly or a rapidly rising lymphocyte count or to correct cytopenias. In the author's experience, splenectomy seems to be the treatment of choice for patients with symptomatic hypersplenism and acceptable surgical risk whilst splenic irradiation represents an alternative in patients with surgical risks. In a series of 50 SLVL reported by our group, 22 patients underwent splenectomy as first or second line therapy and over 90% had prolonged clinical and haematological responses with significant reduction of the WBC and improvement of the cytopenias.[12] Similar results were reported by Spriano et al (1986)[5] in five patients including the reduction of the serum M band. Seven of our patients treated with splenic irradiation, a total of 10 Gy given in several fractions over a period of two weeks, also had good responses.

Chemotherapy with single alkylating agents, e.g. chlorambucil or cyclophosphamide does not seem to be very effective, although one-third of patients may show benefit. There is little or no experience in the treatment of SLVL with alpha-interferon and the new nucleoside analogues 2 deoxycoformycin, 2 chlorodeoxyadenosine and fludarabine. We have treated three patients with deoxycoformycin and two responded. One had a partial response lasting for 5 years with no evidence of recurrence in the last follow-up. The other patient had a short-lived response of the lymphocytosis and bone marrow infiltration but died eventually of sepsis with features suggesting transformation. Fludarabine may also has a potential role in the treatment of SLVL as shown by one patient previously resistant to chlorambucil and who had benefited from splenectomy for 5½ years. This patient achieved a good partial response with fludarabine that lasted more than 1 year but did not respond again after relapse. Another patient with a rather aggressive course did not respond to three courses of fludarabine.

Our current approach to the treatment of SLVL is first to assess the pattern of the disease. If there are no symptoms or progression, we follow a wait policy. We have several patients followed for a number of years without active therapy. If treatment is required, we would consider splenectomy first or splenic irradiation if surgery is contraindicated. In patients with progressive disease, fludarabine may be considered. Combination chemotherapy with an anthracycline, e.g. CHOP, may be indicated in patients with evidence of transformation.

Transformation of SLVL

In 5% of SLVL patients, the disease transforms into a high grade (large cell) NHL, a situation analogous to Richter's syndrome in CLL.

We have documented transformation in four patients. All manifested systemic symptoms, fever, weight loss, sweating, bulky peripheral and/or abdominal lymphadenopathy and in one chest pain, lung infiltrates and persistent cough. The median time from diagnosis to transformation was 4 years (range 2–15 years); three of the patients had been splenectomized. Lymph node histology showed a diffuse infiltration by large lymphoid cells with dispersed chromatin and prominent nucleoli; mitosis were easily seen (Fig. 6). In contrast, the bone marrow and peripheral blood were still consistent with low grade disease. Three of the patients responded (two complete and one partial) to CHOP which had also beneficial effect on the manifestations of the low grade disease. One patient was a non responder and died of progressive disease after three courses of CHOP. The partial response lasted for 10 months and the disease became them refractory to therapy. The two complete remitters, are still alive, one 2 years after transformation and the other having required further combination chemotherapy for a relapse and responded again.

Survival

The median survival in a series of 50 patients with a median follow-up of $3\frac{1}{2}$ years had not been reached with 82% of patients alive at 3 years and 78% at 5 years.[12] Thus, it is apparent that the overall median survival in SLVL is greater than 5 years.

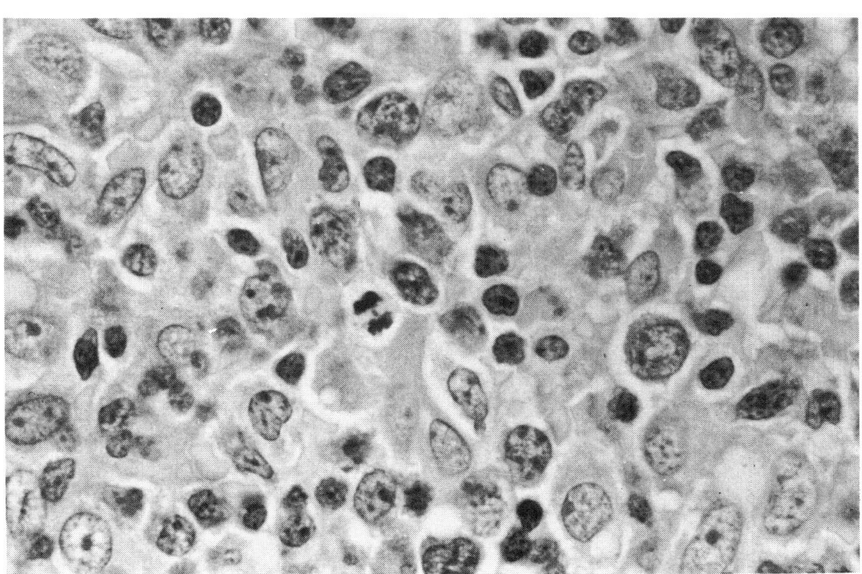

Fig. 6. Lymph node section from an SLVL patient with evidence of transformation to a large-cell lymphoma. Most of the cells are large and have immature nuclear chromatin and one or two prominent nucleoli. Mitotic figures can be identified.

As in early stage CLL, the causes of death in a proportion of SLVL may be unrelated to the disease. Few patients die of disease progression or of complications of the cytopenias.

Conclusions

SLVL constitutes a distinct entity with a characteristic benign clinical course. By careful examination of blood and bone marrow morphology and the use of a selective range of McAb it is possible to distinguish most cases from CLL, HCL and related B-cell diseases. The pathological basis of the disease needs further study of spleen specimens. Although there is no unique chromosome abnormality, a larger number of patients need to be studied to confirm the incidence of the four types of changes already observed. Improvements in diagnosis will facilitate the evaluation of the new generation of therapeutic agents with activity in other low grade lymphoid malignancies.

References

(1) Catovsky D, Foa R. *The lymphoid leukaemias*. London: Butterworth, 1990.
(2) Bennett JM, Catovsky D, Daniel MT et al. The French–American–British (FAB) Cooperative Group. Proposals for the classification of chronic (mature) B and T lymphoid leukaemias. *J Clin Pathol* 1989; 42: 567–84.
(3) Neiman RS, Sullivan AL, Jaffe R. Malignant lymphoma simulating leukemic reticuloendotheliosis. A clinicopathologic study of ten cases. *Cancer*, 1979; 43: 329–42.
(4) Palutke M, Tabaczka P, Mirchandani I, Goldbarf S. Lymphocytic lymphoma simulating hairy cell leukemia: a consideration of reliable and unreliable diagnostic features. *Cancer*, 1981; 48:2047–55.
(5) Spriano P, Barosi G, Invernizzi R et al. Splenomegalic immunocytoma with circulating hairy cells. report of eight cases and revision of the literature. *Hematologica*, 1986; 71: 25–33.
(6) Kraemer BB, Osborne BM, Butler JJ. Primary splenic presentation of malignant lymphoma and related disorders. A study of 49 cases. *Cancer*, 1984; 54: 1606–19.
(7) Kehoe J, Straus DJ. Primary lymphoma of the spleen. Clinical features and outcome after splenectomy. *Cancer*, 1988; 62: 1433–8.
(8) Narang S, Wolf BC, Neiman RS. Malignant lymphoma presenting with prominent splenomegaly. *Cancer*, 1985; 55: 1948–57.
(9) Hanson CA, Gribbin TE, Schnitzer B, Schlegelmilch JA, Mitchell BS, Stoolman LM. CD11c (Leu-M5) expression characterizes a B-cell chronic lymphoproliferative disorder with features of both chronic lymphocytic leukemia and hairy cell leukemia. *Blood*, 1990; 76: 2360.
(10) Wormsley SB, Baird SM, Gadol N, Rai KR, Sobol RE. Characteristics of CD11c+ CD5+ chronic B-cell leukemias and the identification of novel peripheral blood B-cell subsets with chronic lymphoid leukemia immunophenotypes. *Blood*, 1990; 76: 123–30.

(11) Melo JV, Hedge U, Parreira A, Thompson I, Lampert IA, Catovsky D. Splenic B cell lymphoma with circulating villous lymphocytes: differential diagnosis of B cell leukaemias with large spleens. *J Clin Path*, 1987; 40:642–651.
(12) Mulligan S, Matutes E, Dearden C, Catovsky D. Splenic lymphoma with villous lymphocytes: natural history and response to therapy in 50 cases. *Br J Haematol*, 1991; 78: 206–9.
(13) Oscier D, Matutes E, Gardiner A et al. Cytogenetic studies in splenic lymphoma with villous lymphocytes. *Br J Haematol*, 1993; 85: 487–91.
(14) Brito–Babapulle V, Ellis J, Matutes E et al. Translocation t(11;14)(q13;q32) in chronic lymphoid disorders. *Genes, Chromosomes Cancer*, 1992; 5: 158–65.
(15) Matutes E, Morilla R, Owusu-Ankomah K, Houlihan A, Catovsky D. The immunophenotype of splenic lymphoma with villous lymphocytes and its relevance to the differential diagnosis with other B-cell disorders. *Blood*, 1994; 83: 1558–62.
(16) Jadayel D, Matutes E, Dyer MJS, Brito-Babapulle V, Khokhar MT, Catovsky D. Rearrangement within the bcl-1 locus and expression of cyclin D1 gene in splenic lymphoma with villous lymphocytes *Blood*, 1994; 83: 3664–71.
(17) Bates 1, Bedu-Addo G, Rutherford T, Bevan DH. Splenic lymphoma with villous lymphocytes in tropical West Africa. *Lancet*, 1992; 340: 575–7.
(18) Ribeiro I, Costa MM, Fernandes BA, Sousa I, Melo A, Parreira A, Uva LS. Splenic lymphoma with villous lymphocytes in two sisters. J Clin Pathol, 1992; 45: 1111–13.
(19) Bassan R, Neonato MG, Abbate M, Motta T, Barbui T, Rambaldi A. Monoclonal lymphocytosis with villous lymphocytes: a chronic lymphoproliferative disease of CD11c+ B-cells. *Leukemia*, 1991; 5–799–806.
(20) Gale R, Smith OP, Wood M, Mehta AB. Splenic lymphoma with villous lymphocytes complicated by autoimmune haemolytic anaemia. *Lancet*, 1992; 340: 1106.
(21) Bain BJ, Catovsky D, Ewan PW. Acquired angiooedema as the presenting feature of lymphoproliferative disorders of mature B-lymphocytes. *Cancer*, 1993; 72: 3318–22.
(22) Schmid C, Kirkham N, Diss T, Isaacson PG. Splenic marginal zone cell lymphoma. *Am J Sug Pathol* 1992; 16: 455–66.
(23) Matutes E, Owusu–Ankomah K, Morilla R, Houlihan A, Que TH, Catovsky D. The immunological profile of B-cell lymphoproliferative disorders and proposal of a scoring system for the diagnosis of CLL. *Blood*, 1993 (suppl), vol 82, pp 392a, abstract 1551.
(24) Bain B, Morilla R, Monard S, Kokai Y, Catovsky D. Spectrum of reactivity with three monoclonal antibodies- MHM6(CD23), L30 (CD24) and UCHB1 in B-cell leukaemias. *Leuk Lymph*, 1990; 3: 97–102.
(25) Matutes E, Morilla R, Owusu–Ankomah K, Meeus P, Catovsky D. The immunophenotype of hairy cell leukaemia (HCL). Proposal for a scoring system to distinguish HCL from B cell disorders with hairy or villous lymphocytes. *Leuk Lymph*, 1994; 14 (Suppl 1): 57–61.
(26) Sainati L, Matutes E, Mulligan S et al. A variant form of hairy cell leukemia resistant to alpha-Interferon. Clinical and phenotypic characteristics of 17 patients *Blood*. 1990; 76: 157–62.

(27) Cordone I, Matutes E, Catovsky D. The monoclonal antibody Ki-67 identifies B and T cells in cycle in chronic lymphocytic leukemia: correlation with disease activity. *Leukemia*, 1992; 6: 902–6.

Prognostic factors in non-Hodgkin's lymphomas (NHL)

B KOZINER

The NHL include an heterogenous group of lymphoid neoplasias differing in their morphological features, biological behaviour and responsiveness to therapy.[1] Discriminating 'good' and 'poor' prognosis patients has implications in the therapeutic management of NHL and helps in the interpretation of therapeutic results.

In the absence of specific therapy, the NHL show a diversity of natural histories that correlate with their histological appearance.[2] Increasingly, other factors have been brought into the definition of prognostic groups such as those related to the tumour, the patient's clinical condition and the type of treatment administered.

A listing of the factors which will be discussed in this review is shown in Table 1.

Tumour-related prognostic factors

Histology

At least six different histological classifications of clinical relevance proposed by Drs Lennert, Rappaport, Lukes, Dorfman, O'Conor and Henry have been formulated. In 1982, the International Working Formulation was proposed which categorized the NHL in three broad histopathological categories differing in their natural histories.[3] Retrospective analysis has demonstrated that without specific therapy, median survival for low grade NHL could be of several years, months for intermediate grade NHL and only weeks for the high grade NHL (Table 2).

Recently proposed changes involve the inclusion of the diffuse small cleaved and the T cell cutaneous lymphomas in the low grade category

All correspondence to: Dr B Koziner, Unidad de Investigaciones Oncohematológicas, Agrelo 3038, 1221–Buenos Aires, Argentina.

Cambridge Medical Reviews: Haematological Oncology Volume 4

Table 1. *Listing of prognostic factors for intermediate and high grade NHL*

Tumour related
- Histology
- Disease extension
    - Stage
    - Tumour burden
    - Number and localization of nodal and extranodal sites
- B-symptoms
- Serum markers (LDH, beta-2 microglobulin)
- Cytogenetics
- Proliferation markers (S phase, Ki-67)
- Others (absence of HLA-DR expression, lymphocyte homing receptors)

Patient related
- Age
- Performance status

Treatment related
- Regimen used
- Dose intensity

and the immunoblastic lymphoma in the intermediate grade group where also the diffuse intermediate lymphocytic lymphoma[4] has been classified. The T cell leukaemia-lymphoma associated with HTLV-1[5] was justifiably included in the high grade category.

However, this classification has not been free of criticism since newly described lymphomatous subtypes such as the monocytoid, mantle cell, peripheral T-cell, marginal B-cell, anaplastic Ki-1+[6] and MALT-type (discussed elsewhere in this volume) lymphomas have not been included. A recently published Revised European American Classification incorporates these histological types among other proposals.[7]

Disease extension

Stage Although the Ann Arbor classification has established useful criteria for the staging of Hodgkin's disease based on well-documented patterns of tumour spread,[8] it has been shown to be less precise to properly define the extent of disease in NHL, characteristically more systemic and erratic in nature.

Different prognosis have been recognized for similar Ann Arbor stages based on tumor burden, localization and other features. This is particularly important in stage II, where patients with low tumour mass show a clinical course similar to stage I while those presenting with bulky disease (≥10

Table 2. *Characteristics of the subtypes of non-Hodgkin's lymphoma according to the Working Formulation*

Subtypes	Growth pattern	Cell type	Frequency (%)
Low grade			
A. Small lymphocytic	Diffuse	Small round cells	4
B. Follicular small cleaved cell	Follicular	Small cleaved cells	22
C. Follicular mixed cell	Follicular	Small cleaved cells; intermediate number of large cells	8
Intermediate grade			
D. Follicular large cell	Follicular	Many large cleaved and non-cleaved cells	4
E. Diffuse small cleaved cell	Diffuse	Small cleaved or small irregular cells	7
F. Diffuse mixed cell	Diffuse	Mixed small and large cells	7
G. Diffuse large cell	Diffuse	Predominantly large cleaved or non-cleaved cells	20
High grade			
H. Immunoblastic	Diffuse	Predominantly immunoblasts, plasmacytoid, clear, or pleomorphic	8
I. Lymphoblastc	Diffuse	Round or convoluted lymphoblasts	4
J. Small non-cleaved cell	Diffuse	Uniform, intermediate-sized round cells	5

cm) or elevated serum lactate dehydrogenase (LDH) should be considered advanced disease.

The influence of stage in the natural history of intermediate grade NHL has been extensively evaluated. In several analyses carried out at Memorial Sloan Kettering Cancer Center (MSKCC),[11, 12] stage was not an independent prognostic factor, although no cases of stage I were included. In the reports originating from the MD Anderson Cancer Center, stage I cases showed a better prognosis but tumour burden was a more useful parameter in multivariate analysis.[13,14]

According to the NCI group, stage IV disease – including bone marrow and gastro-intestinal involvment – implied a poor prognosis.[9] In the report from Coiffier et al, advanced stage (III and IV) was an important factor, negatively affecting overall survival and together with age and tumour volume entered in the design of the prognostic model proposed.[10]

Undoubtedly, the most detailed evaluation of this parameter came recently from The International NHL Prognostic Factor Project.[15] In this analysis, patients with stages I and II (considered localized disease) showed better prognosis than those with stages III and IV (characterizing advanced disease) in regard to every parameter of the evaluation looked at, such as proportion of complete remission (CR)(83% vs 57%), relapse-free survival (RFS) (70% vs 51%) and overall survival at 5 years (69% vs 44%) ($p < 0.001$). In stage II, differences were observed between those patients showing bulky (>10 cm) vs non-bulky disease (≤10 cm).

Number and localization of sites of disease In studies reported prior to the publication of the International Project, the number of involved sites, particularly extranodal, was emphasized as a prognostic parameter. The MSKCC group also reported that the location of nodal involvment had predictive value for the assessment of response rate and survival.[12] In their report, five levels of site involvment (LSI) were described: (I) peripheral lymph nodes (PLN) ± involvment of Waldeyer's ring ± spleen; (II) extranodal disease (EN) ± PLN; (III) retroperitoneal lymph nodes (RLN) ± PLN; (IV) bulky mediastinal disease (>1/3 of the cardiothoracic diameter ± any other disease group; (V) EN + RLN ± PLN. These five LSI were condensed into two groups to simplify the analysis (I) + (II) vs III+IV+V), keeping their prognostic significance ($p < 0.017$). Tumour bulk was not as strong predictor as tumour location, although those cases with bulky tumour had a worse clinical course in univariate analysis. It should be pointed out that patients in group II which could be staged as IV according to the Ann Arbor scheme, had better prognosis than those patients in group III, correspondingly staged as Ann Arbor III.

In the report from the International Project, although several extranodal sites of involment were associated with poor prognosis (BM, CNS, liver, lung, GI tract) the predictive factor more significant for prognosis, which was incorporated to the model proposed, was number of involved extranodal sites (≤1 vs >1).[15]

Tumour burden Although this parameter is recognized as a significant predictor of outcome in the NHL, it has been difficult to agree on a definition for bulkiness that could be universally accepted.

The MD Anderson Group designed a clinical system based on tumour burden[13,14] and a serological scheme (based on LDH and beta-2 microglobulin)[16] to assign patients to different risk categories. The definition of tumour bulkiness could vary according to the site of involvement. The MD Anderson Group used a 7 cm value to define peripheral nodal masses as bulky, but defined a mediastinal mass as bulky when it was visible on CXR. For abdominal or pelvic masses the definition was broader including any palpable tumour mass displacing organs or a combination of paraaortic and pelvic adenopathy.[14] These empiric rules to define 'tumour' bulkiness reveal the difficulty of measuring with accuracy the diameter of tumour masses in some locations.

In reports from other groups, a more simple definition of bulky tumour mass (>10 cm in diameter) showed to be a significant predictor of poor prognosis in multivariate analysis, although there was no significant correlation with the location of the mass.[9] Use of the 10 cm cutoff value to define bulky tumour mass was sufficient to detect the significance of this parameter according to the International Project in regard to probability of obtaining CR, RFS and overall survival ($p < 0.005$).[15]

Systemic B-symptoms

Although the adverse effect of the presence of fever, night sweats and/or 10% weight loss has been recognized on the achievement of CR and survival duration, its value as an independent prognostic predictor has not been validated.

The presence of B-symptoms had independent prognostic value according to the analysis of Hoskins et al in their population of patients treated with MACOP-B.[17]

According to the International Project,[15] patients presenting with B-symptoms had a lesser probability to achieve a CR (52% vs 75%), to mantain this response (52% vs 62%) and to survive at 5 years (40% vs 61%), at a statistical significant level ($p < 0.001$).

Serum markers

The value of LDH level as prognostic indicator in NHL has been recognized and incorporated into the analysis of treatment results by the MSKCC group, resulting the most significant variable in regard to attainment of CR and survival.[11,12,18] In the univariate analysis carried out by the Dana Farber Cancer Institute (DFCI)[19] and Vancouver groups,[17] LDH level was also found to be a significant prognostic determinant. The MD Anderson group devised a prognostic scheme based only on serum levels of LDH and beta-2 microglobulin.[16] DFS ranged from 100% to 25% when markers were both normal or elevated, respectively. The cutoff levels used have varied in different reports. The M.D. Anderson group used a cutoff level of 250 IU/L and for beta-2 microglobulin 3 mg/l. In the proposed International Index, any elevation of LDH is considered abnormal, showing significance for achievement of CR and survival ($p < 0.001$) Elevated beta-2 microglobulin levels were also significant for similar end points ($p < 0.001$).[15]

With the intent of exploring further the usefulness of serum LDH level as a prognostic parameter, the MSKCC group used three levels of elevation of this enzyme and correlated them with the different LSI previously mentioned for the construction of a four stage scheme differing significantly in their survival at 48 months.[12]

Cytogenetics

The relationship between certain cytogenetic reciprocal translocations and particular histological lymphoma subtypes have been well documented, such as t(8;14) for Burkitt's lymphoma and t(14;18) for follicular lymphomas.[20,21]

Other reports have focused on chromosomal anomalies other than the reciprocal translocations, such as the association of trisomy 3 with high grade histology and abnormalities of chromosomes 3 or 6 with immunoblastic lymphoma. Other kariotypic alterations have shown to have prognostic significance for survival such as trisomies affecting chromosomes 5, 6 and 18, all structural anomalies of chromosomes 5 and 17 and those affecting the breakpoint region of chromosome 14 (q11–12). According to the group at Nebraska,[21] in a multivariate analysis these cytogenetic features were highly significant related to survival which was between 6 and 8 months when they were present, compared with 36 to 42 months when they were absent. Although other clinical characteristics were associated with short survival (elevated LDH, B-symptoms, stage IV and age <70 yrs), abnormal cytogenetics was the most significant predictor. The M.D. Anderson group has reported similar findings for abnormal chromosomes 7 and 17.[22]

Proliferation markers

NHL with a high proliferative fraction (DNA synthesis phase) have been those associated with diffuse histologies. Their natural history has been characteristically short, showing a high initial response to chemotherapy but at the same time developing frequent pharmacological resistance.[23,24]

It has been reported that the determination of proliferative rate has independent value with respect to histological type as measured by the percentage of cells in S phase by flow cytometry, the pulse [^{3}H]-thymidine labelling index or staining with monoclonal antibody (mo ab) Ki-67 of a nuclear antigen present on cells in cycle.

The group at the University of Arizona investigated the usefulness of Ki-67 stain as prognostic indicator in 105 patients with diffuse large cell NHL.[25] In combination with stage, B-symptoms and absence of HLA-DR expression, reactivity with Ki-67 significantly correlated with survival ($p <$

0.003). Proliferation rate was defined as high when the percentage of cells positively stained with Ki-67 was over 60%. In this situation, survival was 8 months vs 39 months with negative or lower percentages of expression of this mo ab.

In the report of Jalkanen et al,[26] the proliferation fraction was inferred from the proportion of cells in S phase by flow cytometry and was considered elevated when was over 12%. This finding was associated with an unfavourable histological type and short survival ($p < 0.0002$) and was a prognostic feature independent of stage and the presence of receptors for lymphocyte homing. These receptors regulate the circulation of lymphocytes through the blood stream to lymphoid sites and could be involved in the dissemination of NHL.

The patients in which no receptors were detected had more localized stages and better survival. Five-year survival was 61% if S phase was < 12% and the receptors were not detected but only 15% in the opposite situation.

Other factors

Immunophenotype There is ongoing debate on its significance. In many studies no relationship was found between B or T cell phenotype and clinical course, independently of histological type.[27] The group of Arizona described the association between T cell phenotype with bulky tumour mass, frequent cutaneous infiltration and shorter DFS (0 vs 55% at 2 years).[28]

Abscence of HLA-DR expression

Also the Arizona Group reported this laboratory characteristic as predictive of short survival (8 months vs 39 months).[29] Although the biological explanation for this phenomenom remains elusive, it has been suggested that the lack of expression of this antigen system could impair cellular host defense mechanisms against the lymphoma. Hypothetically this situation could be corrected by enhancing HLA-DR expression through cytokines, particularly interferon-gamma.

Prognostic factors related to the patient

Two clinical features are associated to treatment efficacy: age and performance status (PS).

Advanced age negatively affects the clinical course, mostly due to the poor patient tolerance to myelosuppressive regimens and the frequent tendency to reduce the dose of chemotherapy fearing this complication.

Even in those series of patients in which the concept of dose intensity (DI) has been applied, worse results than in comparable younger patient populations have been observed due to increased morbi-mortality and relapse rate.[30] In the International Project, 60 years was considered the upper cutoff point for inclusion of patients in the analysis.[15]

The PS is associated with tumour burden since very infrequently patients with localized disease will show impairment of this parameter, although some reports consider it independently of the degree of disease extension. PS was the most important predictor of response and survival in the DFCI analysis,[19,31] observation which was confirmed in the more extensive analysis of the International Project.[15] The survival difference for patients with PS 0–1 vs 2–4 was highly significant ($p < 0.001$).

Prognostic factors related to the treatment

Regimen used Patients that receive suboptimal dosis of chemotherapy, lower than those used in the most frequently prescribed regimens such as CHOP or others, have being considered to have a lesser chance to achieve a CR. However, more recently, there has been considerable debate about the impact of the DI concept in regard to DFS and survival in NHL based on the report from the multi-institutional Southwest and Eastern Cooperative Oncology Group's analysis that included 1138 patients comparing in a randomized phase III study CHOP vs m-BACOD, PROMACE-CYTABOM and MACOP-B. The initial report of this important study failed to reveal any differences in therapeutic efficacy impacting on survival among these different treatments.[32]

Dose intensity The Stanford group reported DI analysis in 115 patients treated with CHOP, m-BACOD or MACOP-B. DI was defined as the amount of drug administered in the first 12 weeks of treatment, calculated as a percentage of the ideal dose standardized for CHOP.[33] With this methodology, the real DI of doxorubicin became a significant prognostic factor for survival and was incorporated in a prognostic model which also included LDH level, PS and extranodal involvment which recognized three different prognostic categories of patients with survival at 3 years of 89%, 63% and 18%. These differences were mantained when DI was analysed relative to the optimal dose for each regimen, and the analysis was restricted to a population of patients < 50 years.

Design of systems of prognostic significance

The main problem with the majority of the reported studies on prognostic factors is their complexity. In general, the number of characteristics considered is excessive for the number of patients being analysed that in most instances have been treated with different programmes and followed for relatively short periods. Many of the features analysed are interconnected with each other and lose their significance in multivariate analysis.

As it has been the case with the histological classifications for NHL, the profusion of prognostic formulations based on complex statistical models attempted against their acceptance. A similar approach to the Working Formulation Party for the histological classification of NHL was taken by The International NHL Prognostic Factors Project that reported on an International Index based on information collected from 16 different institutions and co-operative groups in the United States, Canada and Europe on 3.273 patients with aggresive (intermediate or high grade) NHL treated between 1982 and 1987 with combination chemotherapy regimens including doxorubicin.[15] Among the many reported prognostic predictors for long-term survival, five factors independently significant in univariate analysis were selected (age, tumour stage, serum LDH, PS and number of extranodal sites) and four risk groups were categorized with 5-year survival rates of 73%, 51%, 43% and 26% (Table 3).

Separate analysis of 1.274 patients < 60 years of age, validated the significance of an age-adjusted model that included PS, tumour stage and LDH level for the definition of four risk groups predicting 5-year survival rates of 83%, 69%, 46% and 32%. The prognostic differences in survival observed applying these two indices were not only in relation to the probability of attainment of a CR but also to a greater number of recurrences in the poor risk groups.

Potential candidates for new therapeutic approaches would include those encompassed by the high and high-intermediate definitions according to the international and age-adjusted indices. Although originally designed for aggressive NHL, those indices or variants could help to identify prognostic subgroups among low grade NHL.

Prognostic factors in low grade NHL

Some of the factors that influence the prognosis of aggressive NHLs have been also shown to apply to low grade NHL such as age, tumour bulkiness, B-symptoms, number and localization of extranodal sites of involvment, serum levels of LDH and beta-2 microglobulin.

Gallagher et al[34] in their report of 148 patients with follicular lymphoma reported as features of poor prognosis the presence of B symptoms, hepatosplenomegaly, anaemia (Hbg < 11.5 g%) (which could be considered an indirect sign of bone marrow infiltration), abnormalities in liver enzymes and histological transformation to more aggressive forms of NHL. This event which is observed in at least one-third of the patients was the most significant predictor of prognosis. Median survival of low grade NHL after histological transformation was 10 month.

Table 3. *Outcome according to risk group defined by the international index and the age-adjusted international index*

Risk group	Number of risk factors	Distribution of patients (%)	Complete response rate (%)	Relapse-free survival		Survival	
				2 yr rate (%)	5 yr rate (%)	2 yr rate (%)	5 yr rate (%)
International index, all patients (n=2031)							
Low	0 or 1	35	87	79	70	84	73
Low/intermediate	2	27	67	66	50	66	51
High/intermediate	3	22	55	59	49	54	43
High	4 or 5	16	44	58	40	34	26
Age-adjusted index, patients ≤60 years (n=1274)							
Low	0	22	92	88	86	90	83
Low/intermediate	1	32	78	74	66	79	69
High/intermediate	2	32	57	62	53	59	46
High	3	14	46	61	58	37	32
Age-adjusted index, patients >60 years (n=761)							
Low	0	18	91	75	46	80	56
Low/intermediate	1	31	71	64	45	68	44
High/intermediate	2	35	56	60	41	48	37
High	3	16	36	47	37	31	21

Reproduced from Shipp *et al.*, N Engl J Med 1993; 329: 987–94.

Leonard et al[35] reported a relatively complex prognostic index which allowed discrimination of patients in subgroups of good, intermediate and poor prognosis based on PS, age, stage and haemoglobin level. Age was the most important factor with all patients <70 years being assigned to the high risk group.

The cumulative work in this field attests to the interest in more selectively established treatment strategies for patients with NHL. It is hoped that future investigation will provide more simple and objective means of widespread acceptance to identify prognostic subgroups and that this characterization will not only be useful at presentation but throughout the course of the particular NHL.

Acknowledgement

The author wishes to thank Dr Elena Torello for her contribution in gathering bibliographical data and Mrs Diana Oyhandi for skilful secretarial assistance in the preparation of this manuscript.

References

(1) Armitage JO. Treatment of non-Hodgkin's lymphoma. *N Engl J Med* 1993; 328: 1023–30.

(2) Straus DJ, Filippa DA, Lieberman PH et al. The non-Hodgkin's lymphomas: I. A retrospective clinical and pathologic analysis of 499 cases diagnosed between 1958 and 1969. *Cancer* 1983; 51: 101–9.

(3) Non-Hodgkin's Lymphoma Pathologic Classification Project. National Cancer Institute sponsored study of classifications of non-Hodgkin's lymphomas: summary and description of a working formulation for clinical usage. *Cancer* 1982; 49: 2112–35.

(4) Weisenburger DD, Sanger WG, Armitage JO, Purtilo DT. Intermediate lymphocytic lymphoma: immunophenotypic and cytogenetic findings. *Blood* 1987; 69: 1617–21.

(5) Broder S, Moderator T-cell lymphoproliferative syndrome associated with human T-cell leukemia/lymphoma virus. *Ann Intern Med* 1984: 100: 543–57.

(6) Greer JP. Kinney MC, Collins RD et al. Clinical features of 31 patients with Ki−1 anaplastic large-cell lymphoma. *J Clin Oncol* 1991: 9: 539–47.

(7) Harris NL, Jaffe ES, Stein H et al. A revised European–American classification of lymphoid neoplasms: a proposal from the International Lymphoma Study Group. *Blood* 1994; 84: 1361–92.

(8) Carbone PP, Kaplan HS, Musshoft K, Smithers DW. Tubiana M. Report of the Committee on Hodgkin's Disease Staging Classification. *Cancer Res* 1971; 31: 1860–1.

(9) Fisher RI, Hubbard SM, DeVita VT et al. Factors predicting long-term survival in diffuse mixed, histiocytic, or undifferentiated lymphoma. Blood 1981; 58: 45–51.

(10) Coiffier B, Gisselbrecht C, Vose JM et al. Prognostic factors in aggressive malignant lymphomas: description and validation of a prognostic index that

could identify patients requiring a more intensive therapy. *J Clin Oncol* 1991; 9: 211–19.

(11) Koziner B, Little C, Posse S et al. Treatment of diffuse histiocytic lymphoma: an analysis of prognostic variables. *Cancer* 1982; 49: 1571–9.

(12) Danieu L, Wong G, Koziner B, Clarkson B. Predictive model for prognosis in advanced diffuse histiocytic lymphoma. *Cancer Res* 1986; 46: 5372–9.

(13) Jagannath S, Velasquez WS, Tucker SL et al. Tumor burden assessment and its implication for a prognostic model in advanced diffuse large-cell lymphoma. *J Clin Oncol* 1986; 4: 859–65.

(14) Velasquez WS, Jagannath S, Tucker SL et al. Risk classification as the basis for clinical staging of diffuse large-cell lymphoma derived from 10-year survival data. *Blood* 1989; 74: 551–7.

(15) The International Non-Hodgkin's Lymphoma Prognostic Factors Project. A predictive model for aggresive non-Hodgkin's lymphoma. *N Engl J Med* 1993; 329: 987–94.

(16) Swan F Jr, Velasquez WS, Tucker S et al. A new serologic staging system for large-cell lymphomas based on initial B_2-microglobulin and lactate de hydrogenase levels. *J Clin Oncol* 1989; 7: 1518–27.

(17) Hoskins PJ, Ng V, Spinelli JJ, Klimo P, Connors JM. Prognostic variables in patients with diffuse large-cell lymphoma treated with MACOP-B. *J Clin Oncol* 1991; 9: 220–6.

(18) Al-Katib A, Koziner B, Kurland E et al. Treatment of diffuse poorly differentiated lymphocytic lymphoma. An analysis of prognostic variables. *Cancer* 1984; 53: 2404–12.

(19) Shipp MA, Yeap BY, Harrington DP et al. The m-BACOD combination chemotherapy regimen in large-cell lymphoma: analysis of the completed trial and comparison with the M-BACOD regimen. *J Clin Oncol* 1990; 8: 84–93.

(20) Levine EG, Arthur DC, Frizzera G, Peterson BA, Hurd DD, Bloomfield CD. Cytogenetic abnormalities predict clinical outcome in non-Hodgkin's lymphoma. *Ann Intern Med* 1988; 108; 1420.

(21) Schouten HC, Sanger WG, Weisenburger DD, Anderson J, Armitage JO. Chromosomal abnormalities in untreated patients with non-Hodgkin's lymphoma: associations with histology, clinical chacteristics, and treatment outcome. *Blood* 1990; 75; 1841–7.

(22) Cabanillas F, Pathak S, Grant G et al. Refractoriness to chemotherapy and poor survival related to abnormalities of chromosomes 17 and 7 in lymphoma. *Am J Med* 1989; 87; 167–72.

(23) Hansen H, Koziner B, Clarkson B. Marker and kinetic studies in the non-Hodgkin's lymphomas. *Am J Med* 1981; 71: 107–23.

(24) Cowan RA, Harris M, Jones M, Crowther D. DNA content in high and intemediate grade non-Hodgkin's lymphoma – prognostic significance and clinicopathological correlations. *Br J Cancer* 1989–60–110.

(25) Grogan TM, Lippman SM, Spier CM et al. Independent prognostic significance of a nuclear proliferation antigen in diffuse large cell lymphomas as determined by the monoclonal antibody Ki−67. *Blood* 1988; 71: 1157–60.

(26) Jalkanen S, Joensuu H, Klemi P. Prognostic value of lymphocyte homing

receptor and S phase fraction in non-Hodgkin's lymphoma. *Blood* 1990, 75: 1549–56.
(27) Armitage JO, Vose JM, Linden J et al. Clinical significance of immunophenotype in diffuse aggressive non-Hodgkin's lymphoma. *J Clin Oncol* 1989, 7: 1783–9.
(28) Lippman SM, Miller TP, Spier CM. Slymen DJ. Grogan TM. The prognostic significance of the immunotype in diffuse large-cell lymphoma: a comparative study of the T-cell and B-cell phenotype. *Blood* 1988: 72: 436–41.
(29) Miller TP, Lippman SM, Spier CM, Slymen DJ, Grogan TM. HLA-DR (la) immune phenotype predicts outcome for patients with diffuse large cell lymphoma. *J Clin Invest* 1988; 82: 370–2.
(30) Dixon DO, Neilan B, Jones SE et al. Effect of age on therapeutic outcome in advanced diffuse histiocytic lymphoma: the Southwest Oncology Gtoup experience. *J Clin Oncol* 1986; 4: 295–305.
(31) Shipp MA, Harrington DP, Klatt MM et al. Identification of major prognostic subgroups of patients with large-cell lymphoma treated with m-BACOD or M-BACOD. *Ann Intern Med* 1986; 104: 757–65.
(32) Fisher RI, Gaynor ER, Dahlberg S et al. Comparison of a standard regimen (CHOP) with three intensive chemotherapy regimens for advanced non-Hodgkin's lymphoma. *N Engl J Med* 1993; 328: 1002–6.
(33) Gordon LI, Harrington D, Andersen J et al. Comparison of a second generation combination chemotherapeutic regimen (m-BACOD) with a standard regimen (CHOP) for advanced diffuse non-Hodgkin's lymphoma. *N Engl J Med* 1992; 327; 1342–9.
(34) Gallaher CJ, Gregory WM, Jones AE et al. Follicular lymphoma prognostic factor for response and survival. *J Clin Oncol* 1986; 4: 1470–80.
(35) Leonard RCF, Hayward RL, Prescott RJ, Wang JX. The identification of discrete prognostic groups in low grade non-Hodgkin's lymphoma. *Ann Oncol* 2: 655–62.

Growth factors and peripheral blood progenitor cell transplants

A GRIGG

Historical background

After high dose chemotherapy followed by autologous transplantation with marrow as the source of haemopoietic rescue, there is a prolonged period of neutropenia and thrombocytopenia. This is associated with a small mortality and considerable morbidity from bleeding and infection, as well as a prolonged period of hospitalization.

Various attempts have been made over the last decade to hasten haematological recovery. One approach has been to use haemopoietic growth factors, such as granulocyte colony stimulating factor (G–CSF) and granulocyte macrophage colony stimulating factor (GM–CSF). These factors were first identified by their ability to stimulate the clonal growth of haemopoietic progenitor cells in vitro.[1] The purification and molecular cloning of these factors have allowed study of their effects in various clinical settings. After autologous marrow infusion following high dose chemotherapy, these growth factors shorten the period of severe neutropenia, but not thrombocytopenia,[2] consistent with their lack of action on megakaryocyte colonies in vitro and platelet production in vivo.

A different approach was based on the observation that marrow-derived progenitor cells are mobilized in large numbers into the peripheral blood after myelosuppressive chemotherapy.[3] These cells were subsequently used to reconstitute hemopoiesis after myeloablative chemotherapy. A crucial observation was that, in adequate numbers, these cells resulted in faster platelet as well as neutrophil engraftment than infusion of marrow cells.[4]

Collection of peripheral blood progenitor cells (PBPC) in the steady state was also investigated. However, due to the low basal level of circulating

All correspondence to: Dr A Grigg, Bone Marrow Transplant Service, Department of Medical Oncology and Clinical Haematology, The Royal Melbourne Hospital, Grattan Street, Parkville 3050, Victoria, Australia.

Cambridge Medical Reviews: Haematological Oncology Volume 4

PBPC, it was found that the collection of sufficient progenitors under these conditions required multiple leukaphereses (LP). The infusion of these cells can be quite toxic due to the large amounts of the dimethylsulfoxide used as a cryopreservative.[5] Moreover, haemopoietic recovery was generally no faster than infusion of marrow alone.[6] Accordingly, this technique has not been widely utilized.

In the late 1980s, it was demonstrated that growth factors also increased the number of circulating progenitor cells.[7,8] This led to autografts using cells mobilized in this way, initially with marrow as well,[9] but more recently using PBPC alone.[10] Synergy between chemotherapy and growth factors in PBPC mobilization was also demonstrated in the late 1980s.[11]

The use of PBPC, often without marrow support, is becoming routine in many autologous transplant centres. Nevertheless, there remain many areas of controversy in their use. The aim of this chapter is to review the current status of PBPC autografts and discuss some of the clinical controversies in this area, to review some of the biological issues with their use, to speculate on future uses of growth factor mobilized PBPC, and to discuss the impact of this technology on resource utilisation and disease survival. The main areas of discussion are summarized in Table 1.

Current status of peripheral blood progenitor cell autografts

Haemopoietic recovery after infusion of mobilized progenitor cells

Overview

There is substantial evidence that the infusion of an adequate number of mobilized progenitors results in rapid and durable trilineage recovery. One of the largest single institution experiences is from the Bordeaux group, with 118 patients reported.[12] PBPC were mobilized by chemotherapy $\pm$ growth factor. A median of 9.5×10^4 granulocyte – macrophage colony forming units (CFU-GM) per kg were infused. No growth factors were used post-infusion. The median time to recovery to 0.5×10^9/l neutrophils and 50×10^9/l platelets was 12.5 and 15 days, respectively.

The results of the 1994 Melbourne study[13], in which patients infused with lower numbers of progenitor cells mobilized by G–CSF had slower neutrophil and platelet recovery, is consistent with the hypothesis that the rapid haematopoietic recovery is due to the in vivo maturation and proliferation of large numbers of committed progenitor cells obtained by LP.

Pattern of haemopoietic recovery after PBPC reinfusion

There is a particular pattern of platelet recovery after PBPC transplantation, initially described in patients with acute myeloid leukaemia given chemotherapy mobilized PBPC[14] and more recently after G–CSF mobilized PBPC

Table 1. *Issues in peripheral blood progenitor cell transplantation*

Clinical issues in the use of peripheral blood progenitor cell autografts
- What is the pattern of haemopoietic recovery after infusion of mobilized progenitor cells?
- Is there a preferred growth factor for PBPC mobilization?
- Are growth factors and chemotherapy synergistic in mobilizing PBPC? What degree of myelosuppression is required to exert this effect? What is the optimal time to begin a growth factor after chemotherapy?
- How can the optimal time to begin leukapheresis be predicted?
- What is the minimum number of progenitor cells required for haemopoietic reconstitution? How can the adequacy of a leukapheresis collection be rapidly assessed rapidly?
- Are growth factors needed post-infusion of PBPC?

Biology of peripheral blood progenitor cells and their mobilization
- How do growth factors increase levels of circulating PBPC?
- What are the immunophenotypical and functional characteristics of PBPC?
- Why do PBPC produce rapid haemopoietic recovery?
- Are PBPC capable of long-term haemopoietic reconstitution?
- Are PBPC less contaminated with tumour cells than marrow?
- Is a combination of growth factors more effective at mobilizing progenitors?
- Are any of the newer growth factors likely to be useful?
- Are there differences between PBPC and marrow in the kinetics of immunological recovery after transplantation?

Future uses of growth factor mobilized PBPC
- As the source of cells for CD34+ positive selection.
- *Ex vivo* incubation with cytokines.
- To support multiple rounds of high dose chemotherapy.
- In allogeneic transplantation.

Overview
- What is the impact of PBPC autografts on resource utilization and survival?

autografts.[13] There is usually a rapid rise in platelet count during the second week post-infusion. This is frequently, but not invariably, followed by a secondary fall 3–4 weeks later. This probably reflects polyphasic haemopoiesis with early engraftment of mature but shortlived megakaryocyte progenitors. Ongoing haemopoiesis is probably dependent on the production of mature cells by more primitive progenitors.

Strategies for mobilization of progenitor cells

This section reviews the various mobilization strategies. A summary of the advantages and disadvantages of these strategies is detailed in Table 2.

Table 2. *Collection of peripheral blood progenitor cells by leukapheresis*

Mobilization	Advantages	Disadvantages
Steady state	• ?less tumour contamination	• multiple collections required • toxicity of reinfusion • slow haemopoietic recovery
Chemotherapy	• ?*in vivo* purge	• adequate yield requires significant myelosuppression • difficulty in predicting optimum time for collection in advance • unsuitable for allogeneic transplantation
Growth factors	• able to plan timing of collection • generally well tolerated	• yield often inadequate in heavily pre-treated patients
Chemotherapy and Growth factors	• less leukaphereses and less myelosuppression required for adequate collection • timing of collection may be less critical • may mobilize adequate numbers in heavily pretreated patients	• unsuitable for allogeneic transplantation

Autografts using growth factor only mobilized peripheral blood progenitor cells

G-CSF MOBILIZED PBPC Dührsen et al[7] observed that G–CSF administered at doses up to 10μg/kg/day induced a dose-related rise (10–100 times normal) in PBPC after four days of treatment. In 1992, Sheridan et al[9] reported autografts using G–CSF mobilized PBPC added to marrow. Subsequently, a number of autograft studies using G–CSF mobilized PBPC alone have been reported (Table 3).[10,13,15,16]

The main conclusions from these studies are that the infusion of adequate amounts of PBPC hastens platelet and neutrophil recovery compared with marrow alone, and that, at least in the medium term, the haemopoietic recovery after PBPC only autografts has been durable. The utility of this approach is now well established, although some issues have only recently been resolved or are yet to be fully addressed:

Table 3. *Autografts using G–CSF mobilized PBPC alone*

Author/year/ reference	Dose/route	No. pts	Pt. population	LP volume and schedule	No. LP	Total CFU–GM×10^4/kg median (range)	Engraftment (day) neutrophils >0.5×10^9/l	Engraftment (day) platelets >20×10^9/l	Follow-up (months)
Chao 1992[15]	10 μg/kg IV or SC	4	as above	10–16 litres D4 onwards	4	9.6 (0–32)	8**	9	up to 10 months
Bensinger 1993[10]	16 μg/kg SC	12	BM disease or low cellularity	10 litres D4 onwards	3	9.7 (2.4–97.8)	12.7*	10	4–12
Nademanee 1993[16]	5 μg/kg IV or SC	11	as above	D4 onwards	7	9 (1–47)	10**	15	–
Sheridan[a] 1994[13]	12–24 μg/kg SC	29	lymphoid malignancy	7 litres D4, 6, 8 or D5, 6, 7	3	21 (1–198)	10 (9)**	11 (9)	11–25

LP=Leukapheresis.

* No G–CSF post-infusion.

** G–CSF post-infusion.

[a] Eleven of the 29 patients mobilized >30×10^4 CFU–GM/kg and were reinfused with PBPC only. The rest mobilized <30×10^4 CFU–GM/kg and were reinfused with BM and PBPC. The engraftment data refers to the whole group, with that of the PBPC only group in parentheses.

Method of administration of G–CSF The original reports demonstrated that there was no significant difference between responses following subcutaneous or intravenous administration of G–CSF.[7] In the majority of studies, subcutaneous administration has been associated with a good effect and, as it is generally more convenient, is the preferred option. Single daily subcutaneous injections appear as effective as continuous infusions (AG: personal observation).

The optimal dose In small numbers of patients, Dührsen et al[7] demonstrated a dose-dependent increase in progenitor mobilization with subcutaneous doses up to 10 μg/kg; higher subcutaneous doses were not evaluated. Given intravenously, 10 μg/kg of G–CSF was as good as 30 and 60 μg/kg.

In the largest study using G–CSF mobilized PBPC, there was a trend to better yields in patients receiving 24 μg/kg subcutaneously compared with 12 μg/kg, but the heterogeneity in the degree of pretreatment of these patients makes it difficult to draw definitive conclusions.[17] Doses as low as 5 μg/kg of G–CSF have been used.[16] Of interest, the platelet recovery at this low dose was delayed compared with that observed with progenitors mobilized with higher doses of G–CSF in other studies, but in the absence of prospective randomized studies, definitive conclusions cannot be drawn.

Type of G–CSF While there is evidence that the mammalian-derived glycosylated G–CSF is more biologically potent in vitro than the bacterially synthesized unglycosylated G–CSF,[18] it is not known whether this is clinically relevant in vivo.

GM–CSF MOBILIZED PBPC The effect of GM–CSF at doses between 4 and 64 μg/kg/day by an intravenous continuous infusion has been reported.[8] A median 80-fold increase in CFU–GM numbers was observed. Within the limitations of the small numbers within the study, there was no apparent correlation between the dose of GM–CSF and the response of peripheral blood progenitor cells. Subsequently, a dose-dependent rise in PBPC levels was documented in patients receiving GM–CSF up to 30 μg/kg/day.[19] The level of progenitor cells remained elevated for five days after the last injection, suggesting a proliferative effect of GM–CSF on the marrow.

There are a limited number of studies using GM–CSF only mobilized PBPC with or without marrow after high dose chemotherapy (Table 4).[20–24] The largest study using PBPC alone involved patients with preceding marrow hypoplasia or tumour involvement.[21] A shorter time to neutrophil recovery and platelet and red cell transfusion independence was observed compared with PBPC collected in the steady state in a similar patient group.

Table 4. *GM–CSF only mobilized PBPC*±bone marrow autografts*

Author/year/ reference	Dose/route	No. pts	Pt. population	LP volume and schedule	No. LP	Total CFU–GM×10^4/kg median (range)	Bone marrow infused	G–CSF post-infusion	Engraftment (Median day) neutrophils >0.5	platelets >20
Haas 1990[20]	250 μg/m^2 IV	11	lymphoma; marrow hypoplasia	9.5–10 litres started when WCC>10×10^9/l	6 (3–9)	3 (0.9–9.5)[b]	no	no	28.5 (14–42)[c]	39
Bishop 1993[21]	125–250 μg/m^2 IV	58	heavily pretreated; marrow hypoplasia or tumour	NS	7	NS	no	no	18–23	NS
Kritz 1993[22]	10 μ/kg SC	13	metastatic breast cancer, previously treated	10 litres d4, 6, 8, 10	4	NS	no	no	15 (11–24)	14
Peters 1993[23]	8 μg/kg IV	17	Stage II or IV breast cancer; previously treated	9 litres d6–9	3	12.5	yes[a]	yes	8.9	NS
Janusewicz 1994[24]	10 μg/kg SC	24[d]	predominantly relapsed lymphoma	7 litres d4 or 5 onwards	5 (4–9)	27.3 (8.6–98.6)	no	no	12	14 (8–639)[+]

LP=Leukapheresis. NS=Not specifed.

[a] PBPC given d−1, d+0, d+1. Bone marrow given d+0.

[b] Based on 70 kg patient weight.

[c] Only six patients proceeded to autograft.

[d] Five additional patients were excluded owing to inadequate harvests.

* Only studies with more than ten patients are included.

IS THERE A DIFFERENCE BETWEEN G–CSF AND GM–CSF IN THE EFFICIENCY OF PROGENITOR MOBILIZATION AND ENGRAFTMENT? There are no conclusive data available in this respect. Comparisons have used the CD34 antigen, which identifies haemopoietic precursor cells, to quantify the number of progenitors. The sequential studies of Peters et al[23] showed that, at roughly equivalent doses and using the same LP schedule, G–CSF mobilized more CD34+ PBPC than GM–CSF. However, patient numbers were small (n= 16 and 17 respectively) in each group. In contrast, a prospective study by Bolwell et al[25] in forty-four patients found no significant difference in CD34+ numbers mobilized by G–CSF or GM–CSF.

In the Peters study, the addition of G–CSF primed, but not GM–CSF primed, PBPC reduced the median number of red cell and platelet transfusions, compared with marrow. In the Bolwell study, neutrophil and platelet recovery was significantly faster using the G–CSF primed PBPC. An analysis of the platelet recovery data in Tables 3 to 5, also suggests that G–CSF primed PBPC may be associated with faster platelet recovery than GM–CSF primed PBPC.

There are a number of possible reasons for these observations. The most obvious is that the treatment groups are heterogenous, having received prior radiotherapy and chemotherapy of variable intensity, and hence are not comparable. The route of administration may also be important, particularly for GM–CSF in which daily subcutaneous injections are more effective than short intravenous infusions in ameliorating neutropenia.[26] In the Peters study, G–CSF was given subcutaneously while GM–CSF was given intravenously. The kinetics of progenitor cell mobilization may also differ between the two cytokines, requiring different LP schedules for optimal progenitor cell collection. A dose–response relationship for PBPC mobilization with GM–CSF may exist,[18] and higher doses of GM–CSF than G–CSF may be required for equivalent mobilization. The use of G–CSF vs GM–CSF after infusion may impact on engraftment. Finally, the mobilized progenitors may be qualitatively different between the two cytokines; for example, G–CSF may mobilize more relatively mature megakaryocytic and erythroid progenitors. While the Bolwell study[25] showed a trend (p=0.06) towards higher mobilization of CD34+ cells with an immature phenotype (CD33−) using GM–CSF compared with G–CSF, the Peters study[23] showed the opposite.

TOLERABILITY OF G–CSF AND GM–CSF G–CSF is generally well tolerated. Few significant adverse effects, even at high doses have been observed, with the only common side effect being mild to moderate bone pain.[13]

GM–CSF appears to have more toxicity. A first dose effect consisting of dyspnoea and hypotension has been described.[27] In one autologous transplant study, continuous infusion GM–CSF was associated with persist-

Table 5. *Multi-agent chemotherapy and growth factor mobilization*

Author/year/reference	Disease	No. pts	Pretreatment	Mobilizing chemotherapy	Growth factor/ dose	Median (range) CFU–GM×10^4/ kg per LP	Median days to platelets >20×10^9/l post-transplant
Elias 1992[32]	metastatic breast cancer	16	62% pretreated	doxorubicin 5-fluorouracil methotrexate	GM–CSF 5 μg/kg	NS	12
Shimakazi 1992[33]	heterogeneous	20	NS	HIDAC VP16	G–CSF 500 μg/m²	110 (2–1150)	11
Brugger 1993[34]	heterogeneous	24	62% pretreated	VP16 ifosfamide cisplatinum	G–CSF 5 μg/kg	11.5[a]	9–10
Haas 1993[35]	NHL	8	pretreated	HIDAC, mitoxantrone	IL-3 5 μg/kg GM–CSF 5 μg/kg	2.1 (1.3–13)[a]	14
Ho 1993[36]	metastatic breast cancer	15	none for 6 months	cyclophosphamide epirubicin 5FU	GM–CSF 5 μg/kg	10.2	11
Hohaus 1993[37]	relapsed Hodgkin's and NHL	10	heavily pretreated	dexa BEAM or COP-BLAM or HIDAC, mitoxantrone	G–CSF 5 μg/kg	4.1 (0.8–38)[b]	22[c]
Pettengell 1993[38]	NHL Hodgkin's	34 10	untreated pretreated	VAPEC-B	G–CSF 300 μg	270 (70–11 900) 52 (13–1840)	9 13
Lickliter 1994[39]	NHL	7	pretreated no RT	MTX, ara-C, VP16, cyclophosphamide, dexamethasone	G–CSF 300–600 μg	99 (19–800)	8

[a] Assuming 70 kg body weight.
[b] The total of a median of six leukaphereses.
[c] Days to platelets >50×10^9/l.
NS=Not specified.

ent fever, despite neutrophil engraftment and antibiotic therapy, in 69% of patients; side effects prevented half the patients from completing the entire course.[28] In another study using GM–CSF alone to mobilize PBPC, 79% of patients developed fever.[24]

There are limited data directly comparing the toxicity of the two cytokines. In one study, 45 consecutive patients received high dose cyclophosphamide followed by either G–CSF or GM–CSF.[29] Side effects occurred in 17 and 41% of patients, respectively. Fever, fluid retention and venous thrombosis were only observed in GM–CSF patients. A multi-centre double blinded trial compared yeast-derived GM–CSF with G–CSF after chemotherapy.[30] Both were well tolerated and had comparable toxicity except for more fever in the GM–CSF group.

In summary, while the frequency of side effects may depend on the derivation of the growth factor, the dose and the method of administration, it appears that G–CSF is generally better tolerated than GM–CSF. Severe side effects are, however, uncommon with either cytokine.

Growth factor plus chemotherapy mobilization of progenitors

OVERVIEW There are now plenty of data to suggest that the combination of growth factors and chemotherapy is superior to either treatment alone in the capacity to mobilize PBPC. In one study using patients as their own controls, a 5.5-fold increase in CFU–GM was obtained by adding G–CSF to chemotherapy.[31]

In practice, many centres now appear to be utilizing the synergy between chemotherapy and growth factors to mobilize PBPC in preference to using either alone. This approach has the additional advantages of reducing the disease bulk prior to transplant and, perhaps, acting as an in vivo purge (q.v.).

Table 5 details some of the studies in adults using multi-agent chemotherapy in combination with a growth factor for PBPC mobilization.[32–40]

The conclusions that can be drawn from these studies are as follows:

1. the quantity of progenitors mobilized using this combination generally far exceeds the quantity able to be mobilized by either chemotherapy or a growth factor alone.
2. in many patients, a single LP can collect sufficient progenitor cells to proceed safely to a transplant. Nevertheless, there is substantial interindividual difference in the mobilization of progenitors[35] and in occasional patients mobilization is poor. This may reflect intrinsic biological differences between individuals, the extent of marrow infiltration with tumour, or stem cell damage from prior treatment. Radiotherapy in particular appears to compromise marrow reserve.

In the study of Hohaus[37], in which mobilization was poor and platelet recovery relatively slow, seven of the ten patients had received previous radiotherapy. Progenitor release may be delayed by sepsis and be lower in patients with a poor performance status at presentation.[40]

There is one report of poor PBPC mobilization using high dose cyclophosphamide and GM–CSF in patients with myeloma with extensive marrow plasma cell infiltration.[41] This contrasted with the uniformly high levels seen in patients with lymphoma or breast cancer mobilized by the same regimen at the same institution. Whether this reflects local secretion of suppressive cytokines by plasma cells and hence is unique to myeloma, or occurs in any disease with heavy marrow involvement, is unknown.

3. when infused in sufficient numbers, the progenitors mobilized by this technique result in rapid and durable trilineage engraftment.

HOW MYELOSUPPRESSIVE DOES CHEMOTHERAPY HAVE TO BE TO MOBILIZE PBPC IN COMBINATION WITH A GROWTH FACTOR? The number of PBPC mobilized in the rebound phase after chemotherapy alone reflects the intensity of the preceding myelosuppression.[42] However, at the chemotherapy doses required to mobilize sufficient PBPC there is considerable clinical toxicity. The synergy between growth factor and chemotherapy in PBPC mobilization has allowed investigators to use lower doses of chemotherapy which are less myelosuppressive and better tolerated.

Table 6 details the results of studies using doses of cyclophosphamide ranging between 1.5 and 7 g/m^2 in combination with either G–CSF or GM–CSF.[43–49] There are a number of observations which emerge. At higher doses the incidence of febrile neutroenia is substantial. In one study with 7 g/m^2, patients spent a median of 22 days in hospital.[44] In contrast, at the lower doses there is minimal clinical toxicity, but sufficient progenitors are still mobilized in the majority of patients to safely proceed to a transplant. If growth factors are used post chemotherapy, a low nadir neutrophil count may not be a prerequisite for the release of PBPC.[40] These results suggest that the administration of chemotherapy, subsequent patient care and PBPC collections can potentially all be performed on an outpatient basis.

The kinetics of PBPC release seem to be different at the lower doses. Maximum circulating progenitor levels generally occur around day 9–10 post cyclophosphamide at doses $\leqslant$ 4 g/m^2, and around day 12–15 at 7 g/m^2 (Table 6). While more data are required, and accepting that the kinetics may vary somewhat due to biological differences both between patients and diseases, this reasonably predictable time of progenitor cell release enables the collection to be scheduled at a convenient time.

Table 6. *Mobilization of progenitors using cyclophosphamide and a growth factor*

Author/year/ reference	Cyclo. dose (g/m^2)	Disease	No. pts	Growth factor/ dose	LP: median no.	Febrile neutropenia (%)	Median (range) total CFU–GM×10^4/kg	Day peak CD34+ or CFU–GM	Neutrophil recovery >0.5×10^9/l post-infusion	Platelet recovery post-infusion
Gianni 1989[43]	7	lymphoma	7	GM–CSF 5.5 μg/kg	2–4	NS[a]	121 (33–201)	NS	9[c]	10.7[d]
Boiron 1993[44]	7	myeloma	10	GM–CSF 5 μg/kg	6	NS[b]	53.2	12–15	11.5	13[d]
Craig 1993[45]	4	lymphoma	17	G–CSF 5 μg/kg	3–5	22	21.2 (0–262)	12.5	NS	NS
Dale 1993[46]	5	various	16	G–CSF 5 μg/kg	5	60	50	12	NS	NS
Jones 1993[47]	1.5	lymphoma	26	G–CSF 10 μ/kg (*n*=21) 5 μg/kg (*n*=5)	1	0	31 (3–126)	9–10	11[c]	13[g]
Liberti 1993[48]	4	lymphoma	6	G–CSF 5–10 μg/kg	3	0	42 (8–105)	9	13	14[d]
Passos-Coelho 1993[49]	4	advanced breast cancer	9	GM–CSF 5 μg/kg	1[e]	55	38 (0.6–170)	NS	14	10[f]

[a] Neutrophils <0.5×10^9/l for approx. 6 days.
[b] Neutrophils <0.5×10(9/l for 14 days.
[c] Some patients received growth factor post-transplant.
[d] Platelets >50×10^9/l.
[e] Large volume (36 l) apheresis.
[f] Day of last platelet transfusion.
[g] Platelets >20×10^9/l.
NS=Not specified.

Chemotherapy drugs other than cyclophosphamide may also be useful for PBPC mobilization. Etoposide, which also spares stem-cells, has been used successfully as a single agent for this purpose.[41]

OPTIMAL DOSE AND TIME TO BEGIN GROWTH FACTOR ADMINISTRATION AFTER CHEMOTHERAPY FOR MOBILIZATION OF PBPC In most studies, growth factors have been commenced the day after the completion of chemotherapy. In patients receiving cyclophosphamide this results in a clearcut neutrophil nadir, at a time dependent on the dose of cyclophosphamide.

It is possible, however, that this may not be the optimal timing of administration. The effects of 10 μg/kg vs 5 μg/kg of G–CSF beginning one day after 1.5 g/m^2 cyclophosphamide, as well as delaying the G–CSF to four days post-treatment, have been evaluated.[47] The preliminary observations were that a reduced dose or delayed administration of G–CSF was associated with less severe neutropenia without apparently compromising progenitor yields. It was hypothesized that the maturational effect of G–CSF causes post-mitotic cells that survive the cyclophosphamide to leave the marrow more rapidly and die more quickly. However, the absence of a clear neutrophil nadir and recovery phase made it more difficult to judge when to perform a leukapheresis.

These results are very preliminary and need confirmation with larger patient numbers. Moreover, whether these phenomena occur at higher doses of cyclophosphamide is unknown. If they do, there are potential substantial financial advantages both in drug costs and reduction in the incidence of febrile neutropenia.

Prediction of optimal time of leukaphereses

Investigators have used various means of predicting when best to collect progenitor cells by LP. The preferred test should be one which gives a reliable result available on the same day. Colony assays are impractical as results take two weeks to become available.

PBPC mobilized by chemotherapy and a growth factor The following rapidly available peripheral blood cell parameters have been used to predict the optimal timing of LP in this situation.

WHITE CELL COUNT (WCC) There is not a particularly close relationship between WCC and circulating CFU–GM and CD34 numbers.[50] Nevertheless, this may not matter clinically, as the *kinetics* of progenitor cell release in relation to changes in the WCC are probably more important.

A number of investigators have examined this relationship. In patients with lymphoma receiving chemotherapy (VAPEC-B) and G–CSF, the release of circulating colony cells precedes the rise in WCC by 24 hours and is maximal when the recovering WCC reaches 5–10 × 10^9/l.[40] In patients with myeloma receiving chemotherapy and G–CSF, maximal numbers of CD34 levels were collected on the third and fourth days after the WCC exceeded 2 × 10^9/l.[51]

A similar pattern is observed in patients receiving chemotherapy and GM–CSF.[36] PBPC levels reach their maximum level 2 days after the WCC exceeds 2 × 10^9/l post nadir. This level is sustained for 4–5 days with the continuation of GM–CSF, but falls thereafter despite a sustained increase in the WCC.

The observation that high levels of PBPC are maintained for long periods after chemotherapy and growth factor mobilization has implications for the ease of LP collection. For example, weekend collections may be avoided and greater flexibility of timing of collections during normal working hours is available.

MONONUCLEAR CELL COUNT In patients receiving chemotherapy and G–CSF, a close correlation has been observed between the number of mononuclear cells and both $CD34^+$ cells (r=0.80)[52] and CFU-GM (r=0.7)[53] in peripheral blood. Synchronization of the peak levels of monocytes and circulating CFU–GM has been reported.[54] Hence sequential examination of absolute monocyte counts may be useful in evaluating when best to perform a LP.

$CD34^+$ LEVELS Daily monitoring of the peripheral blood $CD34^+$ levels has also been used to guide the appropriate time to start PBPC collection.

An analysis from Haas et al[52] suggests that after chemotherapy and G–CSF the peak level of $CD34^+$ in the peripheral blood is highly predictive for the total $CD34^+$ harvest. In their experience, patients autografted with more than 2.5 × 10^6 $CD34^+$ cells/kg achieve complete engraftment and rapid platelet recovery. Patients who were able to have this $CD34^+$ quantity collected, often by a single LP, had peripheral blood $CD34^+$ cells above 20/μl. Patients who did not mobilize this quantity (despite a median of 7 LP) had <20/μl ($p<0.001$); these patients were more heavily pretreated with chemotherapy and radiotherapy.

However, it must be stressed that what applies in one institution may not apply in another using different laboratory techniques. In addition, more data are required to establish any correlation between $CD34^+$ numbers in PB, the number of CFU–GM collected by LP on that day and engraftment. In the absence of uniform standards for assessing $CD34^+$ numbers and performing colony assays, it is inappropriate at this point to recommend specific guidelines based on these results.

PBPC mobilized by chemotherapy alone The optimal time for LP appears to be different for PBPC mobilized by chemotherapy. The peak peripheral blood CFU–GM after induction therapy in acute myeloid leukaemia coincides with that of circulating immature myeloid cells and monocytes, and regularly occurs a few days after the platelet counts exceed 100 × 10^9/l.[55]

PBPC mobilized by a growth factor alone Using G–CSF alone at doses of 12 or 24 μg/kg for 6 days, progenitor cell yields are maximal with collections towards the end of G–CSF administration.[56] The preferred schedule for harvesting the maximal number of CFU–GM appears to be days 5, 6 and 7, with maximal yields on day 5.[56] It is not known whether continuing G–CSF beyond six days results in sustained and/or increasing progenitor yields.

The kinetics of progenitor release with GM–CSF alone are not well characterized. Similarly, the optimal time for LP using cytokine combinations such as interleukin three (IL–3)/GM–CSF and stem cell factor (SCF)/G–CSF is the subject of ongoing studies.

Leukapheresis time Leukaphereses have generally been performed for three hours, on each occasion processing 7–10 litres of blood. Prolonging the LP time may be more efficient, tolerable and cost effective. There are preliminary data to suggest that, after G–CSF stimulation, a single six hour LP produces similar yields and quality of PBPC compared with two 4.5 hour LP and three 3-hour LP on consecutive days.[57] In one study, a single 14 litre apheresis in patients receiving chemotherapy and G–CSF collected sufficient progenitors to proceed to an autograft.[58]

Minimum number of peripheral blood progenitor cells required for rapid engraftment

Variables correlating with engraftment Investigators have attempted to correlate a number of clinical and laboratory parameters with engraftment after PBPC infusion. Clinical factors such as leukaemia as the underlying diagnosis[12] and total body irradiation in the conditioning regimen[59] have been associated with slower engraftment.

The laboratory parameters evaluated in this respect include the number of white cells, mononuclear cells (MNC), CFU–GM and $CD34^+$ cells. Various investigators have found no correlation of WCC and platelet recovery with the number of MNC infused.[36,60] However, there are reports of a negative exponential relationship between CFU–GM and the time to platelet recovery (W. Sheridan: personal communication), and a similar relationship between $CD34^+$ numbers and platelet recovery.[36]

Provided sufficient PBPC are infused, the mobilizing stimulus does not seem to be a major factor affecting engraftment. Platelet recovery generally occurs 9–10 days after infusion of G–CSF mobilized PBPC and 9–11 days after infusion of large numbers of G–CSF and chemotherapy mobilized

PBPC (tables 3, 5). The infusion of GM–CSF and chemotherapy mobilized PBPC or GM–CSF alone mobilized PBPC may result in platelet engraftment slightly later.

The concept of a threshold

OVERVIEW The exponential relationship between CFU–GM/CD34+ numbers and engraftment suggests that, beyond a certain threshold, engraftment is not hastened by infusion of extra progenitors. There appears to be an obligate time, between eight and eleven days, for early white cell and platelet recovery which cannot be overcome by increasing the dose of PBPC infused.

COLONY ASSAYS Traditionally, CFU–GM assays have been the gold standard in assessing the adequacy of PBPC collections. A threshold of 30×10^4 CFU–GM/ kg for rapid platelet recovery using G–CSF only mobilized PBPC has been suggested, but infusion with as low as 10×10^4 CFU–GM/ kg has resulted in rapid engraftment.[13] A threshold of 5×10^4 CFU–GM/ kg has been reported using chemotherapy and G–CSF mobilized PBPC.[60] A safe threshold using chemotherapy only mobilized PBPC is not well established. A minimum level of 50×10^4 CFU–GM/ kg in acute myeloid leukaemia (AML) has been recommended.[61] The threshold may vary between diseases, with the suggestion that the level is lower in non-AML patients than in patients with AML.[62]

Using colony assays, the threshold is likely to vary between different laboratories due to technical differences in performing the assay. Considerable differences in the growth supporting ability exist between batches of serum and meticulous pre-testing is required just to maintain reproducibility in each laboratory. There is no commonly agreed standard for the colony stimulating factors used in the assay and there are differences between single or multiple cytokine stimulated cultures. *Hence, each institution needs to determine its own threshold if CFU–GM assays are to be used.*

CD34 NUMBERS Various authors have described a variably close linear correlation between CD34+ numbers and day 14 CFU–GM in LP products (Table 7).[12,36,50,63–65] These results suggest that CD34+ estimations on LP samples may be useful in assessing adequacy of the collection. The closeness of the relationship may depend on technical aspects such as the type of antibody used,[36,65] the method of colony assay detection, and perhaps on the mobilising stimulus.[66]

However, there are data to suggest that CD34+ assays are *independently* predictive for rapid engraftment. Table 8 depicts the results of representative studies[36,52,60,63,67–69] which suggest that there is a CD34+

Table 7. *Relationship between CD34⁺ and CFU–GM in leukapheresis products*

Author/year/reference	Mobilization	No. pts	*r* value
Sienna 1991[50]	CT+GM–CSF	16	0.89
Bitran 1993[63]	CT+GM–CSF	14	0.92
Ho 1993[36]	CT+G–CSF	15	0.77
Jouault 1993[64]	growth factor±CT	13	0.75
O'Kane Murphy 1993[65]	GM–CSF	25	0.63
Reiffers 1993[12]	growth factor±CT	118	'no correlation'

CT=Chemotherapy.

threshold below which platelet recovery is delayed. The variance in CD34+ threshold again most likely reflects the differences in assay techniques between different laboratories.

Additional data suggests that the correlation of CD34+ cells with parameters of engraftment is better for flow cytometrically defined phenotypical subsets than the total CD34+ pool. Haemopoietic recovery may be predicted most accurately by the more mature CD34+/CD33+ numbers rather than by total numbers of nucleated cells, CFU–GM or CD34+/CD33− cells.[50] The correlation for platelet recovery has been reported to be best defined by CD34+ subsets expressing platelet specific antigens (CD41, CD61) and the adhesion antigen L-selectin.[67] These observations are consistent with functional heterogeneity of the CD34+ population and suggest that different cells contribute to haemopoietic reconstitution.

MONONUCLEAR CELL NUMBERS A minimum of 4 × 10^8 MNC/kg has been recommended for engraftment using mobilized PBPC, higher than the

Table 8. *Threshold to slow platelet recovery**

Author/year/reference	No. pts evaluated	Mobilization stimulus	Threshold: $CD34^+ \times 10^6$/kg
Akard 1993[60]	35	CT and G–CSF	<8
Bitran 1993[63]	14	CT and GM–CSF	<2
Dercksen 1993[67]	27	NS	<5
Ho 1993[36]	15	CT and G–CSF	<2.3–4.9
Raptis 1993[68]	60	NS	<1
Schwartzberg 1993[69]	13	CT and G–CSF	<2.5
Haas 1994[52]	35	CT and G–CSF	<2.5

* The definition of 'slow' platelet recovery is not specified in all of these reports. NS=Not specified.

1–2 × 10^8 MNC/kg recommended for an adequate marrow harvest.[58] However, on the basis that mobilized PBPC have in vitro engraftment potential equivalent to that of marrow,[70] it has been suggested that the same criterion be used for both sources of cells.[58] In a recent study from the Manchester group, in which progenitors were mobilized by chemotherapy and GCSF, infusion with as few as 1.1 × 10^8 MNC/kg produced successful engraftment.[58]

The Manchester study also noted a correlation between the numbers of MNC/kg and $CD34^+$ cells/kg (r=0.65), suggesting that MNC numbers in the LP product may by themselves be sufficient to predict adequate engraftment. However, further information is needed before MNC numbers become widely accepted for this purpose, including the correlation of MNC numbers with engraftment using other types of mobilized PBPC, and confirmation from other centres of a MNC threshold for rapid trilineage engraftment. If confirmed, use of MNC numbers will have advantages over $CD34^+$ and colony assays, including speed, cost and ease of standardization. Depending on the automated cell counter used, the machine differential may be as accurate as a manual differential in estimating MNC numbers.[71]

The number of peripheral blood mononuclear cells in DNA synthesis phase has also been reported to closely predict the total CFU–GM obtained by LP, and may be useful both to determine the optimal day of LP and the richness of the LP product.[72]

Are growth factors needed after progenitor cell infusion?

Preliminary results of two randomized studies to evaluate this question have been reported.[73,74] In one of these,[73] 37 patients were infused with growth factor mobilized PBPC and randomized to receive either G–CSF *and* GM–CSF or no growth factor thereafter. There was a significantly ($p<0.001$) faster recovery to a neutrophil count of 0.1 × 10^9/l (nine vs eleven days) and 0.5 × 10^9/l (ten vs sixteen days), respectively. No difference in platelet recovery was observed. The growth factor patients were discharged two days earlier ($p=0.01$), but did not have fewer febrile days, smaller transfusion requirements or less bacteraemia.

In the second study,[74] patients infused with PBPC were randomized to receive G–CSF or not. The time to reach a neutrophil count of 0.5 × 10^9/l was five days shorter (thirteen vs eighteen days; $p=0.01$) in the G-CSF group who were discharged four days (twenty vs twenty-four days; $p=0.05$) earlier.

A non-randomized study also documented a 3–4 day shortening of neutrophil recovery to 0.5 × 10^9/l by the addition of G–CSF, with a corresponding reduction in days of antibiotics and hospitalisation.[69] The use of GM–CSF post-infusion of chemotherapy and GM–CSF mobilized

PBPC also appears to hasten neutrophil recovery to $0.5 \times 10^9/l$ by three days.[75]

It is possible that the reduced antibiotic use and duration of hospitalization reflects the common practice of waiting until a particular neutrophil count (often $1–2 \times 10^9/l$) is reached before ceasing antibiotics and discharging patients after 1–2 afebrile days thereafter. It is also possible that this approach is too conservative and cessation of antibiotics earlier, particularly in the context of a rising neutrophil count, may be equally effective. Studies evaluating this latter approach are desirable before the cost-effectiveness of growth factors after PBPC infusion can be properly ascertained. At present, the addition of growth factors does not appear to produce a major clinical benefit.

Biology of peripheral blood progenitor cells and their mobilization

This section discusses the basic biology of PBPC and some of the clinical issues relevant to this area.

How does the administration of growth factors result in increased progenitor levels in peripheral blood?

It is likely that multiple mechanisms are involved. These include an increased rate of cycling of marrow progenitors, redistribution of progenitors from marrow into the circulation, and a reduced exit of progenitors from the bloodstream.

The rate of cycling of marrow progenitors may increase under the direct influence of growth factors.[8] Growth factors may also act indirectly in this respect. For example, G–CSF stimulates monocytes in vivo to release IL-6[54] and in vitro G–CSF and IL-6 stimulate multipotential progenitor cells in G_0 phase to enter the cell cycle.[76] Of interest, however, is the observation that mobilized CD34+ cells show less CD71 expression than steady-state bone marrow CD34+ cells, suggesting that they are not actively cycling.[77]

Redistribution of progenitor cells as a possible mechanism is supported by the observation that administration of growth factors generally does not lead to an increase in the number of marrow progenitor cells. This redistribution may be mediated by down-regulation of the expression of adhesion molecules on mobilized progenitors. The leucocyte function antigen-1 (LFA-1) is an adhesion molecule belonging to the integrin superfamily and expressed on myeloid and erythroid progenitors. Möhle et al[78] found LFA-1 expression on 88% of steady state peripheral blood CD34+ cells and 75% of resting marrow CD34+ cells, but on only 60% of peripheral blood CD34+ cells (and with low fluorescence intensity) after growth factor administration. Reduced expression of LFA-1 may facilitate the egress of cells from the bone marrow and prolong the period they remain in the circulation.

Immunophenotypic and functional characteristics of mobilized progenitor cells

CD34⁺ cell subsets The CD34 antigen has been used to identify haemopoietic precursor cells. CD34+ cells represent approximately 1–4% of normal bone marrow mononuclear cells[11,79] and 0.2% of resting peripheral blood cells.[79] The majority of these cells have a mature phenotype (CD38+ DR+) characteristic of committed lineage progenitors. However, slightly more of the CD34+ cells in resting peripheral blood than marrow (6 vs 1%) express the primitive phenotype CD38- DR-.[80]

The majority of mobilized $CD34^+$ also have a mature phenotype,[81–83] and contain a lower percentage of cells with a primitive phenotype than in the marrow.[80] The antigenic profile is relatively consistent, independent of the mobilizing regimen. However, there may be a degree of phenotypic and functional heterogeneity according to the mobilizing stimulus. For example, G–CSF mobilized $CD34^+$ cells appear to have a higher proportion of cells with a more primitive phenotype[77,84] and a lower cloning efficiency (CFU–GM per $CD34^+$ cells) than cells mobilized by a combination of chemotherapy and G–CSF.[77]

The calculated cloning efficiency of chemotherapy and growth factor mobilized PBPC in one report[85] was 5–6%, indicating that only one out of 18 $CD34^+$ cells gave rise to colonies. This is consistent with the phenotypical data and suggests that mobilized $CD34^+$ cells consist mainly of mature precursors without clonogenic capacity in vitro.

Colony assays Mobilizing stimuli result in substantial increases in the more mature differentiated colony-forming cells of the CFU–GM and erythroid (BFU–E) type[9] More immature colonies are also detected, such as CFU–Mix and long-term culture-initiating cells (LTC–IC).[70]

LTC–IC are thought to be derived from the subpopulation of $CD34^+$ cells with an immature phenotype and to represent those cells responsible for restoring long-term hemopoiesis in vivo. In vitro, the capacity of mobilized PBPC to repopulate irradiated marrow stroma is at least as effective as bone marrow cells on a cell per cell basis and much more effective than peripheral blood mononuclear cells collected in the steady state.[70,86] The release of LTC–IC into the circulation after chemotherapy and a growth factor roughly parallels, or may slightly precede, that of more mature progenitor cell release.[70,87,88]

Why do mobilized PBPC result in faster engraftment than marrow cells?

RAPID NEUTROPHIL RECOVERY A likely explanation is that mobilized PBPC contain large numbers of relatively mature cells, and the results of immunophenotyping studies support this. Compared with unstimulated bone marrow CD34+ cells, mobilized peripheral blood CD34+ cells more frequently express CD13 and CD33[89] a phenotype characteristic of myeloid lineage committed progenitors. These cells may contribute to rapid neutrophil recovery.

RAPID PLATELET RECOVERY Many investigators have been unable to detect megakaryocyte colony (CFU–Meg) forming cells in PBPC collections. This may reflect the difficulty with this assay. One notable recent exception is the report[90] of a several hundred-fold increase in megakaryocyte burst-forming units (BFU–Meg) and the more mature CFU–Meg, with a prevalence of the latter, after high dose cyclophosphamide and growth factors

Two recent reports offer an alternative explanation, viz. that mobilized PBPC contain a considerable number of mature megakaryocyte precursor cells which may not be clonogenic in vitro, but in vivo are capable of rapidly producing platelets after engraftment. Brugger et al[54] detected circulating GPIIb IIIa positive megakaryocyte precursor cells, without clonogenic capacity in vitro. Storozynsky et al[91] observed a 10–20-fold increase in the proportion of CD34+ cells expressing the early megakaryocytic antigen CD41a on mobilized PBPC compared with resting bone marrow. These cells were weakly positive for both CD41b (GpIIb) and CD61 (GpIIIa). They noted that CD34+ CD41a− cells could form CFU–GM, BFU-e and CFU–Meg in vitro but that CD34+ CD41a+ cells had only limited proliferative potential.

These findings are consistent with the frequent observation of a secondary dip in platelet count occurring 3–6 weeks after a stem cell infusion; it is possible that the mature megakaryocytes expire at this time with the characteristically gradual and sustained subsequent rise in platelet count representing thrombopoiesis by more immature but durable megakaryocytic progenitors.

Are mobilized progenitor cells capable of long-term haemopoietic reconstitution?

There is evidence that PBPC collected after chemotherapy and G-CSF are able to generate and sustain haemopoiesis in long term culture at a level comparable or superior to that of normal bone marrow.[70] However, gene marking studies are necessary to establish unequivocally that autologous PBPC can reconstitute long-term haemopoiesis in vivo, as conditioning regimens prior to transplantation may not be completely myeloablative. Using a retroviral marker, infused exogenous marrow cells can be identified as the source of haemopoietic recovery after autologous transplantation.[92,93]

Gene marking studies using PBPC have not been reported. In their absence, the only evidence that these cells are capable of durable engraftment consists of medium term follow up of patients receiving PBPC only transplants. Thus far, there are no reports of late onset graft failure. The longest survivor of patients with acute myeloid leukaemia transplanted with PBPC collected in the recovery phase after chemotherapy[94] is now 6.5 years post-infusion (C Juttner: personal communication). The longest surviving patient from the Sheridan study[13] using G–CSF mobilized PBPC alone is now 3.5 years post-transplant, and has a normal blood count.

Of interest is recent work from Manchester examining colony-forming progenitor cells and LTC–IC in the peripheral blood of patients with breast cancer receiving chemotherapy and G–CSF.[95] After repeated cycles of chemotherapy, the release of LTC–IC was decreased to a far greater extent than progenitor cells. This suggests that the number of progenitors per ml blood does not necessarily reflect the marrow repopulating ability of peripheral haemopoietic cells at a given time point.

Are peripheral blood progenitor cells less contaminated with tumour than marrow? This has been the subject of a recent review.[96] Various issues are discussed below.

STEADY-STATE PBPC VS BONE MARROW Circulating tumour cells have been detected in the steady state in a variety of tumours including breast cancer,[97] non-Hodgkin's lymphoma (NHL), particularly follicular type,[98] ovarian cancer[99] and neuroblastoma.[100] In NHL, there is a suggestion that the steady-state peripheral blood is less involved than bone marrow,[99] but the clinical relevance of this is uncertain. Preliminary results of a prospective randomized trial comparing bone marrow with non-mobilized PBPC as the source of hemopoietic reconstitution after high dose chemotherapy have been reported.[101] Patients with chemotherapy responsive NHL or Hodgkin's disease with a morphologically clear bone marrow were eligible. Thus far there is no difference in the incidence of relapse, overall survival or relapse-free survival.

MOBILIZED VS STEADY STATE PBPCS If there is marrow involvement with tumour, theoretically, mobilization of haemopoietic progenitors may also release malignant cells into the peripheral blood.

This issue has been examined recently in patients with breast cancer and small cell lung cancer.[97] In this study, PBPCs were mobilized with chemotherapy and G–CSF. Tumour cells detected by immunohistochemistry were found among the PBPC of all patients with stage IV breast cancer and half of those with extensive small cell lung cancer. Tumour cells post-mobilization were found in patients in whom such cells were not detected in the steady state, and at a higher level after mobilization in patients with detectable steady-state tumour. Tumour cells were also found in patients without detectable marrow involvement, suggesting that they may be mobilized from sites other than marrow, and raising the concern that mobilizing stimuli may hasten metastatic spread. Clearance of circulating tumour cells was observed after further chemotherapy in the majority of patients, suggesting that it may be best in these diseases to administer induction chemotherapy before PBPCs are mobilized and collected.

Tumour cell contamination of mobilized PBPC has also been documented in patients with haematological malignancies such as NHL[102] and myeloma.[103,104]

MOBILIZED PBPC VS BONE MARROW As steady-state aphereses result in poor PBPC yields and generally are not used in autografting, a more relevant question is whether, for each tumour type and perhaps for each mobilising stimulus, mobilized PBPC are less contaminated than bone marrow.

Breast cancer contamination appears to be less in mobilized PBPC collections than in bone marrow,[105] and there are emerging data on other tumour types. Preliminary evidence from small numbers of patients with lymphoma using clone specific probes suggests that PCR negative PBPC harvest may be obtained in patients with marrow involvement with lymphoma or myeloma after chemotherapy and G–CSF.[106] Similar results using cytogenetic analysis have been observed in chronic myeloid leukemia and acute lymphoblastic leukaemia.[107, 108] There is a suggestion that early collections (i.e. at low white cell counts) may be less contaminated than later collection,[103,107] perhaps due to preferential earlier release of normal haemopoietic progenitors.

ARE THE PBPC TUMOUR CELLS CAPABLE OF CAUSING RELAPSE AFTER INFUSION? To contribute to relapse, the tumour cells must survive cryopreservation and be clonogenic in vivo. There are little data available in this respect. Breast cancer cells in PBPC are capable of clonogenic growth in vitro.[105] Gene-marking studies suggest that infusion of marrow acute myeloid leukaemia cells can contribute to relapse.[109]

DOES EFFECTIVE PURGING OF TUMOUR CELLS FROM PBPC ALTER TRANSPLANT OUTCOME? As yet, there are no randomized data available to evaluate this proposition. It has been speculated that a substantial burden of circulating tumour cells may reflect biologically bad disease and prognosis is related essentially to the underlying disease rather than the number of reinfused tumour cells.[97] Of note, in a study of marrow autografting in T–ALL, the log kill efficacy of purging and the remaining numbers of leukaemic progenitors in the purged autografts did not correlate with disease free survival.[110] While not necessarily comparable to PBPC autografting for other tumours, it suggests that treatment failure more often than not may be due to inadequate eradiation of disease in the patient by pretransplant radiochemotherapy.

GROWTH FACTOR STIMULATION OF TUMOUR CELL GROWTH There are little available data on in vivo effects of growth factors on tumour cell proliferation or differentiation. One recent report suggests that these effects may be clinically relevant.[111] In this case, a patient with prior marrow involvement with t(14;18) positive 1gM-kappa follicular lymphoma cells underwent a marrow autograft. IL-3 was given post-transplant and was associated with the development of a transient monoclonal plasmacytosis with the same immunophenotype and translocation, which resolved after cessation of the cytokine. IL-3 has been shown to be an in vitro growth and differentiation factor for follicular lymphoma cells.[112]

SUMMARY Tumour contamination of mobilized PBPC is common, and the degree may be influenced by the timing of collection. The biological significance of this contamination is unknown.

Progenitor mobilization by combinations of growth factors

G–CSF and GM–CSF Preliminary results of a phase I/II clinical trial in patients with breast cancer or lymphoma have recently been reported.[113] The addition of a second growth factor (G–CSF or GM–CSF) on day 7–12 after day 1–6 treatment with the alternate cytokine was evaluated. The CFU–GM obtained by LP during the combined treatment was greater than that collected on day five of single growth factor administration. The enhanced mobilization persisted for the six days of combined treatment. Whether *concomitant* administration of G–CSF and GM–CSF from the outset is as effective as *sequential* administration, is unknown.

Interleukin three and GM–CSF IL–3 by itself induces only modest increases in the number of circulating PBPC.[114–116] However, because IL–3 acts on an earlier progenitor cell population than GM–CSF,[117] sequential use of IL–3/GM–CSF has been examined in an attempt to synergize the action of the two cytokines.

Synergy was demonstrated initially in non-human primates.[118] Subsequent human studies have shown that IL–3 given sequentially with GM–CSF is more effective in mobilising PBPC than IL–3 alone in the steady state[117] and GM–CSF alone post-chemotherapy.[119] IL–3 at 5 μg/kg for seven days followed by three days of GM–CSF resulted in a 22-fold increase in mobilising PBPC compared with the baseline.[120] The efficacy of sequential versus overlapping IL–3/GM–CSF is currently under evaluation.[121] Complete engraftment has been observed in five of six patients (one had early relapse) autografted with IL–3/GM–CSF mobilized PBPC.[35]

It is unknown whether this regimen will prove superior to the use of single growth factors or growth factor combinations. Dose escalation studies of IL–3 and GM–CSF may be limited by side effects such as fever and chills[117] which may impact also on their widespread clinical use.

Stem cell factor ± G–CSF mobilization SCF, the ligand for c-kit, by itself does not significantly promote colony formation, but synergistically enhances the ability of other growth factors such as erythropoietin, G–CSF, GM–CSF and IL–3 to augment the in vitro proliferative capacity of both primitive and differentiated progenitor cells in humans.[122] Administration of SCF to humans exerts a similar effect on *marrow* cells.[123]

The ability of SCF to mobilize *PBPC* has also been evaluated. An increase in both primitive and mature circulating progenitors was observed in baboons at doses at, or above, 50 μg/kg/day.[124] In humans, PBPC mobilization has been observed at doses between 10 and 50 μg/kg/day.[125] At the highest dose, without prophylaxis with antihistamines, dose-limiting respiratory toxicity consistent with mast cell degranulation was observed.

Based on murine and baboon experiments demonstrating synergy between SCF at lower doses and G–CSF in increasing the number of blood-borne spleen colony-forming cells[126–128] and the ability of these cells to repopulate the marrow of lethally irradiated mice,[128] human studies using this combination have been initiated.[129,130] One of these studies[129] evaluated patients with breast cancer, some of whom had received previous chemotherapy. SCF was administered for 13 days at doses from 5–20 μg/kg with concomitant G–CSF at 10 μg/kg. Harvesting was performed on days 11–13. SCF was well tolerated at these doses using premedication with antihistamines and β adrenergic agonists. The preliminary results suggest that, compared with G–CSF alone, yields of PBPC may be increased with SCF/G–CSF. A dose-dependent increase in both mature and primitive megakaryocytic progenitors was observed with SCF/G–CSF compared with G–CSF alone,[130] which may explain the trend in this study to more rapid platelet recovery after high dose chemotherapy in patients infused with PBPC mobilized by SCF/G–CSF vs G–CSF alone.

The second study enrolled untreated patients with poor prognosis breast cancer.[131] SCF was given at 5–10 μg/kg for 7 days in combination with G–CSF 12 μg/kg, with aphereses on days 5–7. A control group received G–CSF alone. Progenitor levels in the peripheral blood remained higher for a longer period in the SCF patients, perhaps reflecting a longer lag time for SCF-induced mobilization, and suggesting that sequential administration of SCF followed by G–CSF may be an effective strategy.

Progenitor mobilization using newer growth factors

The ability to mobilize PBPC does not appear to be restricted to the well-investigated growth factors such as G–CSF and GM–CSF and, to a lesser extent, IL-3.

In humans, erythropoietin is able to mobilize CFU–GM and megakaryocyte progenitors and these have been used clinically for transplantation.[132]

In mice, the administration of interleukin-7 post chemotherapy results in an increase in total spleen CFU–GM four to seven times that of the control,[133] and both interleukin-1 and interleukin-8 induce rapid mobilization of progenitor cells capable of rescuing lethally irradiated murine recipients.[134, 135] Interleukin-11 (IL-11) in non-human primates mobilizes PBPC.[136] However, in human studies 2 weeks of IL-11 up to a maximum of 75 mg/kg/day did not increase PBPC,[137] apart from modest increases in megakaryocyte progenitors at the highest dose. IL-11 and G–CSF have synergistic effects on progenitor cell mobilization in mice.[138]

Immune reconstitution after progenitor cell transplants

The limited data available suggest that the kinetics of immune recovery after autologous PBPC transplants and autologous marrow transplants are similar.[139, 140] In both, lymphocyte counts recover quickly, reaching 1×10^9/l 2–3 weeks following infusion.[140] Most of the lymphocytes are CD8+. NK cells (CD56+) remain in the normal range throughout the post-transplant period in both groups. In one study,[140] chemotherapy mobilized PBPC resulted in faster CD3 recovery and faster CD4 recovery to the 'safe' minimum level of 0.2×10^9/l, perhaps reflecting the increased numbers of mononuclear cells infused and indicating that the infusion of mature lymphoid cells may contribute to circulating lymphocytes post-transplant.

Future uses of mobilized progenitor cells

Allogeneic peripheral blood progenitor cell transplants

Interest in the use of mobilized PBPC in allogeneic transplantation has been provoked by the rapid trilineage engraftment characteristic of PBPC in the autologous setting, together with the avoidance of general anaesthesia in the donor.

The excellent safety profile of G–CSF makes it an obvious candidate for use in normal donors. In a murine model, G–CSF mobilized PBPC are capable of restoring hemopoiesis in lethally irradiated recipients.[141] There is an emerging, albeit predominantly anecdotal, experience of the use of these cells alone[142,143] or in combination with marrow[144] in human allogeneic transplantation. In all cases thus far, trilineage and durable medium-term engraftment has been demonstrated.

This area of research and clinical practice is likely to be the focus of much effort over the next few years. There are a number of issues which need to be addressed. The optimal cytokine(s), and its (their) dose and duration for PBPC mobilization is under investigation. The possible impact of methotrexate, commonly used as graft versus host disease prophylaxis, on heamopoietic recovery after PBPC infusion needs evaluation. Perhaps most importantly, there is the potential for an increased incidence and severity of graft versus host disease due to the infusion of large numbers of immunocompetent T cells collected from the circulation. If this is true, adjustment of T cell dose may be required.

Ex vivo expansion of PBPC

There are many potential uses of ex vivo expansion of progenitor cells. These include providing sufficient progenitors to support multiple cycles of high dose chemotherapy, providing candidate cells for therapeutic gene transfer and the avoidance of aphereses by expanding progenitors contained in a unit of blood.[145] The feasibility of large-scale expansion of PBPCs starting from small numbers of peripheral blood $CD34^+$ cells has been established.[145,146]

Another potential use of ex vivo expanded PBPC would be to abrogate completely the severe cytopenia after high dose chemotherapy. Work thus far has focused on producing an expanded post-progenitor cell population that can provide mature functional end cells within days of infusion.[147] To do so, ex vivo culture using $CD34^+$ cells from PBPC collections or marrow has been performed, with delineation of the optimal cytokine combination to produce mature neutrophils and megakaryocytes.[147]

The results of clinical trials using ex vivo expanded PBPC have yet to be published. These will be necessary to establish whether these cells are biologically equivalent to unmodified PBPCs[145] and whether neutropenia can be ameliorated sufficiently to produce clinical benefit.

Peripheral blood progenitor cells to support multiple cycles of high-dose chemotherapy

Using progenitors collected by leukapheresis Multiple cycles of intensive chemotherapy with PBPC support are now being used in an attempt to improve the cure rate of tumours of intermediate chemosensitivity such as metastatic breast cancer and advanced ovarian cancer (Table 9).[148–153]

Preliminary results suggest this approach is feasible and rapid haemopoietic reconstitution occurs even after multiple cycles of treatment. In untreated breast cancer patients, sufficient PBPC were mobilized by G–CSF alone to support three cycles of intensive treatment.[149] Of note, however, is the initial observation from this study of a slight delay in recovery of blood counts after the third cycle of intensive treatment. This suggests that cumulative marrow stromal damage may occur.

Whether the ability to deliver more intensive chemotherapy impacts on the survival of patients with tumours of intermediate chemosensitivity, or

Table 9. *Studies of multiple intensive chemotherapy cycles with peripheral blood progenitor cell support**

Author/year/ reference	Disease	Chemotherapy per cycle	No. cycles delivered	Support
Shea 1992[148]	Various	Carboplatin 1–2 g/m^2	2.5 (mean)	PBPC and GM–CSF
Basser 1993[149]	High risk breast cancer	Epirubicin 200 mg/m^2 Cyclophosphamide 4 g/m^2	3	PBPC and G–CSF
Chao 1993[150]	Metastatic breast cancer; refractory NHL	Cyclophosphamide 4.5–5 g/m^2 Thiotepa 150–200 mg/m^2 Mitoxantrone 18 g/m^2	4	PBPC and G–CSF
Crown 1993[151]	Metastatic breast cancer	Carboplatin 1.5 g/m^2 Etoposide 1.2 g/m^2 Cyclophosphamide 5 g/m^2	3	PBPC and GM–CSF
Tepler 1993[152]	Ovarian cancer	Carboplatin 600 mg/m^2 Cyclophosphamide 600 mg/m^2	4	PBPC and GM–CSF
Wheeler 1993[153]	Relapsed lymphoma	Ifosfamide 3.3 g/m^2 Carboplatin 133 mg/m^2 Etoposide 200 mg/m^2	2**	PPBC and G–CSF

* This list does not include all such studies; it is representative only.
** Responding patients proceeded to ABMT.

even those with highly sensitive tumours such as lymphomas and germ cell tumours, is unknown.

Using progenitors from unprocessed whole blood Peripheral blood may be so enriched for progenitor cells that sufficient cells may be obtainable from a unit of blood to hasten haematological recovery after high dose chemotherapy. Based on CFU–GM yields from patients with lymphoma primed with chemotherapy and G–CSF, it has been predicted that mononuclear cells from 5 ml/kg body weight peripheral blood would be sufficient for successful engraftment.[39]

This approach has been evaluated in six patients receiving high dose melphalan for myeloma.[154] A litre of autologous whole blood was collected after six days of G–CSF, kept unprocessed at room temperature, and reinfused 24 hours after chemotherapy followed by G–CSF. Neutrophil and platelet recovery was substantially faster, and antibiotic use, number of transfusions and length of hospital stay were significantly reduced in these patients compared with a control group receiving no reinfusion.

Issues which need to be addressed for this approach to be successful include:

(i) defining the most appropriate conditions (temperature, medium) for progenitor survival and how long the majority of progenitors remain viable under these conditions. Alternatives may include cryopreservation of a buffy coat preparation or short-term culture of cells in the presence of growth factors to enhance their viability.
(ii) ensuring that cytotoxic metabolites have been cleared before infusion of the progenitors after chemotherapy.
(iii) determining the feasibility of administering multiple cycles of chemotherapy at short intervals using this technique.

CD34 positive selection and PBPC transplantation

Background The CD34 antigen is expressed on 1–4% of human marrow cells and is present on virtually all unipotent and multipotent colony-forming cells and the precursors of colony forming cells in long term marrow culture.[155]

Positive $CD34^+$ selection has been achieved by a variety of techniques. Using a biotin-avidin immunoadsorption column, 50–90% pure $CD34^+$ cells with >50% recovery of colony assay activity can be achieved.[156] The vast majority (>94%) of these cells coexpress CD33, CD38 and HLA–DR, indicating a committed progenitor phenotype. However, more immature $CD34^+$ HLA–DR- cells and LTC–IC are also demonstrable.[157] Large scale preparation of $CD34^+$ HLA–DR- cells by immunoadsorption followed by fluorescence-activated cell sorting has recently been reported.[158]

Autologous transplantation The use of $CD34^+$ selected cells in autologous transplantation has potential advantages. These include (a) reduction of tumour contamination, based on the observation that most malignant cells, including lymphoma, multiple myeloma and breast cancer, do not express CD34[159] and (b) volume reduction to a smaller aliquot resulting in less toxicity with infusion, and providing a concentrated population of cells suitable for (i) ex vivo expansion, (ii) gene marking and gene therapy and (iii) further purging.

MARROW STUDIES It was initially demonstrated that enriched populations of autologous marrow $CD34^+$ cells could engraft lethally irradiated baboons.[160]

Subsequently, the ability to reconstitute humans after high dose chemotherapy with CD34+ autologous marrow cells has been demonstrated.[161]

PERIPHERAL BLOOD PROGENITOR STUDIES Recently, preliminary results of a number of studies of the effect of CD34+ selected mobilized PBPC on engraftment and tumour contamination have been reported.[157,162–164] The results can be summarized as follows.

Engraftment: The rate of haemopoietic recovery after high dose chemotherapy appears comparable between CD34+ selected mobilized PBPC or unprocessed mobilized PBPC.[157,162]

The influence of autologous CD34+ PBPC and/or CD34+ marrow and growth factors on engraftment after high dose chemotherapy in 44 patients with breast cancer has also been evaluated by Shpall et al.[163] CD34+ PBPC were mobilized by G–CSF. No acute toxicity was detected during the infusion of the small volume (5–10 ml) CD34+ fractions. Neutrophil engraftment was no different between marrow and G–CSF, marrow and PBPC and G–CSF, and PBPC and G–CSF alone, but platelet engraftment was significantly faster in patients receiving PBPC. No granulocyte engraftment failure was observed (median follow-up 9 months: range 2–24), but one patient who received CD34+ marrow remained platelet dependent 5 months post-transplant.

These observations suggest that CD34+ selection generally does not deplete PBPC of cells responsible for both the early transient and later durable phases of engraftment which are characteristic of PBPC reinfusions.

Tumour contamination: Immunohistochemical staining was used in the Shpall study to detect breast cancer cell contamination.[163] In patients with tumour initially detected in marrow or blood, a 1 – >4 logs of breast cancer cell depletion occurred after CD34+ selection.

A purging effect in myeloma may also occur. Using patient-specific lg gene primers, PCR analysis of CD34+ PBPC mobilized by chemotherapy and G–CSF in patients with myeloma showed no tumour contamination.[164]

Further studies are required to confirm this purging effect in larger number of patients and in other diseases. Moreover, the clinical relevance of purging remains to be established.

ALLOGENEIC TRANSPLANTS CD34+ selection of allogeneic donor cells may be useful by depleting those mature T cells capable of causing graft versus host disease. This may be particularly relevant in unrelated or haplotype-mismatched related donor allografts. It has been shown that isolated allogeneic CD34+ marrow cells devoid of T and B lymphocytes can engraft and reconstitute stable long-term myelopoiesis and lymphopoiesis in lethally irradiated baboons.[165] CD34+ selection may be particularly important if growth factor-stimulated PBPC collections are used with the intention of speeding haematological recovery, as unmanipulated these collections will contain large numbers of T cells. As with any method of T cell depletion, the impact on the graft versus leukaemia effect of allogeneic cells will need to be evaluted.

Another use of $CD34^+$ selection may be to augment engraftment after counterflow elutriation, a process which results in the partial loss of progenitor cells and delayed engraftment. A preliminary report suggests that the addition of $CD34^+$ cells obtained from the lymphoid fraction reduces the duration of cytopenia after transplantation of elutriated marrow, without increasing the risk of graft versus host disease.[166]

Overview and conclusion

Impact of peripheral blood progenitor cells on resource utilization of autografts

There is now strong evidence from at least three institutions to suggest that, compared with marrow, PBPC autografts are better tolerated, require less transfusion and antibiotic support, and are usually cheaper.

In sequential non-randomized trials in patients receiving identical high dose chemotherapy, the effect of the addition of G–CSF or GM–CSF primed PBPC to marrow on haemopoietic reconstitution and resource utilization was evaluated.[23] The use of both types of PBPCs led to a highly significant reduction in the duration of severe neutropenia and use of antibiotics compared with marrow plus growth factor or marrow alone. The use of G–CSF primed PBPCs was associated with reduced red cell and platelet transfusions, reduced number of days in hospital and discounted hospital charges.

In another large retrospective analysis, autografting with PBPC followed by growth factors was associated with a statistically significant reduction both in the duration of neutropenia and the incidence of infection compared with marrow only autografts.[167]

The Adelaide group compared patients receiving chemotherapy mobilized PBPC or autologous marrow transplants.[168] No growth factors were used. The PBPC group had faster neutrophil and platelet recovery, a shorter hospital stay, fewer febrile days and lower antibiotic, red cell and platelet usage.

The consumable and labour costs of bone marrow harvesting and three LP are roughly comparable.[23] Any substantial savings therefore must be derived from a shorter hospital stay and reduction in transfusions and reduced antibiotic use. As neutrophil recovery after marrow infusion or PBPC infusion followed by G–CSF is roughly comparable (10 vs 9 days)[9] theoretically, at least, infection and antibiotic usage should not differ substantially between these two methods. The rapid platelet recovery seen with PBPC autografts is probably a major factor in cost reduction, due both to less blood product usage and the ability to discharge patients earlier who are platelet transfusion independent.

In addition, it is possible that PBPC autografts generally are better tolerated. The group from Omaha has examined organ dysfunction after autologous transplantation using PBPC or marrow transplants.[169] Independent of underlying disease or conditioning regimen, PBPC autografts were associated with a significantly lower incidence of pulmonary and liver dysfunction, and coagulation factor deficiency.

In future, other issues will need to be factored into assessing the resource utilization of PBPC transplants. These include:

(i) the savings from having to perform only one LP by collecting at the optimal time after chemotherapy and growth factor mobilization.
(ii) the savings by not using a growth factor post PBPC infusion.
(iii) the increased cost of administering multiple cycles of high dose chemotherapy with PBPC support.
(iv) outpatient transplantation. Autologous transplantation with PBPC is now being practised predominantly as an outpatient procedure in some centres, resulting in substantial cost savings.[170] Care of patients involves the use of prophylactic antibiotics, which appear to reduce the incidence of infection,[171] and daily review in a dedicated outpatient facility where transfusions can be performed. This approach may, however, be limited in practice to transplants using conditioning regimens not commonly associated with substantial non-haematological toxicity such as mucositis and diarrhoea.

Does the use of peripheral blood progenitor cells impact on survival?

While it is clear that the use of mobilized PBPC reduces the cost and morbidity of autografting, there is no evidence to suggest that they alter survival rates after autografting. Early transplant-related mortality is now uncommon and may well reflect earlier patient referral and better transfusion and antibiotic support as much as enhanced hematological recovery with growth factors and/or PBPC. The overwhelming cause of treatment failure remains persistent or relapsing disease. There is no evidence that the possibly lower tumour contamination seen with mobilized PBPC compared with marrow is clinically relevant. Studies thus far have not shown any reduction in disease-free survival using PBPC compared with marrow autografts.[101,172]

Various post-transplant immunomodulatory approaches, designed to reduce the rate of relapse, are the subject of current studies. These include the use of cyclosporin,[173] linomide,[174] interleukin 2[175,176] or interferon.[177]

Table 10. *Advantages of mobilized progenitor cells versus bone marrow*

1. No general anaesthesia required for collection.
2. Faster haemopoietic recovery.
3. Sufficient progenitors obtainable to support multiple rounds of high dose chemotherapy.
4. Able to be collected despite pelvic hypocellularity or replacement with tumour.

Cyclosporin is postulated to act by impairing thymic deletion of autoreactive T cell clones generated by the recapitulation of lymphocyte ontogeny after engraftment.[178] Interleukin 2 and linomide act to increase lymphokine-activated killer cell and natural killer cell numbers and activity. The impact, if any, of using PBPC versus marrow on these processes is unknown, although the similar kinetics of immune reconstitution after PBPC and marrow transplants suggest that any difference is unlikely to be substantial.

Conclusions

The advantages of mobilized PBPC over marrow (Table 10) are such that most centres are now routinely using PBPC as the source of autologous haemopoietic rescue after high dose chemotherapy. There is, however, still much to be researched. Issues such as determining the optimal mobilization regimen and the most cost effective and convenient method of assessing when to start and stop LP, the whole area of $CD34^+$ selection, the role of PBPC in allogeneic transplantation, the most cost effective use of growth factors pre-collection and post-infusion, the impact on resource utilization and overall survival of patients with malignant disease, and the impact of the recent identification of a cytokine with powerful thrombopoietic activity[179] all need to be addressed.

References

(1) Metcalf D. *The hemopoietic colony stimulating factors*. Elsevier, Amsterdam 1984.

(2) Sheridan W, Morstyn G, Wolf M et al. Granulocyte colony-stimulating factor and neutrophil recovery after high-dose chemotherapy and autologous bone marrow transplantation. *Lancet* 1989; ii: 891–5.

(3) To LB, Haylock DN, Kimber RJ, Juttner CA. High levels of circulating haemopoietic stem cells in very early remission from acute non-lymphoblastic leukaemia and their collection and cryopreservation. *Br J Haem* 1984; 58: 399–410.

(4) To LB, Dyson P, Branford AL et al. Peripheral blood stem cells collected in very early remission produce rapid and sustained autologous hemopoietic

reconstitution in acute non-lymphoblastic leukaemia. *Bone Marrow Transpl* 1987; 2: 103–8.

(5) Kessinger A, Schmit–Pokorny, Smith D et al. Cryopreservation and infusion of autologous peripheral blood stem cells. *Bone Marrow Transpl* 1990; 5 (suppl 1): 25–7.

(6) Lobo F, Kessinger A, Landmark LD et al. Addition of peripheral blood stem cells collected without mobilization techniques to transplanted autologous bone marrow did not hasten marrow recovery following myeloablative therapy. *Bone Marrow Transpl* 1991; 8: 389–92.

(7) Dührsen U, Villeval J-L, Boyd J et al. Effects of recombinant human granulocyte colony-stimulating factor on hematopoietic progenitor cells in cancer patients. *Blood* 1988; 72: 2074–81.

(8) Socinski MA, Elias A, Schnipper L et al. Granulocyte-macrophage colony stimulating factor expands the circulating haemopoietic progenitor cell compartment in man. *Lancet*, 1988; ii: 1194–8.

(9) Sheridan W, Begley C, Juttner C et al. Effect of peripheral-blood progenitor cells mobilized by filgrastim (G–CSF) on platelet recovery after high-dose chemotherapy. *Lancet* 1992; 339: 640–4.

(10) Bensinger W, Singer J, Appelbaum F et al. Autologous transplantation with peripheral blood mononuclear cells collected after administration of recombinant granulocyte stimulating factor. *Blood* 1993; 81: 3158–63.

(11) Siena S, Bregni M, Brando B, Ravagnani F, Bonadonna G, Gianni AM. Circulation of CD34+ hematopoietic stem cells in the peripheral blood of high-dose cyclophosphamide-treated patients: enhancement by intravenous recombinant human granulocyte-macrophage colony-stimulating factor. *Blood* 1989: 74: 1905–14.

(12) Reiffers J, Faberes C, Boiron JM et al. Peripheral blood progenitor cell transplantation in 118 patients with hematological malignancies: analysis of factors affecting the rate of engraftment [Abstract]. *Blood* 1993; 82 (suppl 1): 166a.

(13) Sheridan WP, Begley CG, To LB et al. Phase ll Study of autologous filgrastim (G–CSF)-mobilized peripheral blood progenitor cells to restore haemopoiesis after high-dose chemotherapy for lymphoid malignancies. *Bone Marrow Transpl* 1994; 14: 105–11.

(14) To LB, Haylock DN, Dyson PG et al. An unusual pattern of hemopoietic reconstitution in patients with acute myeloid leukaemia transplanted with autologous recovery phase peripheral blood. *Bone Marrow Transpl* 1990 6: 109–14.

(15) Chao NJ, Long GD, Negrin RS et al. G–CSF and peripheral blood progenitor cells. *Lancet* 1992; 339: 1410.

(16) Nademanee A, Schmidt GM, Sniecinski IR et al. G–CSF primed peripheral blood stem cell autografts in patients with advanced lymphoid malignancies [Abstract]. *Proceedings of ASCO* 1992; 11: 317.

(17) Sheridan W, Begley G, Juttner C et al. Effect of different doses and schedules of r–met–HuG–CSF (Filgrastim) on mononuclear cell and PBPC collections and haematopoietic recovery after high dose chemotherapy (HDC) and infusion of r–metHuG–CSF mobilized peripheral blood progenitor cells (PBPC) without bone marrow [Abstract]. *Blood* 1992; 80 (suppl 1): 331a.

(18) Nissen C, Dalle Carbonare V, Moser Y. In vitro comparison of the biological potency of glycosylated versus nonglycosylated rG–CSF. *Drug Invest* 1994; 7: 346–52.

(19) Villeval JL, Dührsen U, Morstyn G, Metcalf D. Effect of recombinant human granulocyte–macrophage colony stimulating factor on progenitor cells in patients with advanced malignancies. *Brit J Haem* 1990; 74: 36–44.

(20) Haas R, Ho AD, Bredthauer U et al. Successful autologous transplantation of blood stem cells mobilized with recombinant human granulocyte–macrophage colony-stimulating factor. *Exp Haematol* 1990; 18: 94–8.

(21) Bishop MR, Anderson JR, Jackson JD et al. Effects of granulcoyte–macrophage colony-stimulating factor in mobilization and engraftment of peripheral blood progenitor cells [Abstract]. *Blood* 1993; 82 (suppl 1): 627a.

(22) Kritz A, Crown JP, Motzer RJ et al. Beneficial impact of peripheral blood progentior cells in patients with metastatic breast cancer treated with high-dose chemotherapy plus granulocyte–macrophage colony-stimulating factor. *Cancer* 1993; 71: 2515–21.

(23) Peters WP, Rosner G, Ross M et al. Comparative effects of granulocyte–macrophage colony-stimulating factor (GM–CSF) and granulocyte colony-stimulating factor (G–CSF) on priming peripheral blood progenitor cells for use with autologous bone marrow after high-dose chemotherapy. *Blood* 1993; 81: 1709–19.

(24) Januszewicz H, Wolf M, Cooper IA et al. Autotransplantation with peripheral blood stem cells mobilized by granulocyte–macrophage colony stimulating factor (GM–CSF) (submitted for publication).

(25) Bolwell B, Dannley R, Goormastic M et al. A comparison of G–CSF with GM–CSF for mobilisation of peripheral blood progenitor cells and for enhancement of marrow recovery post autologous bone marrow transplant [Abstract]. *Blood* 1993; 82 (suppl 1): 83a.

(26) Edmonson JH, Hartmann LC, Jong et al. Granulocyte–macrophage colony-stimulating factor. Preliminary observations on the influences of dose, schedule and route of administration in patients receiving cyclophosphamide and carboplatin. *Cancer* 1992; 70: 2529–39.

(27) Lieschke GJ, Maher D, O'Connor M et al. Phase I study of intravenously administered bacterially synthesized granulocyte–macrophage colony-stimulating factor and comparison with subcutaneous administration. *Cancer Res* 1990; 50: 606–14.

(28) O'Day S, Rabinowe S, Neuberg D et al. A Phase II Study of continuous infusion recombinant human granulocyte–macrophage colony-stimulating factor (rhGM-CSF) as an adjunct to autologous bone marrow transplantation (ABMT) for non-Hodgkin's lymphoma (NHL) in first remission. *Blood* 1993; 82 (suppl 1): 145a.

(29) Bregni M, Siena S, Di Nicola M et al. RhGM–CSF or rhG–CSF to enhance circulation of hematopoietic progenitors and to ameliorate the hematologic toxicity of high-dose cyclophosphamide (HD–CTX) cancer therapy [Abstract]. *Blood* 1993; 82 (suppl 1): 495a.

(30) Beveridge RA, Kales AN, Binder RA, Robert NJ, Miller JA. Comparison of toxicities of G–CSF and yeast derived GM–CSF [Abstract]. *Blood* 1993; 82 (suppl 1): 495a.

(31) Teshima T, Harada M, Takamatsu Y et al. Granulocyte colony-stimulating factor (G–CSF)-induced mobilisation of circulating haemopoietic stem cells. *Br J Haem* 1993; 84: 570–3.

(32) Elias AD, Ayash L, Anderson KC et al. Mobilisation of peripheral blood progenitor cells by chemotherapy and granulocyte–macrophage colony-stimulating factor for hematologic support after high-dose intensification for breast cancer. *Blood* 1992; 11: 3036–44.

(33) Shimazaki C, Oku N, Ashihara E et al. Collection of peripheral blood stem cells mobilized by high-dose Ara-C plus VP-16 or aclarubicin followed by recombinant human granulocyte–colony stimulating factor. *Bone Marrow Transplant* 1992; 10:341–6.

(34) Brugger W, Birken R, Bertz H et al. Peripheral blood progenitor cells mobilized by chemotherapy plus granulocyte-colony stimulating factor accelerate both neutrophil and platelet recovery after high-dose VP16, ifosfamide and cisplatin. *Br J Haematol* 1993; 84: 402–7.

(35) Haas R, Ehrhardt R, Witt B et al. Autografting with peripheral blood stem cells mobilized by sequential interleukin-3/granulocyte–macrophage colony-stimulating factor following high-dose chemotherapy in non-Hodgkin's lymphoma. *Bone Marrow Transplant* 1993; 12: 643–9.

(36) Ho AD, Glück S, Germond C et al. Optimal timing for collections of blood progenitor cells following induction chemotherapy and granulocyte–macrophage colony-stimulating factor for autologous transplantation in advanced breast cancer. *Leukaemia* 1993; 7: 1738–46.

(37) Hohaus S, Goldschmidt H, Ehrhardt R, Haas R. Successful autografting following myeloablative conditioning therapy with blood stem cells mobilized by chemotherapy plus rhG-CSF. *Exp Haematol* 1993; 21: 508–14.

(38) Pettengell R, Morgenstern G, Change J et al. Peripheral blood progenitor cell (PBPC): The single apheresis transplant [Abstract]. *Fifth International Conference on Malignant Lymphoma*, Lugano, 1993: 39.

(39) Lickliter JD, Begley CG, Boyd AW, Szer J, Grigg AP. Combined chemotherapy and granulocyte colony-stimulating factor (G–CSF) mobilize large numbers of peripheral blood progenitor cells in pretreated patients. *Leukaemia and Lymphoma* 1994 (in press).

(40) Pettengell R, Testa NG, Swindell R, Crowther D, Dexter TM. Transplantation potential of hematopoietic cells released into the circulation during routine chemotherapy for non-Hodgkin's lymphoma. *Blood* 1993; 82:2239–48.

(41) Tarella C, Boccadoro M, Omedé P et al. Role of chemotherapy and GM–CSF on hemopoietic progenitor cell mobilization in multiple myeloma. *Bone Marrow Transpl* 1993; 11:271–7.

(42) Rowlings PA, Rawling CM, To LB, Bayly JL, Juttner CA. A comparison of peripheral blood stem cell mobilisation after chemotherapy with cyclophosphamide as a single agent in doses of 4 g/m^2 or 7 g/m^2 in patients with advanced cancer. *Aust NZ J Med* 1992; 22:660–4.

(43) Gianni AM, Siena S, Bregni M et al. Granulocyte–macrophage colony-stimulating factor to harvest circulating haemopoietic stem cells for autotransplantation. *Lancet* 1989; 580–5.

(44) Boiron J-M, Marit G, Fabéres C et al. Collection of peripheral blood stem cells in multiple myeloma following single high-dose cyclophosphamide with and without recombinant human granulocyte–macrophage colony–stimulating factor (rhGM–CSF). *Bone Marrow Transpl* 1993; 12:49–55.
(45) Craig JI, Anthon RS, Stewart A, Thomson EB, Gillon J, Parker AC. Peripheral blood stem cell mobilisation using high-dose cyclophosphamide and G–CSF in pretreated patients with lymphoma. *Br J Haem* 1993; 85:210–12.
(46) Dale BM, Kotasek D, Sage RE, Norman JE, Bolton A. Peripheral blood stem cell (PBSC) mobilisation with and without granulocyte colony stimulating factor (G–CSF). A comparison of three mobilising regimens [Abstract]. *Proceedings of the 31st Annual Scientific Meeting of the Haematology Society of Australia* 1993; 124, and B Dale, personal communication.
(47) Jones HM, Jones SA, Watts MJ et al. The effects of variation of the dose and schedule of G–CSF administration after low dose cyclophosphamide (1.5 g/m^2) on both neutrophil and peripheral blood haemopoietic progenitor cell levels [Abstract]. *Blood* 1993; 82 (suppl 1):233a.
(48) Liberti G, Indovina A, Buscemi F et al. Single intermediate-dose (4 g/m^2) cyclophosphamide and G–CSF for mobilisation of circulating stem cells on an outpatient basis [Abstract]. *Fifth International Conference on Malignant Lymphoma*, Lugano 1993; 171.
(49) Passos–Coelho JL, Braine H, Davis JM et al. Primed peripheral blood stem cells collected in a single large volume leukaperesis accelerate hematopoietic recovery after high-dose chemotherapy [Abstract]. *Blood* 1993; 82 (suppl 1):84a.
(50) Siena S, Bregni M, Brando M et al. Flow cytometry for clinical estimation of circulating hematopoietic progenitors for autologous transplantation in cancer patients. *Blood* 1991; 77: 400–9.
(51) Cottler–Fox M, Sink BS, Yu M, Leitman SF, Dunbar CE. Mobilization and collection of peripheral blood stem cells (PBSC) for autologous transplant in multiple myeloma using intravenous G–CSF and cyclophosphamide [Abstract]. *Blood* 1993; 82: 265a.
(52) Haas R, Möhle, Fruehauf S, Pförsich M, Witt B, Hunstein W. Mobilisation of peripheral blood stem cells with cytotoxic chemotherapy and granulocyte colony-stimulating factor (G–CSF) in malignant lymphoma. *Hematopoietic Stem Cells: The Mulhouse Manual* 1994; 113–21.
(53) Kanz L, Brugger W, Mertelsmann R. Haematopoietic growth factors and peripheral blood stem cells as supportive agents in dose intensification. *Eur J Cancer* 1993; 29A: S23–6.
(54) Liu K-Y, Akashi K, Harada M, Takamatsu Y, Niho Y. Kinetics of circulating haematopoietic progenitors during chemotherapy-induced mobilization with or without granulocyte colony-stimulating factor. *Br J Haematol* 1993; 84: 31–8.
(55) Tilly H, Vannier JP, Jean P, Bastit D, Monconduit M, Piguet H. Daily evaluation of circulating granulocyte-monocyte progenitors during bone marrow recovery from induction therapy in acute leukaemia. *Leuk Res* 1986; 10: 353–6.

(56) De Luca E, Sheridan WP, Watson D, Szer J, Begley CG. Prior chemotherapy does not prevent effective mobilisation by G–CSF of peripheral blood progenitor cells. *Br J Cancer* 1992; 66: 893–9.
(57) Vredenburgh JJ, Waters-Pick B, Kurtzberg J et al. A single 6-hour steady state leukapheresis is sufficient for collection of peripheral blood progenitor cells (PBPC) after G–CSF [Abstract]. *Blood* 1993; 82: 349a.
(58) Pettengell R, Morgenstern GR, Woll PJ et al. Peripheral blood progenitor cell transplantation in lymphoma and leukemia using a single apheresis. *Blood* 1993; 82: 3770–7.
(59) Brice P, Marolleau JP, Dombret H et al. Autologous peripheral blood stem cell transplantation after high dose therapy in patients with advanced lymphomas. *Bone Marrow Transpl* 1992 9: 337–42.
(60) Akard L, Lane J, Wiemann M et al. Hematopoietic reconstitution following peripheral stem cell (PBSC) transplant [Abstract]. *Blood* 1993; 82: 428a.
(61) To LB, Dyson PG, Juttner CA. Cell-dose effect in circulating stem-cell autografting. *Lancet* 1986; ii: 404–5.
(62) Juttner CA, To LB, Haylock DN et al. Approaches to blood stem cell mobilisation. Initial Australian clinical results. *Bone Marrow Transpl* 1990; 5 (suppl 1): 22–4.
(63) Bitran JD, Martinec J, Okuno T et al. Autologous bone marrow transplantation using peripheral blood hematopoietic progenitor cells. The total number of $CD34^+$ cells/kg predicts for hematologic engraftment [Abstract]. *Blood* 1993; 82: 288a.
(64) Jouault J, Beaujean F, Leforestier C, Bayle C, Jarry MT, Imbert M. Quantitation of peripheral blood progenitor cells (PBPC) for autologous transplantation: Comparison between flow cytometric measurement of $CD34^+$ cells and CFU–GM assay in 13 patients [Abstract]. *Blood* 1993; 82 (suppl 1): 294a.
(65) O'Kane Murphy B, Jackson JD, Bociek G et al. CD34 analysis of GM–CSF mobilized peripheral blood stem cells [Abstract]. *Blood* 1993; 82 (suppl 1): 488a.
(66) Möhle R, Haas R, Hunstein W. Filgrastim-mobilized $CD34^+$ peripheral blood stem cells (PBSC) contain more primitive hematopoietic progenitor cells during steady-state hematopoiesis than post-chemotherapy [Abstract]. *Blood* 1993; 82 (suppl 1): 14a.
(67) Dercksen MW, Gerritsen WR, Rodenhuis S et al. Additional phenotyping of CD34 positive cells improves correlation with hematopoietic recovery after PBSC [Abstract]. *Blood* 1993; 82: 298a.
(68) Raptis G, Vahdat L, Fennelly D et al. Peripheral blood progenitor supported high-dose chemotherapy: determination of a threshold number of $CD34^+$ cells for reliable engraftment [Abstract]. *Blood* 1993; 82 (suppl 1): 289a.
(69) Schwartzberg L, Birch R, Heffernan M, West W. G–CSF is an effective supportive modality in peripheral blood stem cell (PBSC) transplantation [Abstract]. *Blood* 1993; 82 (suppl 1): 286a.
(70) Demuynck H, Pettengell R, de Campos E, Dexter TM, Testa NG. The capacity of peripheral blood stem cells mobilized with chemotherapy plus G–CSF to repopulate irradiated marrow stroma in vitro is similar to that of bone marrow. *Eur J Cancer* 1992; 28: 381–6.

(71) Tarosky T, Gremba C, Rosenfeld CS. Determination of mononuclear cells in mobilized peripheral blood stem cell collections. *Bone Marrow Transpl* 1994; 13: 670.

(72) Legros M, Fleury J, Curé H et al. A new method of stem cell quantification: Practical applications in the management of PBPC transplantation [Abstract]. *Blood* 1992; 81 (suppl 1): 82a.

(73) Spitzer G, Spencer V, Dunphy F et al. Are growth factors (GF) needed after peripheral blood stem cell (PBSC) transplantation? A randomised study to evaluate the question [Abstract]. *Blood* 1993; 82 (suppl 1): 288a.

(74) Klumpp TR, Mangan KF, Goldberg SL et al. The effect of granulocyte colony-stimulating factor (G–CSF) on neutrophil engraftment following autologous peripheral blood stem cell (PBSC) transplantation: A prospective, randomised study [Abstract]. *Blood* 1993; 82 (suppl 1): 285a.

(75) Elias A, Ayash L, Anderson K et al. GM–CSF-mobilized peripheral blood progenitor cells (PBPC) support after high dose chemotherapy for breast cancer: Effect of GM–CSF post reinfusion [Abstract]. *Blood* 1991; 78 (suppl 1): 400a.

(76) Ikebuchi K, Wong GG, Clark SC, Ihle JN, Hirai Y. Interleukin-6 enhancement of interleukin-3 dependent proliferation of multipotential hemopoietic progenitors. *Proc Natl Acad Sci USA* 1987; 84: 9033–7.

(77) To LB, Haylock DN, Dowse T, Simmons PJ, Ashman LK, Juttner CA. Phenotype and proliferative capacity of peripheral blood $CD34^+$ cells mobilized by four different protocols. *Blood* 1993; 82 (suppl 1): 493a.

(78) Möhle R, Haas R, Hunstein W. Expression of adhesion molecules and c-kit on $CD34^+$ hematopoietic progenitor cells: comparison of cytokine-mobilized blood stem cells with normal bone marrow and peripheral blood. *J Hematotherapy* 1993; 2: 483–9.

(79) Bender JG, Unverzagt KL, Walker DE et al. Identification and comparison of CD34 positive cells and their subpopulations from normal peripheral blood and bone marrow using multicolor follow cytometry. *Blood* 1991; 77: 2591–6.

(80) Pincus SM, Nimgaonkar M, Roscoe RA, Patel A, Ball ED, Winkelstein A. A comparative study of blood and marrow derived $CD34^+$ cells: subset analysis reveals differences in the frequencies of primitive hematopoietic stem cells [Abstract]. *Blood* 1993; 82 (suppl 1): 12a.

(81) Siena S, Bregni M, Brando B et al. Flow cytometry for clinical estimation of circulating hematopoietic progenitors for autologous transplantation in cancer patients. *Blood* 1991; 77: 400–9.

(82) Bender JG, Unverzagt KL, Walker DE et al. Characterisation of $CD34^+$ cells mobilized to the peripheral blood during the recovery from cyclophosphamide chemotherapy. *Int J Cell Cloning* 1992; 10 (suppl 1): 23–5.

(83) Haas R, Ehrhardt R, Witt B et al. Autografting with peripheral blood stem cells mobilized by sequential interleukin-3/granulocyte–macrophage colony-stimulating factor following high-dose chemotherapy in non-Hodgkin's lymphoma. *Bone Marrow Transplant* 1993; 12: 643–9.

(84) Möhle R, Haas R, Hunstein W. Filgrastim-mobilized $CD34^+$ peripheral blood stem cells (PBSC) contain more primitive hematopoietic progenitor cells during steady-state hematopoiesis than post-chemotherapy [Abstract]. *Blood* 1993; 82 (suppl 1): 14a.

(85) Kanz L, Brugger W, Mertelsmann R. Haematopoietic growth factors and peripheral blood stem cells as supportive agents in dose intensification. *Eur J Cancer* 1993; 29A: S23–6.

(86) Neben S, Marcus K, Mauch P. Mobilisation of hematopoietic stem and progenitor cell subpopulations from the marrow to the blood of mice following cyclophosphamide and/or granulocyte colony-stimulating factor. *Blood* 1993; 81: 1960–7.

(87) Sutherland HJ, Eaves CJ, Lansdorp PM, Phillips GL, Hogge DE. Peripheral blood long-term culture-initiating cell (LTC–IC) numbers rebound early after chemotherapy and GM–CSF [Abstract]. *Blood* 1991; 80 (suppl 1): 250a.

(88) Dooley D, Spurgin P, Hansen K, Hansen L, Lanier K, Maziarz R. Mobilisation of human long-term culture initiating cells (LTC–IC) into peripheral blood (PB) by granulocyte-colony stimulating factor (G–CSF) [Abstract]. *Blood* 1993; 82 (suppl 1): 292a.

(89) Inaba T, Shimazaki C, Hirata T et al. Phenotypic differences of CD34-positive stem cells harvested from peripheral blood and bone marrow obtained before and after peripheral blood stem cell collection. *Bone Marrow Transplant* 1994; 13:527–32.

(90) Siena S, Bregni M, Bonsi L et al. Increase in peripheral blood megakaryocyte progenitors following cancer therapy with high-dose cyclophosphamide and hematopoietic growth factors. *Exp Hematol* 1993; 21:1583–90.

(91) Storozynsky E, Frediani K, Bray P, Dang C, DiPersio J. Identification and characterisation of $CD34^+$, $CD33^-$, $CD41a^+$ (gpIIb/IIIa) progenitors in the peripheral blood in patients undergoing cytoxan and cytokine-induced PBPC mobilisation [Abstract]. *Blood* 1993; 82 (suppl 1):70a.

(92) Rill DR, Holladay MS, Heslop HE et al. The contribution of autologous marrow infusion to the restoration of long-term hemopoiesis in cancer patients: a study using gene marking. *Blood* 1993; 82 (suppl 1):86a.

(93) Deisseroth A, Zu A, Claxton D et al. Retroviral marking studies show that infused exogenous marrow cells give rise to hematopoietic recovery after autologous transplant, and that relapse after autologous transplant in CML may arise from Ph^+ cells present in marrow at the time of transplant [Abstract]. *Blood* 1993; 82 (suppl 1): 454a.

(94) To LB, Dyson P, Branford AL et al. Peripheral blood stem cells collected in very early remission produce rapid and sustained autologous hemopoietic reconstitution in acute non-lymphoblastic leukaemia. *Bone Marrow Transplant* 1987; 2:103–8.

(95) Baumann I, van Hoeff M, Swindell R et al. The peak numbers of colony forming cells and of $CD34^+$ cells released into peripheral blood after G–CSF with or without chemotherapy may not be correlated with the capacity of harvested blood cells to repopulate bone marrow. *Christie Hospital NHS Trust, Annual Research Report* 1993:56.

(96) Shpall EJ, Jones RB. Release of tumour cells from bone marrow. *Blood* 1994; 83:623–5.

(97) Brugger W, Bross KJ, Glatt M, Weber F, Mertelsmann R, Kanz L. Mobilization of tumour cells and haematopoietic progenitor cells into peripheral blood of patients with solid tumours. *Blood* 1994; 83:636–40.

(98) Berinstein NL, Reis MD, Ngan BY, Sawka CA, Jamal JJ, Kuzniar B. Detection of occult lymphoma in the peripheral blood and bone marrow of patients with untreated early-stage and advanced-stage follicular lymphoma. *J Clin Oncol* 1993; 11:1344–52.
(99) Sharp JC, Kessinger A, Mann S et al. Detection and clinical significance of minimal tumour cell contamination of peripheral blood stem cell harvests. *Int J Cell Cloning* 1992; 10 (suppl 1):92.
(100) Moss TJ, Saunders DG, Lasky LC, Bostrom B. Contamination of peripheral blood stem cell harvests by circulating neuroblastoma cells. *Blood* 1990; 76:1879–83.
(101) Weisdorf K, Daniels K, Miller W et al. Bone Marrow vs peripheral blood stem cells for autologous lymphoma transplantation: a prospective randomized trial [Abstract]. *Blood* 1993; 82 (suppl 1):444a.
(102) Hardingham JE, Kotasek D, Sage RE, Dobrovic A, Gooley T, Dale BM. Molecular detection of residual lymphoma cells in peripheral blood stem cell harvests and following autologous transplantation. *Bone Marrow Transpl* 1993; 11:15–20.
(103) Bird JM, Bloxham D, Russell NH, Samson D, Apperley JF. Detection of clonally rearranged cells in pbsc harvests in multiple myeloma by immunoglobulin gene fingerprinting [Abstract]. *Blood* 1993; 82 (suppl 1):265a.
(104) Dreyfus F, Melle J, Quarre MC, Pillier C. Contamination of peripheral blood by monoclonal B cells following treatment of multiple myeloma by high-dose chemotherapy. *Br J Haematol* 1993; 85:411–12.
(105) Ross AA, Cooper BW, Lazarus HM et al. Detection and viability of tumour cells in peripheral blood stem cells collections from breast cancer patients using immunocytochemical and clonogenic assay techniques. *Blood* 1993; 82:2605–10.
(106) Anthony RS, Craig JIO, Langlands K, Parker AC. Tumour contamination of peripheral blood stem cells collected from patients with leukaemia and lymphoma [Abstract]. *Blood* 1993; 82 (suppl 1):349a.
(107) Carella AM, Frassoni F, Podesta M et al. Intensive chemotherapy and G–CSF are capable in CML patients of recruiting CD34+ DR− cells with high proliferative potential and sustain Ph-negative polyclonal haematopoiesis [Abstract]. *Blood* 1993; 82 (suppl 1):297a.
(108) Carella AM, Pollicard N, Carlier P et al. 'Normal' peripheral blood stem cell mobilisation by myelosuppressive chemotherapy in very high-risk acute lymphoblastic leukaemia with cytogenetic translocations. *Leukaemia and Lymphoma* 1992; 7:19–21.
(109) Brenner MK, Rill DR, Moen RC et al. Gene-marking to trace origin of relapse after autologous bone-marrow transplantation. *Lancet* 1993; 341:85–6.
(110) Uckun FM, Kersey JH, Vallera DA et al. Autologous bone marrow transplantation in high-risk remission T-lineage acute lymphoblastic leukaemia using immunotoxins plus 4-hydroperoxycyclophosphamide for marrow purging. *Blood* 1990; 76:1723–33.
(111) Kramer MHH, Kluin-Nelemans, Kluin Ph. M, Fibb. WE. Occurrence of t(14; 18)-positive monoclonal plasma cells following treatment with IL-3 in

a patient with follicular lymphoma. *Fifth International Conference on Malignant Lymphoma*, Lugano 1993; 60.

(112) Clayberger C, Luna–Fineman S, Lee JE et al. Interleukin 3 is a growth factor for human follicular B cell lymphoma. *J Exp Med* 1992; 175:371–6.

(113) Winter JN, Mangan C, Byrd K et al. Combined r-G- and GM–CSF priming of peripheral blood stem cell harvests [Abstract]. *Blood* 1993; 82 (suppl 1):293a.

(114) Ottman OG, Ganser A, Seipelt G et al. Effects of recombinant human interleukin-3 on human hematopoietic progenitor and precursor cells in vivo. *Blood* 1990; 76:1494–502.

(115) D'Hondt V, Weynants P, Humblet Y et al. Dose dependent interleukin-3 stimulation of thrombopoiesis and neutropoiesis in patients with small-cell lung carcinoma before and following chemotherapy: A placebo-controlled randomized phase lb study. *J Clin Oncol* 1993; 11:2063–71.

(116) Huhn R, Yurkow EJ, Clarke L et al. Clinical and hematopoietic effects of recombinant human Interleukin-3 administered by daily subcutaneous injection to healthy normal volunteers [Abstract]. *Blood* 1993, 82 (suppl 1): 500a.

(117) Ganser A, Lindemann A, Ottman OG et al. Sequential in vivo treatment with two recombinant human hematopoietic growth factors (interleukin-3 and granulocyte-macrophage colony-stimulating factor) as a new therapeutic modality to stimulate hematopoiesis: Results of a phase I study. *Blood* 1992; 79:2583–91.

(118) Geissler K, Valent P, Mayer P et al. Recombinant Human interleukin-3 expands the pool of circulating hemopoietic stem cells in primates. Synergism with recombinant human granulocyte/macrophage colony-stimulating factor. *Blood* 1990; 75:2305–10.

(119) Brugger W, Bross K, Frisch J et al. Mobilization of peripheral blood progenitor cells by sequential administration of interleukin-3 and granulocyte-macrophage colony-stimulating factor following polychemotherapy with etoposide, ifosfamide and cisplatin. *Blood* 1992; 79:1193–200.

(120) Mason J, Ho A, Mullen M et al. High-dose carboplatin with peripheral blood stem cells and sequential interleukin-3 and GM–CSF [Abstract]. *Blood* 1993; 82 (suppl 1): 365a.

(121) To LB, Rawling C, Andary C et al. The efficacy of sequential/combined IL3/GM-CSF administration in peripheral blood progenitor mobilisation [Abstract]. *Blood* 1993; 82 (suppl 1): 83a.

(122) Andrews RG, Knitter GH, Bartelmez SH et al. Recombinant human stem cell factor, a c-kit ligand, stimulates hematopoiesis in primates. *Blood* 1991; 78:1975–80.

(123) Tong J, Gordon MS, Srour EF et al. In vivo administration of recombinant methionyl human stem cell factor expands the number of human marrow hematopoietic stem cells. *Blood* 1993; 82:784–91.

(124) Andrews RG, Bartelmez S, Knitter GH et al. A c-*kit* ligand, recombinant human stem cell factor, mediates reversible expansion of multiple $CD34^+$ colony-forming cell types in blood and marrow of baboons. *Blood* 1992; 80:920–7.

(125) Demetri G, Costa J, Hayes D et al. A phase I trial of recombinant methionyl human stem cell factor (SCF) in patients with advanced breast carcinoma pre

and post-chemotherapy with cyclophosphamide and doxorubicin [Abstract]. *Proceedings of ASCO* 1993; 12:142.
(126) Molineux G, Migdalska A, Szmitkowski M, Zsebo K, Dexter TM. The effects on hematopoiesis of recombinant stem cell factor (ligand for *c-kit*) administered in vivo to mice either alone or in combination with granulocyte colony-stimulating factor. *Blood* 1991; 78:961-6.
(127) Andrews RG, Briddell, Knitter GH et al. Low dose recombinant human stem cell factor has a synergistic interaction with recombinant human granulocyte colony-stimulating factor in vivo for stimulating the circulation of progenitor cells of multiple types in the peripheral blood of baboons [Abstract]. *Blood* 1993; 82 (suppl 1): 232a.
(128) Briddell RA, Hartley CA, Smith KA, McNiece IK. Recombinant rat stem cell factor synergizes with recombinant human granulocyte colony-stimulating factor in vivo in mice to mobilize peripheral blood progenitor cells that have enhanced repopulating potential. *Blood* 1993; 82: 1720–3.
(129) Glaspy J, McNiece I, LeMaistre F et al. Effects of stem cell factor (rhSCF) and filgrastim (rhG–CSF) on mobilisation of peripheral blood progenitor cells (PBPC) and on hematological recovery post transplant: early results from a phase I/II study [Abstract]. *Proceedings of ASCO* 1994; 13: 68.
(130) Briddell R, Glaspy J, Shpall EJ, LeMaistre F, Menchaca D, McNiece I. Mobilisation of myeloid, erythroid and megakaryocyte progenitors by recombinant human stem cell factor (rhSCF) plus filgrastim (rhG-CSF) in patients with breast cancer [Abstract]. *Proceedings of ASCO* 1994; 13: 77.
(131) Basser R, Begley CG, Maher D et al. The use of peripheral blood progenitor cells mobilized by stem cell factor and filgrastim to support multiple cycles of high-dose chemotherapy in untreated women with poor prognosis breast cancer [Abstract]. *Br J Haematol* 1994; 87 (suppl 1): 91.
(132) Kessinger A, Bishop M, Jackson J et al. Erythropoietin for mobilisation of circulating progenitor cells in patients with previously treated malignancies [Abstract]. *Blood* 1993; 82 (suppl 1): 227a.
(133) Jackson JD, Yan U, Kelsey L, Faltynek C, Talmadge JE. Mobilisation of hematopoietic progenitors following IL-7 administration post chemotherapy [Abstract]. *Blood* 1993; 82 (suppl 1): 368a.
(134) Fibbe WE, Hamilton MS, Laterveer LL et al. Sustained engraftment of mice transplanted with IL-1-primed blood-derived stem cells. *J Immunol* 1992; 148: 417–21.
(135) Laterveer L, Hamilton M, Lindley I, Willemze, Fibbe WE. A single dose of Interleukin-8 induces mobilisation of myeloid progenitor cells with radio-protective capacity [Abstract]. *Blood* 1993; 82 (suppl 1): 293a.
(136) Goldman SJ. Hematologic effects of rhIL-11 in nonhuman primates [Abstract]. *First International Symposium: Cytokines in Bone Marrow Transplantation*, Christchurch 1993; 103.
(137) Orazi A, Cooper R, Tong J et al. Recombinant human Interleukin-11 has multiple profound effects on human hematopoiesis [Abstract]. *Blood* 1993; 82 (suppl 1): 369a.
(138) Quinto CM, Leonard JP, Kozitza MK, Goldman SJ. Synergistic interactions between rhIL-11 and G-CSF in the mobilisation of hematopoietic prognenitors [Abstract]. *Blood* 1993; 82 (suppl 1): 369a.

(139) Henon Ph R, Liang H, Beck-Wirth G et al. Comparison of hematopoietic and immune recovery after autologous bone marrow or blood stem cell transplants. *Bone Marrow Transpl* 1992; 9: 285–91.
(140) Roberts MM, To LB, Gillis D et al. Immune reconstitution following peripheral blood stem cell transplantation, autologous bone marrow transplantation and allogeneic bone marrow transplantation. *Bone Marrow Transpl* 1993; 12: 469–75
(141) Molineux G, Pojda Z, Hampson IN, Lord Bl, Dexter TM. Transplantation potential of peripheral blood stem cells induced by granulocyte colony-stimulating factor. *Blood* 1990; 76: 2153–8.
(142) Dreger P, Suttorp M, Haferlach T, Loffler H, Schmitz N, Schroyens W. Allogeneic granulocyte colony-stimulating factor-mobilised peripheral blood progenitor cells for treatment of engraftment failure after bone marrow transplantation. *Blood* 1993; 81: 1404–7.
(143) Russell NH, Hunter A, Rogers S, Hanley J, Anderson D. Peripheral blood stem cells as an alternative to marrow for allogeneic transplantation. *Lancet* 1993; 341: 1482.
(144) Nemunaitis, Rosenfeld C, Collins R et al. Pilot trial of allogeneic transplant combining peripheral blood and bone marrow in patients with refractory hematologic malignancy [Abstract]. *Blood* 1993; 82 (suppl 1): 417a.
(145) Brugger W, Möcklin W, Heimfeld S et al. Ex vivo expansion of enriched peripheral blood CD34+ progenitor cells by stem cell factor, interleukin 1b, IL–6, IL–3 interferon-γ, and erythropoietin. *Blood* 1993; 81: 2579–84.
(146) Sato N, Sawada K, Koizumi K et al. In vitro expansion of human peripheral blood CD34+ cells. *Blood* 1993; 12: 3600–39.
(147) Haylock DN, To LB, Dowse TL et al. Ex vivo expansion and maturation of peripheral blood stem and progenitor cells for transplantation [Abstract]. *Blood* 1993; 82 (suppl 1): 483a.
(148) Shea TC, Mason JR, Storniolo AM et al. Sequential cycles of high-dose carboplatin administered with recombinant human granulocyte-macrophage colony-stimulating factor and repeated infusions of autologous peripheral-blood progenitor cells: a novel and effective method for delivering multiple courses of dose-intensive therapy. *J Clin Oncol* 1992; 10: 464–73.
(149) Basser R, To B, Green M et al. Rapid hematopoietic reconstitution following 3 cycles of high dose chemotherapy with filgrastim (G-CSF)-mobilized peripheral blood progenitor cells (PBPC) and filgrastim in patients with high risk breast cancer [Abstract]. *Blood* 1993; 82 (suppl 1): 233a.
(150) Chao NJ, Long GD, Negrin RS et al. Multiple high dose chemotherapy cycles supported by peripheral blood progenitor cells and G – CSF [Abstract]. *Blood* 1993; 82 (suppl 1): 349a.
(151) Crown J, Kritz A, Vahdat L et al. Rapid administration of multiple cycles of high-dose myelosuppressive chemotherapy in patients with metastatic breast cancer. *J Clin Oncol* 1993; 11: 1144–9.
(152) Tepler I, Cannistra SA, Frei III E et al. Use of peripheral-blood progenitor cells abrogates the myelotoxicity of repetitive outpatient high-dose carboplatin and cyclophosphamide chemotherapy. *J Clin Oncol* 1993; 11: 1583–91.
(153) Wheeler C, Shulman LN, Elias A et al. Sequential ifosfamide, carboplatin,

etoposide with steroids and cyclophosphamide/G-CSF mobilized peripheral blood progenitor cell support in relapsed lymphoma [Abstract]. *Blood* 1993; 82 (suppl 1): 144a.

(154) Ossenkopple GJ, Jonkhoff AR, Huijgens PC et al. Peripheral blood progenitors mobilized by G–CSF (filgrastim) and reinfused as unprocessed autologous whole blood shorten the pancytopenic period following high-dose melphalan in multiple myeloma. *Bone Marrow Transpl* 1994; 13: 37–41.

(155) Andrews RG, Singer JW, Bernstein ID. Monoclonal antibody 12–8 recognizes a 115–kd molecule present on both unipotent and multipotent colony-forming cells and their precursors. *Blood* 1986; 67: 842–5.

(156) Heimfeld S, Andrews R, Bensinger W et al. Peripheral blood stem cell mobilisation: rapid enrichment of progenitor cells using a unique biotin–avidin immunoaffinity separation system. *Blood* 1991; 78 (suppl 1): 16a.

(157) Brugger W, Henschler R, Heimfeld S et al. Hematopoietic recovery after high-dose chemotherapy is identical with positively selected peripheral blood CD34+ Cells and unseparated peripheral blood progenitor cells (PBPCs) [Abstract]. *Blood* 1993; 82 (suppl 1): 455a.

(158) Körbling M, Drach J, Champlin RE et al. Large-scale preparation of highly purified, frozen/thawed CD34+ HLA–DR- hematopoietic progenitor cells by sequential immunoadsorption (CEPRATE SC) and fluorescence-activated cell sorting: implications for gene transduction and/or transplantation. *Bone Marrow Transpl* 1994; 13: 649–54.

(159) Berenson RJ, Bensinger WI, Andrews RG et al. Hematopoietic Stem Cell Transplants, in Gale RP, Golde DW (eds): Recent advances in leukaemia and lymphoma, *UCLA Symposia on Molecular and Cellular Biology*, New Series. New York, NY, Liss, 1987, 61: 527–33.

(160) Berenson RJ, Andrews RG, Bensinger WI. Antigen CD34+ marrow cells engraft lethally irradiated baboons. *J Clin Invest* 1988; 81: 951–5.

(161) Berenson RJ, Bensinger WI, Hill RS et al. Engraftment after infusion of CD34+ marrow cells in patients with breast cancer or neuroblastoma. *Blood* 1991; 77: 1717–22.

(162) Adkins D, Berenson R, Bowers C et al. CD34+ concentrated peripheral blood stem cells (CPBSC) infused after high-dose chemotherapy (HDCT) result in equivalent hematopoietic engraftment kinetics as compared to unconcentrated PBSC and autologous bone marrow transplantation (ABMT) [Abstract]. *Blood* 1993; 82 (suppl 1): 290a.

(163) Shpall EJ, Jones RP, Bearman SI et al. Transplantation of enriched CD34-positive autologous marrow into breast cancer patients following high-dose chemotherapy: influence of CD34-positive peripheral-blood progenitors and growth factors on engraftment. *J Clin Oncol* 1994; 12: 28–36.

(164) Schiller G, Vescio R, Lee M et al. Transplantation of autologous CD34-positive peripheral blood stem cells as treatment for multiple myeloma [Abstract]. *Blood* 1993; 82 (suppl 1): 198a.

(165) Andrews RG, Bryant EM, Bartelmez SH et al. CD34+ marrow cells, devoid of T and B lymphocytes, reconstitute stable lymphopoiesis and myelopoiesis in lethally irradiated allogeneic baboons. *Blood* 1992; 80: 1693–701.

(166) Wagner JE, Filipovich A, McGlave P et al. Transplantation of allogeneic

CD34+ stem and progenitor cells: Results of a phase I–II study [Abstract]. *Blood* 1993; 82 (suppl 1): 290a.
(167) Mossad S, Longworth D, Goormastic M, Serkey J, Keys T, Bolwell B. Decreased incidence of early infectious complications in autologous bone marrow transplantation using growth factors and peripheral blood progenitor cells [Abstract]. *Blood* 1993; 82 (suppl 1): 1679.
(168) To LB, Roberts MM, Haylock DN et al. Comparison of haematological recovery times and supportive care requirements of autologous recovery phase peripheral blood stem cell transplants, autologous bone marrow transplants and allogeneic bone marrow transplants. *Bone Marrow Transpl* 1992; 9: 277–84.
(169) Gordon B, Haire W, Ruby E, Kotulak G, Stephens L, Kessinger A. Factors predicting morbidity following hematopoietic stem cell transplantation [Abstract]. *Blood* 1993; 82 (suppl 1): 165a.
(170) Peters WP, Ross M, Vredenburgh J et al. Role of cytokines in autologous bone marrow transplantation. *Hematology/Oncology Clinics of North America* 1993; 7: 737–47.
(171) Gilbert C, Meisenberg B, Vredenburgh J et al. Sequential prophylactic oral and empiric once-daily parenteral antibiotics for neutropenia and fever after highdose chemotherapy and autologous bone marrow support. *J Clin Oncol* 1994; 12: 1005–11.
(172) Reiffers J, Körbling M, Labopin M, Hénon P, Gorin NC. Autologous blood stem cell transplanation versus autologous bone marrow transplantation for acute myeloid leukaemia in first complete remission. *Int J Cell Cloning* 1992; 10 (suppl 1): 111–13.
(173) Yeager AM, Vogelsang GB, Jones RJ et al. Induction of cutaneous graft-versus-host disease by administration of cyclosporine to patients undergoing autologous bone marrow transplantation for acute myeloid leukaemia. *Blood* 1992; 79: 3031–5.
(174) Rowe J, Ryan D, Dipersio J et al. Autografting in chronic myelogenous leukaemia followed by immunotherapy. *Stem Cells* 1993; 11 (suppl 3): 34–42.
(175) Hamon MD, Prentice HG, Gottlieb DJ et al. Preliminary Report: Immunotherapy with interleukin 2 after ABMT in AML. *Bone Marrow Transpl* 1993; 11: 399–401.
(176) Benyunes MC, Massumoto C, York A et al. Preliminary report: Interleukin 2 with or without lymphokine-activated killer cells as consolidative immunotherapy after autologous bone marrow transplantation for acute myelogenous leukemia. *Bone Marrow Transpl* 1993; 12: 159–63.
(177) Klingemann H-G, Grigg AP, Wilkie–Boyd. Treatment with recombinant interferon (Alpha-2B) early after bone marrow transplantation in patients at high risk of relapse. *Blood* 1991; 78: 3306–11.
(178) Jenkins MK, Schwartz RH, Pardoll DM. Effects of cyclosporin A on T cell development and clonal deletion. *Science* 1988; 241: 1655–8.
(179) Kaushansky K, Lok S, Holly RD et al. Promotion of megakaryocyte progenitor expansion and differentiation by the c-Mpl ligand thrombopoietin. *Nature* 1994; 369: 568–71.

Magnetic resonance imaging of lymphoma within the bone marrow

A F SHIELDS and B A PORTER

Accurate staging is critical in determining the prognosis and appropriate therapy for patients with lymphoma. As diagnostic and therapeutic methods evolve, the optimal staging evaluation is also constantly changing. An essential part of lymphoma staging is determining whether tumour is present within the bone marrow. The most widely used approach has been aspiration and biopsy of marrow from the posterior iliac crests. While this technique easily detects disseminated disease (as in leukaemia), it is less reliable with lymphoma. Marrow biopsies in patients with lymphoma are subject to sampling errors, and lymphoma is often a focal process. Routine use of bilateral iliac aspirations and biopsies improves the sampling of the bone marrow. When two biopsies are obtained in patients with non-Hodgkin's lymphoma (NHL), 17 to 23% of the time tumour will be found in only one the specimens.[1–3] This confirms that scattered, multifocal, marrow involvement is commonly seen in lymphoma. This also suggests that an imaging technique to non-invasively assess a larger volume of marrow could improve the routine staging of malignant marrow disease and complement conventional marrow aspirations and biopsies.

Staging procedures

The staging procedures used in patients with lymphoma vary depending on the tumour histology and the results of routine physical exam and laboratory studies. For example, in patients with well-differentiated lymphocytic lymphoma, a simple examination of the peripheral blood may demonstrate widespread disease. At the opposite end of the spectrum, in Hodgkin's disease complete staging may entail an extensive evaluation including splenectomy. A variety of imaging studies are used for the

All correspondence to: Dr A F Shields, Medical Center (111), 1660 South Columbia Way, Seattle, WA 98108, USA.

Cambridge Medical Reviews: Haematological Oncology Volume 4

assessment of nodal as well as extranodal disease. Routine staging protocols now include chest X-rays, occasional lymphangiograms, and computed tomography (CT) from the neck to pelvis. While each of these supply information on the extent of disease within the nodes and soft tissues, they provide little information regarding marrow involvement. Plain X-rays and CT provide some information to indicate bony disease only when there is substantial cortical and trabecular bone destruction. Replacement of marrow by tumour usually does not alter the electron density of the tissue sufficiently to produce a detectable change in the CT or plain X-ray. Although bone scans or bone marrow scintigraphy are frequently able to detect marrow lesions,[4,5] they can miss marrow infiltrating tumours without cortical or trabecular bone destruction.[6]

Bone marrow imaging with ^{99m}Tc sulphur colloid, an agent similar to that used for liver and spleen scans, is occasionally used to image the marrow space. The colloid is actively taken up in reticuloendothelial (RE) cells. Detection of marrow tumour, requires displacement of the normal RE cells sufficiently for the limited resolution of nuclear medicine studies to detect them (often 1–2 cm or greater). This has lead to limited use of these studies for lymphoma and other tumour involving the marrow.

With the introduction of magnetic renonance (MR) imaging a new method for direct imaging of tumour within the marrow space became available.[6–11] MR techniques do not rely on bone destruction or repair to detect tumour involvement, but rather depict the marrow tumour directly with high contrast and spatial resolution. Furthermore, the ability to image in many planes, without intravenous contrast of ionizing radiation, yields excellent and practical assessment of large volumes of the marrow space, while simultaneously assessing nodal and soft tissue disease.

MRI of the marrow

Pulse sequences

Unlike CT images which are based on electron density of tissue, MR images reflect the proton density and relaxation times (T1 and T2) of tissues under the influence of their local magnetic fields. Depending on the radiofrequency pulse sequence chosen, the tissue contrast of MR can be manipulated to highlight certain tissue characteristics. T1 weighted sequences result in anatomic appearing images with a high signal from fat. This produces a strong signal within the normal marrow which contains a preponderance of fat in adults. The marrow thus appears bright (Table 1, Fig. 1(*a*)) and lesions within the marrow appear as dark defects within the normal, high-signal, fat (Fig. 2(*a*)). T1-weighted images are produced with short pulse repetition times (TR) from 450 to 650 ms and an short echo delay times of 10 to 20 ms. We currently employ these parameters

Table 1. *MR signal scale*

Signal intensity	Scale
Diffuse change (T1-SE ↑ , STIR ↓) (fatty, aplastic, irradiated marrow)	−2
Patchy change (T1-SE ↑ , STIR ↓) (fatty, hypoplastic, irradiated marrow)	−1
Normal	0
Mild heterogeneous change (T1-SE ↓ , STIR ↑) Males, non-menstruating females, and elderly: recovering marrow Menstruating females (15–45 years old): considered normal	+1
Scattered miliary (3 to 5 mm) (T1-SE ↓ , STIR ↑)	+2
Focal larger (>5 mm) lesions (T1-SE ↓ , STIR ↑)	+3
Marked signal abnormality (T1-SE ↓ , STIR ↑)	+4

Abbreviations: ↑ , increased signal intensity; ↓ , decreased signal intensity.

on a 0.5 tesla system, but any MR field strength can be used if the TE and TR are kept as short as possible to maximize T1 weighting. The TR should be the minimum necessary to produce adequate numbers of slices for anatomic coverage.

Other MR techniques, such as chemical shift and short TI inversion recovery (STIR)-based sequences, also suppress the signal from fat and are useful for marrow imaging.[12,13] These sequences produce low signal in most of the normal fat containing marrow space (Fig. 1(*b*)). With such techniques, marrow lesions are very bright and conspicuous, particularly with STIR (Fig. 2(*b*)). Since it is easier for the eye to detect a bright lesion on a dark background, rather than the reverse, such a technique improves detection of small marrow lesions. The STIR sequence we employ is TR2000/TE30/TI110 at 0.5 tesla. The TR time is varied to provide the number of slices required to image the desired anatomic area and a 128 by 256 imaging matrix is used to diminish imaging time.

Marrow space imaging

Intrinsically, routine marrow aspirations and biopsies provide only a tiny and possibly non-representative portion of the bone marrow for pathologic analysis. While MRI images a much larger volume of the marrow space, practical limitations remain in choosing the regions to be imaged. Most investigators have predominantly imaged the vertebral marrow in the sagittal plane. However, the coronal plane simultaneously images the pelvic and femoral marrow, as well as the lumbar vertebrae (Fig. 1). Similarly, coronal images of the chest include the humuri, ribs, scapula, sternum,

1(*a*)

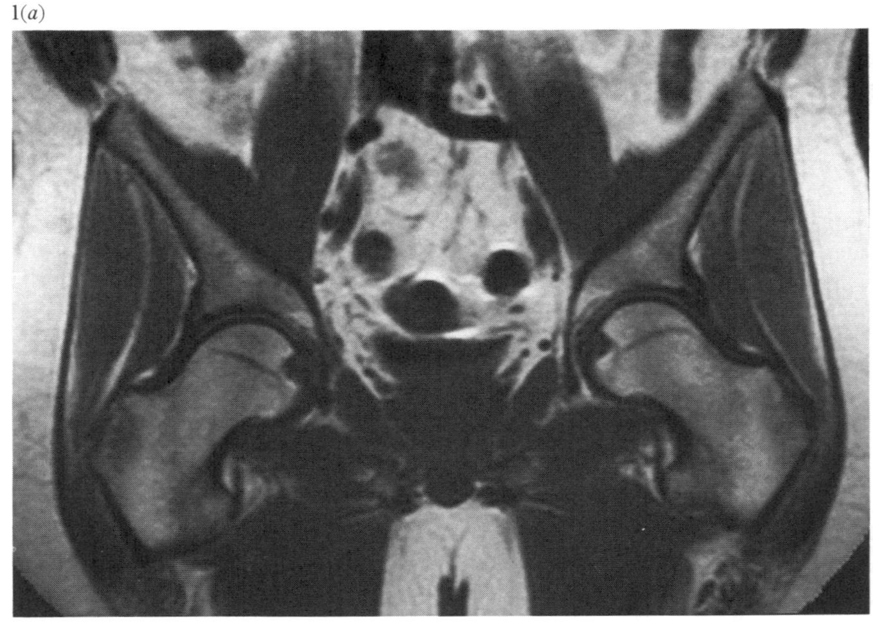

1(*b*)

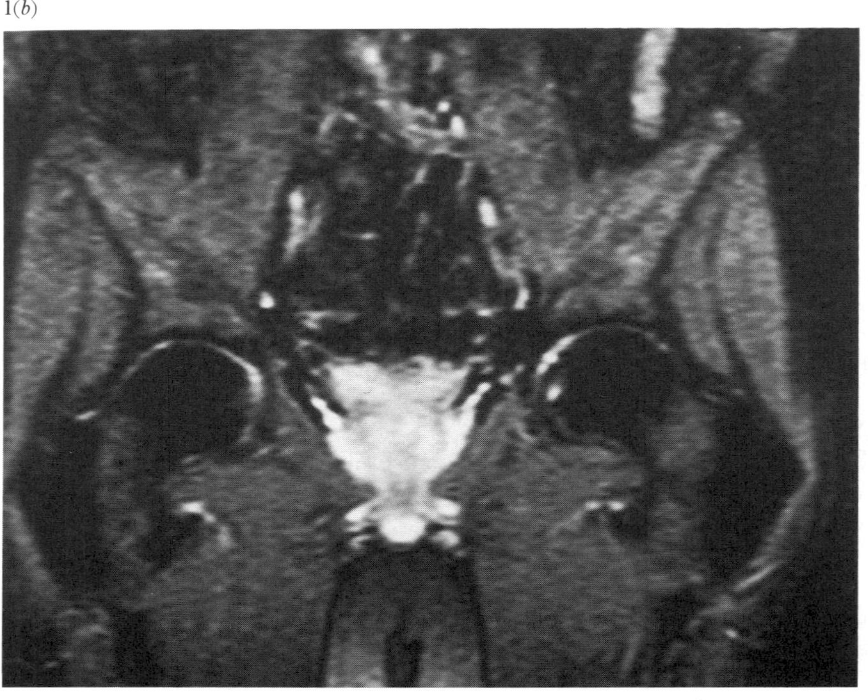

and clavicles. This approach provides an assessment of the majority of the red marrow space. The calvarium and distal extremities are not routinely imaged by this protocol, but can be if symptoms indicate. Furthermore, the ribs are not ideally imaged with any orthogonal sections since they course obliquely downward, although the high contrast of STIR compensates for this substantially. An additional benefit of MR is sensitive detection of lymph node, soft tissue and hepatic tumor without IV contrast material.

Image interpretation

Analysis of MR studies involves detailed as well as general visual inspection of each of the images. Tumour appears as a dark area on T1 weighted images and with STIR the marrow is dark and tumor bright. The overall pattern of marrow tumour may vary greatly from diffuse marrow replacement to focal large lesions, or some combination of both. We have generated a rating scale (Table 1) for these variable patterns of marrow involvement. While focal lesions are generally conspicuous, diffuse, homogenous marrow tumour can be more difficult to diagnose with MR, and is often better detected by marrow sampling. For example, hyperplastic marrow, as seen in marrow recovering from chemotherapy, may show a diffusely increased STIR signal and a low signal intensity on T1 weighted images. Such studies need to be read with caution. Work on evaluating marrow T1 images using quantitative methods may assist in such situations. Smith et al measured mean marrow T1 and T1 variation and found that T1 prolongation correlated with diffuse marrow involvement in patients with Hodgkin's disease.[14] Characteristic signal patterns may be definable with pattern recognition techniques under development. These approaches may someday improve detection of diffuse marrow involvement and help to monitor therapy. For now, these are research techniques, but there is a great deal of promise for future applications of MR in assessing marrow-based and other malignancies.

Efficacy of MR marrow imaging

Low grade non-Hodgkin's lymphoma

Low grade NHL most commonly presents with disseminated disease (about 85%).[15] This includes marrow involvement in about 30–70% of patients.

Fig. 1 (*a*). Normal marrow MR images obtained using coronal T1-weighted spin-echo imaging of the pelvis in a 56 year old male. The signal intensity of pelvic and proximal femoral marrow is slightly less than that of subcutaneous and peritoneal fat. (*b*). The corresponding normal marrow STIR image of the same patient (TR 1800, TE 30, TI 110) suppresses the fat signal, as seen in the normally yellow (fatty) marrow of the femoral epiphyses and greater trochanters. The red marrow of the iliac bone and proximal femurs is slightly higher in signal (grey), reflecting its greater cellularity and water content. The signal of normal red marrow is similar to muscle on STIR.

2(*a*)

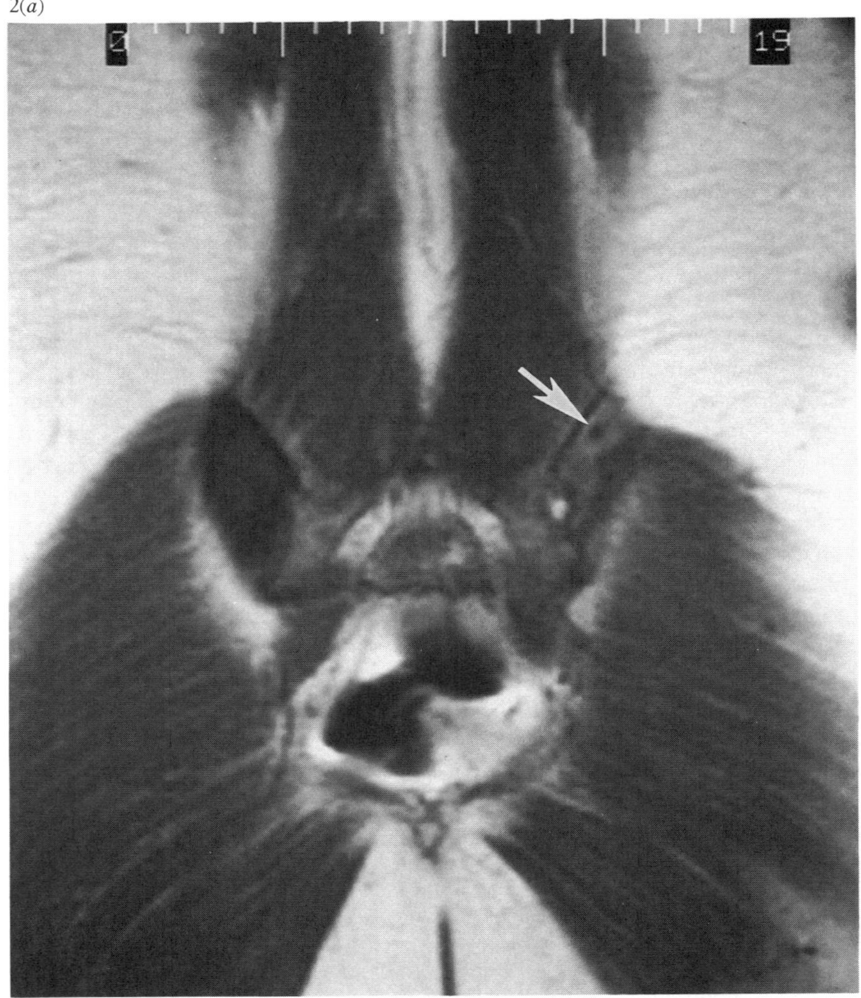

Fig. 2 (*a*). Pre-bone marrow transplant coronal T1 spin-echo image of the posterior iliac crests from a 39 year old male with Hodgkin's disease. A left posterior crest biopsy (arrow) was normal and the marrow imaged adjacent to the biopsy appears normal. The right posterior iliac crest (not biopsied), however, demonstrates confluent signal abnormalities. (*b*) Corresponding STIR image reveals the biopsy site (arrow) with a small amount of bright adjacent edema. The MR appearance of the marrow is normal in this area, whereas the right posterior iliac crest is diffusely hyperintense owing to tumour infiltration.

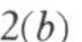

2(*b*)

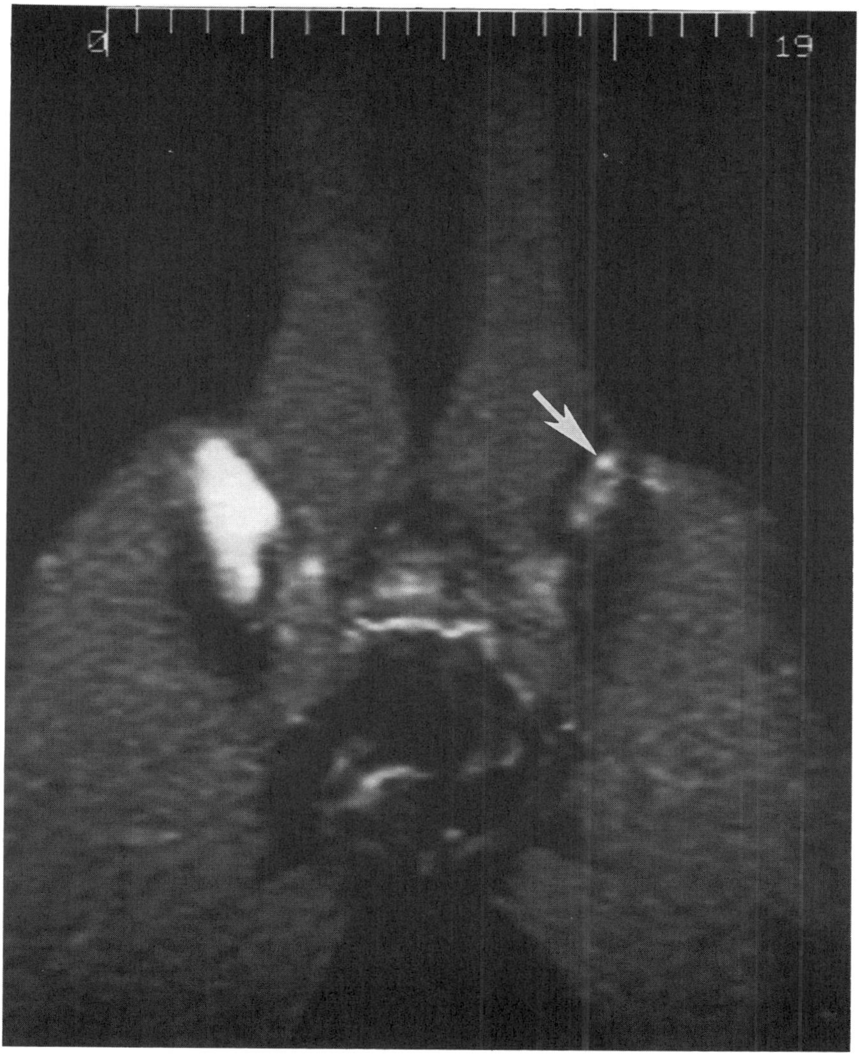

Marrow tumour, is more common in patients with small lymphocytic subtype and least common with follicular, mixed, small cleaved and large cell subtype. In about a third of patients with low grade NHL, abnormal peripheral blood lymphocytes can document the marrow involvement. When marrow disease is present, it is often diffuse. The detection of marrow lymphoma in these patients, therefore, is often accomplished by

Table 2. *Low grade lymphoma; marrow biopsy vs MR*

Biopsy	MR scan +	MR scan −
+	7	5
−	2	13

a simple blood test. When this is not sufficient, routine aspirates and bilateral biopsies are generally adequate for detecting marrow involvement. As a result there is little additional advantage for the routine use of MR in the staging of the marrow in low grade NHL. In our previous comparison of MR and marrow biopsy in 27 patients with low grade lymphoma, 12/27 (44%) had positive marrows by biopsy whereas 9/27 (33%) had marrow tumour detected by MR (Table 2).[13] Five patients had disease detected by biopsy and missed by MR. Conversely, biopsy missed two patients with abnormalities detected by MR. In one of these, the patient had previously documented marrow involvement, but the marrow biopsy at the time of the MR study was negative, with no intervening treatment. The other patient missed by biopsy had previous irradiation to the pelvis. Hence, it appears that imaging plays a lesser role in the routine staging of low grade lymphoma. However, it may find use in selected symptomatic patients in whom soft tissue, extranodal disease is suspected.

Intermediate grade non-Hodgkin's lymphoma

Intermediate grade lymphomas are less likely to have marrow involvement than are low grade tumours. On the other hand, when present (10% of cases), marrow disease is often focal, heterogeneous, and less reliably detected with bone marrow sampling.[2,13] In our previous study, marrow disease was found by biopsy in 25% of patients with advanced disease, while MR detected disease in 41% (Table 3).[13] These techniques appear quite complementary since five patients had disease found only with biopsy and ten had disease detected only by MR.

Table 3. *Intermediate grade lymphoma; marrow biopsy vs MR*

Biopsy	MR scan +	MR scan −
+	3	5
−	10	14

Table 4. *High grade lymphoma and Hodgkin's disease marrow biopsy vs MR*

	MR scan	
Biopsy	+	−
+	3	0
−	14	22

High grade non-Hodgkin's lymphoma

High grade lymphomas are substantially more likely to have scattered, often multi-focal marrow lesions, than are intermediate and low grade disease.[13] In a comparative evaluation of patients with high grade disease, 12% (7/17) had tumour detected by biopsy while 41% had disease evident on MR (Table 4).[13] This is an indication for the complementary use of large field of view MR to assess the marrow space.

Hodgkin's disease

Hodgkin's disease in the marrow is characteristically multifocal (Figs. 3, 4).[16] Our studies found a marked discrepancy between MR and marrow biopsy in these patients. Localized marrow lesions were seen by MR in 45% (10/22) patients with Hodgkin's disease, while only 5% had detectable disease on biopsy Table 4.[13] No Hodgkin's patient with a positive marrow biopsy had a normal MR study. These results where obtained in patients with advanced disease, but even in newly diagnosed patients, MR found focal marrow lesions in 2/12 patients with negative biopsies.[17]

Changes after therapy

One must be mindful of the clinical status and treatment history when interpreting MR images of lymphoma patients. Aggressive chemotherapy, radiation, or combined therapy may significantly complicate image interpretation (Figs. 3, 4). Also, focal marrow lesions may take months to resolve after successful therapy. For example, lesions detected on T1 weighted or STIR images, will not appear normal until the tumour debris has been resorbed and normal marrow fat had reentered the region. The timing of this process is variable and can take several months, as has been demonstrated in patients imaged after successful marrow transplants for leukaemia.[7] Additionally, T2 weighted or STIR images may depict recently treated focal tumour with markedly increased signal, which reflects the water-like nature of necrotic but unresorbed marrow tumour. Similar problems are encountered in following the response of nodal disease to successful treatment. Serial observations usually clarify the situation since

3(*a*)

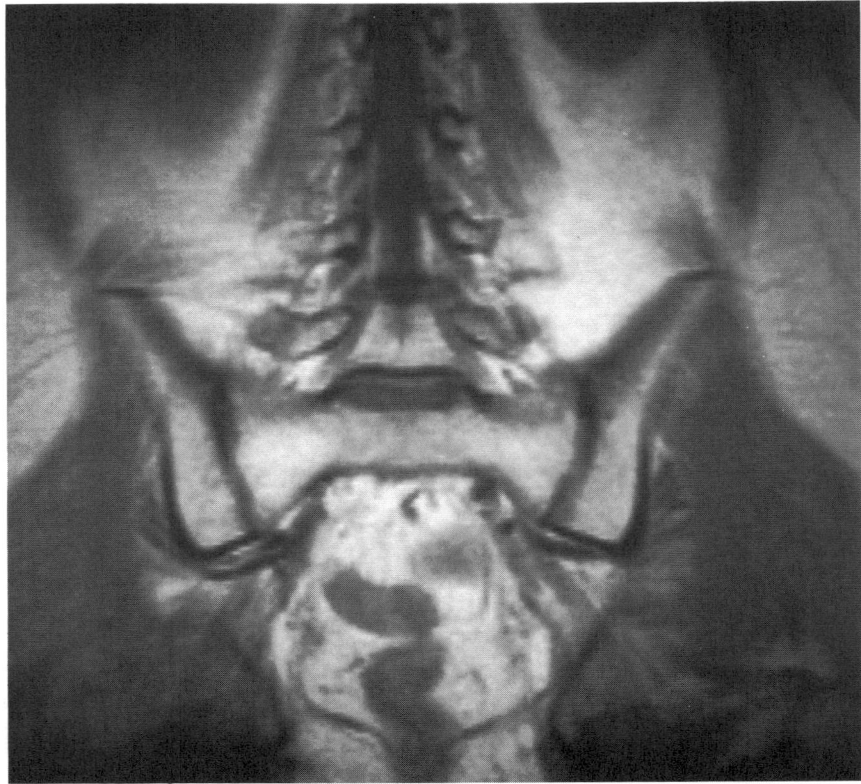

Fig. 3. Images from a 36 year-old male with Hodgkin's disease. (*a*) Coronal T1 spin-echo image of sacrum and posterior iliac crests at approximately 80 days after bone marrow transplant reveals no focal abnormality in the marrow and diffuse subtle hyperintensity of the marrow. (*b*) The corresponding coronal STIR image shows a diffuse marked decrease in signal intensity, reflecting the hypocellular (fatty) marrow typically seen after aggressive chemotherapy and radiation. (*c*) Nine months following images A and B, repeat T1SE examination shows a subtle low signal intensity in the left posterior iliac crest (arrows) as well as mild heterogeneity in the midbody of the sacrum. (*d*) The corresponding coronal STIR image reveals red marrow repopulation in the midbody of the sacrum, with a typically heterogeneous pattern of low to moderate signal intensity. Multifocal marrow relapse of Hodgkin's disease is also depicted in the left sacrum and left iliac crest (arrows) with substantially higher contrast.

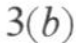

3(*b*)

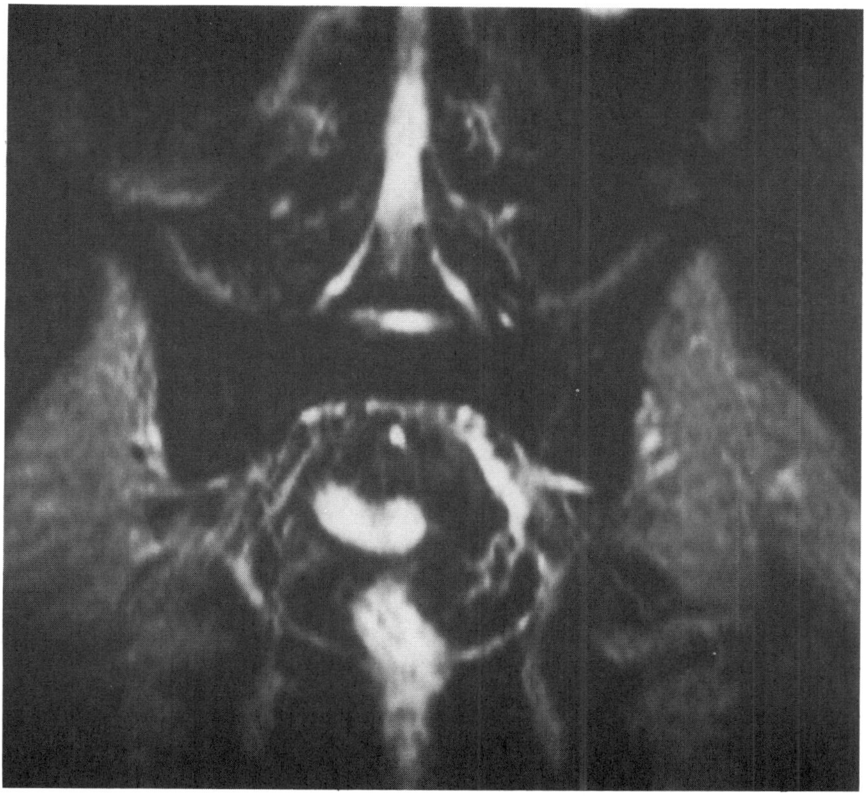

recurrent tumour usually progresses and necrotic residual is resorbed or remains stable.

Clinical use and limitations

Limitations

As discussed above, MR assesses a much greater volume of marrow than is analysed by biopsy. Nevertheless the marrow space of the calvarium and distal extremities is not included in the routine scans of the chest, abdomen, and pelvis. For diseases with diffuse marrow involvement this is not a major drawback, since in such situations biopsy should be adequate. For tumour with scattered marrow involvement MR is likely to be more useful, but it may still miss lesions in portions of the skeleton not in the

3(*c*)

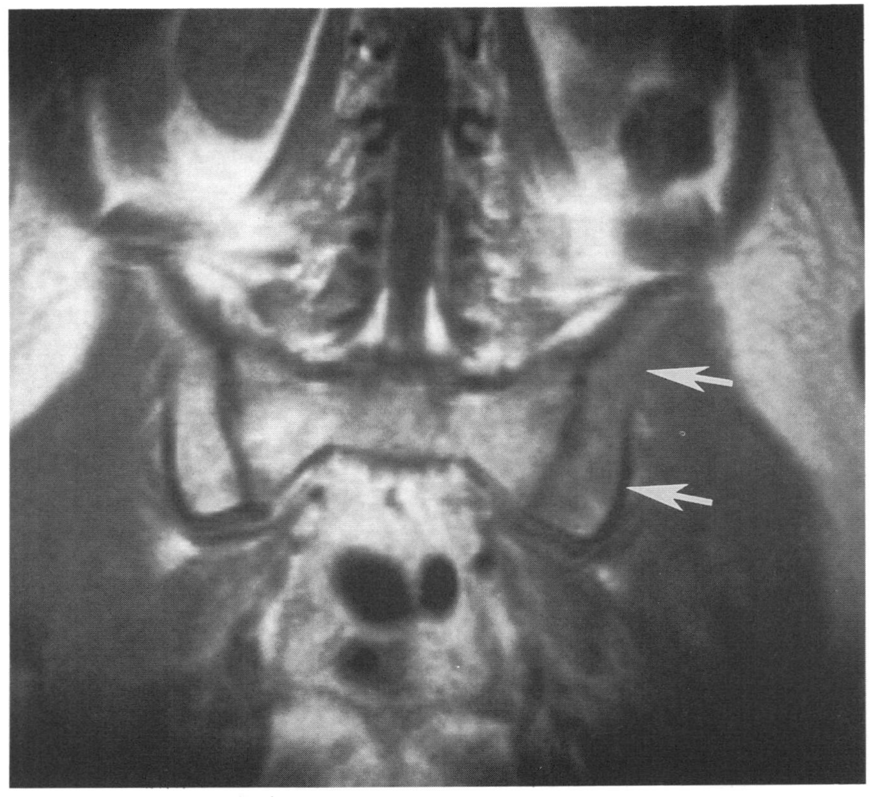

imaging volume. The calvarium and distal extremities, are, however, areas of low probability for isolated disease.

MR imaging must still be considered an indirect and complementary measure of tumour marrow involvement. It does not replace pathological examination. A variety of benign processes can produce focal lesions within the marrow space by MR, which may be falsely diagnosed as tumour. This can be a problem if images are not analysed within their clinical context. For example, recent marrow aspirates, biopsies, and marrow harvests are frequently visualized with MR imaging of the pelvis. These may be erroneously interpreted as focal tumours by an inexperienced observer without appropriate and relevant history. When pathological confirmation of isolated or solitary lesions is required, it should be obtained with CT used to direct marrow biopsies at the sites detected by MR. As

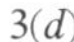

3(*d*)

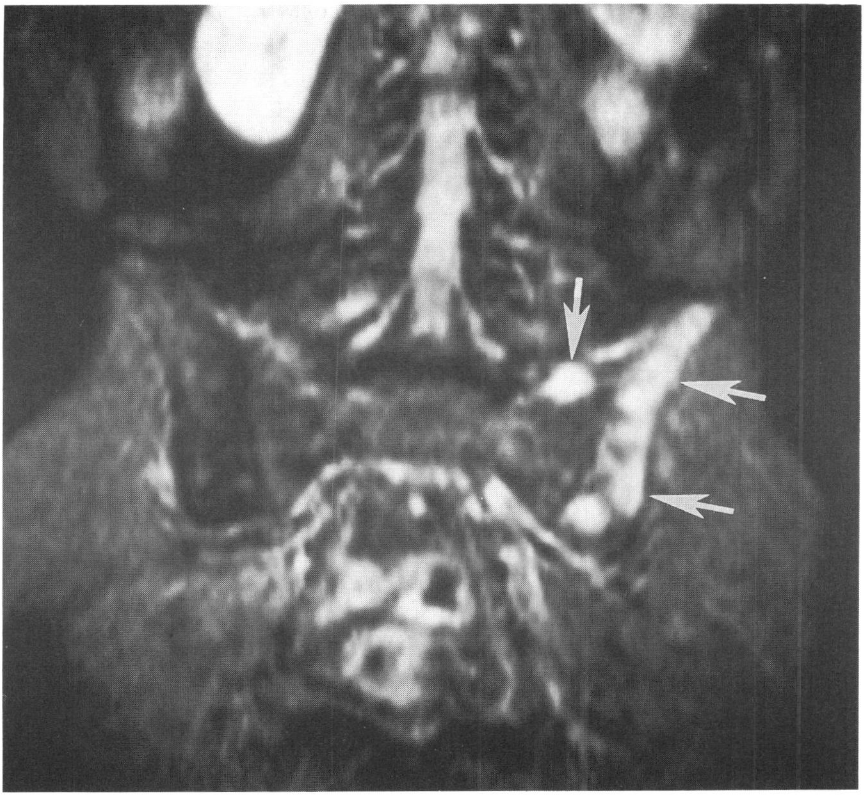

previously discussed recovering marrow after chemotherapy may appear diffusely abnormal; the treatment history must be kept in mind when interpreting marrow MR. The marrow also changes with age.[18] Children's marrow is normally much more cellular and less fatty than that of adults, where fat predominates. Therefore, one must also be aware of age-related differences in red marrow when interpreting MR marrow studies, to avoid over-diagnosis.

MR image appearance is also affected by differences in the magnetic field strength used, as well as, the pulse sequences employed. MR machines in routine clinical use vary from 0.064 to 2.0 tesla. This affects the tissue contrast and pulse sequence availability. Marrow imaging as described here is not currently a routine procedure at all MR centres. The MR system and imaging protocols in every centre may not be tailored or optimized

4(*a*)

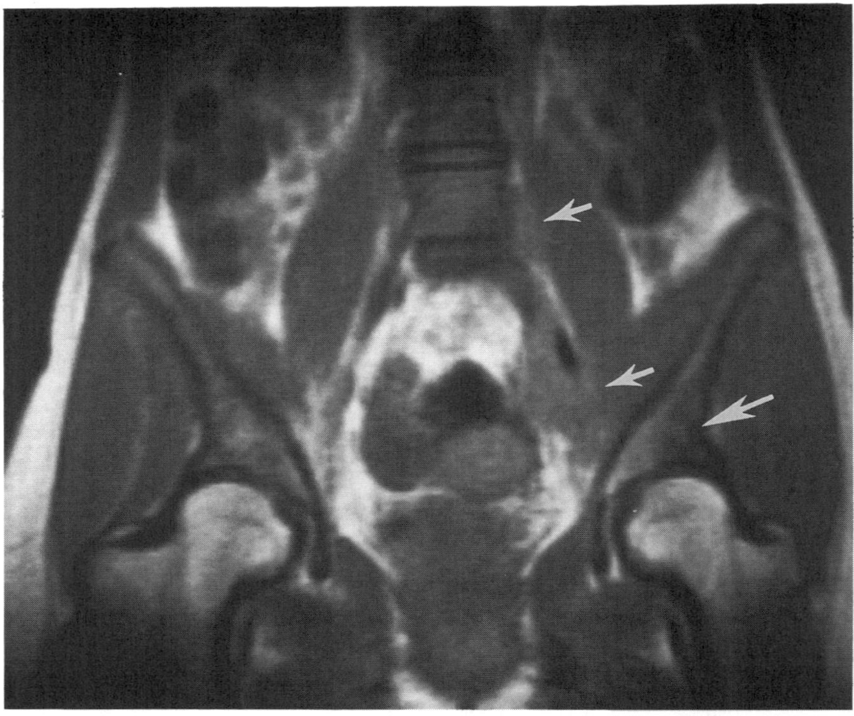

Fig. 4 (*a*). Coronal TISE image of the mid-pelvis in a 21 year old female with Hodgkin's disease. The coronal T1SE image reveals diffuse heterogeneity and low T1 signal of the lumbar marrow. The signal intensity of the vertebral marrow is approximately equal to the intervertebral discs, indicating prolonged T1 due to diffuse marrow tumour. Decreased signal intensity in the left supra-acetabular marrow (large arrow) is indicative of tumour infiltration. Left external iliac adenopathy is also present (small arrows). (*b*) The corresponding coronal STIR image reveals the background pattern of diffusely hyperintense (bright) marrow tumour involving the pelvis but not the femurs. The untreated lymphadenopathy is also typically hyperintense (small arrows). (*c*) Follow-up examination, following chemotherapy, at 8 months, T1SE images show an increase in marrow signal intensity of the supra-acetabular marrow, which now approaches normal. The lymphadenopathy has now cleared. (*d*) The corresponding STIR images confirm the normalization of the marrow signal intensity. A slightly exaggerated red/yellow marrow differential is noted, which is frequent in patients after chemotherapy. Red marrow will usually fill in areas of previous tumour involvement following effective therapy, although the timing and pattern is unpredictable. No signal abnormality is seen adjacent to the external iliac artery and vein, indicating resolution of the lymphadenopathy.

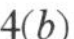

4(*b*)

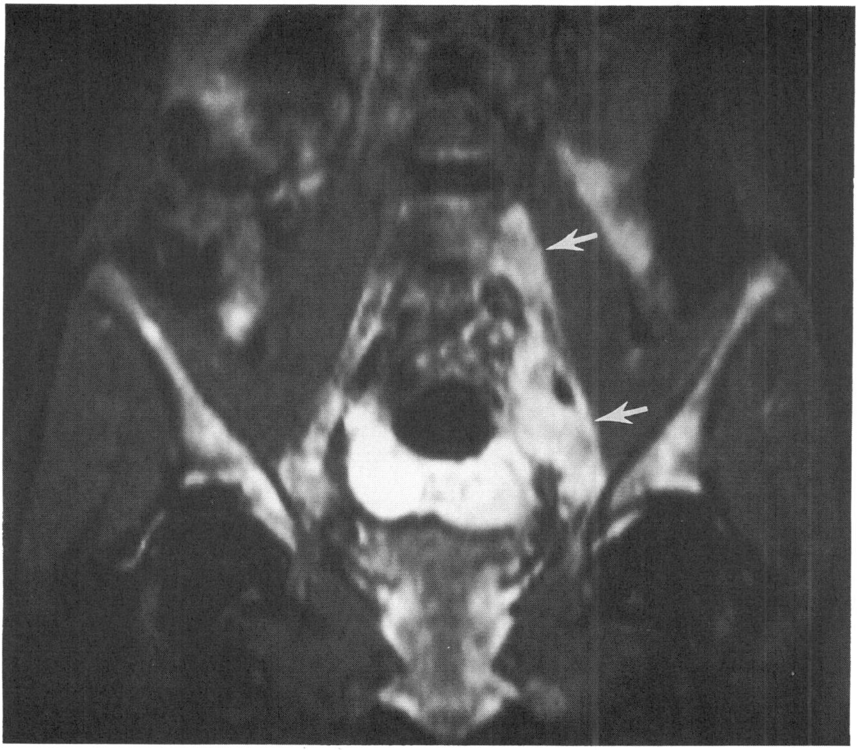

for marrow assessment, and the radiologist may not be experienced with marrow MR. Therefore, physicians should be aware of variations in the local experience when using imaging results to decide individual patient treatment.

Marrow and nodal MR in clinical practice

It is clear that MR imaging capably detects focal or distant marrow involvement by lymphoma not found on routine bilateral marrow aspirations and biopsies. Given this background, for MR to be routinely used, it must provide significant additional information which alters final staging and treatment of the patients. We have compared CT, marrow biopsy, and MR in the initial staging of 23 patients with newly diagnosed lymphoma.[17] Although the MR protocol used was specifically designed for marrow tumour detection, nodal assessment was also done during image interpretation. Six patients (23%) were increased in stage by MR compared

4(*c*)

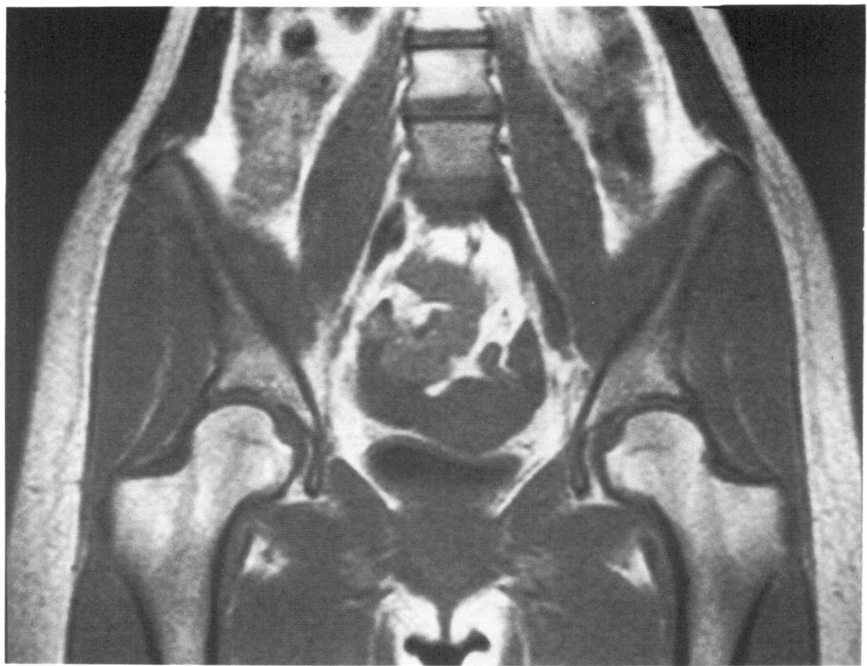

to CT. Two patients with thoracic disease detected by both modalities, were found to have nodal disease below the diaphragm on MR but not CT. Four patients had marrow involvement by MR, while CT did not detect any of these; two had NHL and their marrow disease was confirmed by biopsy. Two of these four patients had Hodgkin's disease with marrow involvement detected by MR but not by marrow biopsy. These results indicate MR has the potential to replace CT in the staging of lymph nodes, while providing the additional benefit of marrow assessment. Although staging with MR is somewhat more costly and less readily available than CT, the detection of marrow involvement, with its effect on tumour staging, appears to justify its use in patients at high risk for marrow involvement.

Patient selection and conclusions

What patients are most likely to benefit from MR imaging? The above results indicate that in low grade lymphoma marrow aspirates and biopsies are usually adequate for detecting marrow disease, while MR does rather poorly at detecting diffuse, but low level marrow involvement. On the

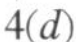
4(*d*)

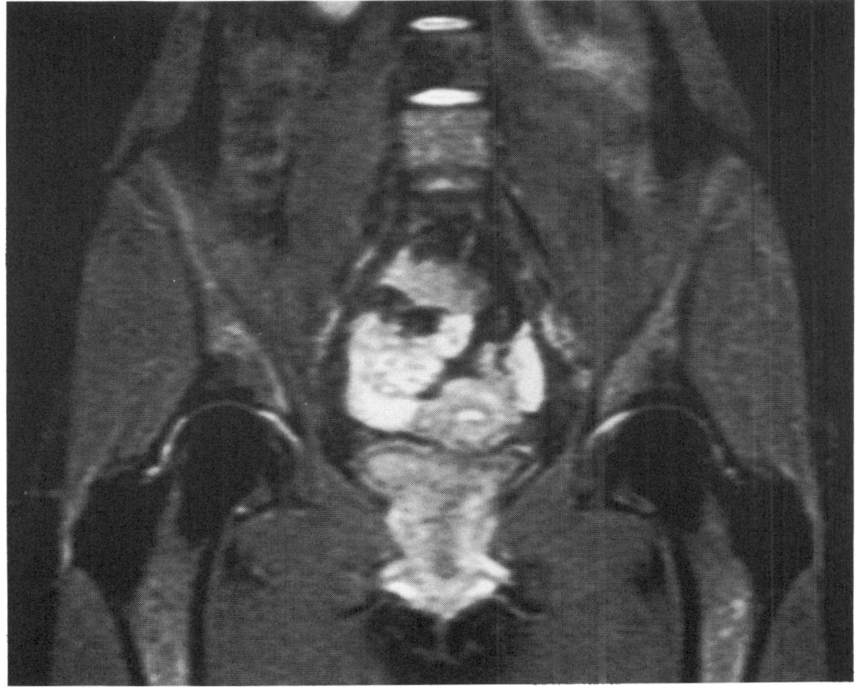

other hand, in patients with intermediate grade disease, MR often detected lesions missed by biopsy. This was an even more frequent finding in patients with high grade lymphoma or Hodgkin's disease where MR missed none of the patients with positive biopsies and detected an additional 40% of marrow tumour missed by biopsy. This suggests that MR provides additional information needed in the accurate staging of such patients. It is of note that no prospective study looking at the contribution of MR to all patients with high grade lymphoma and Hodgkin's disease has been completed. Nevertheless, one could reasonably argue that MR could be used instead of the routine CT scans now employed in staging of lymphoma. The present results indicate that a significant number of patients will have MR detectable marrow disease, which would be occult on CT and conventional staging.

We routinely image patients being considered for autologous marrow transplantation. The MR detection of marrow disease affects the decision on the source of marrow used in transplantation. If the marrow MR is positive then the use allogeneic marrow may be preferred if it is available. As peripheral stem cell transplants have become available, they also offer another option in those with documented marrow involvement.

The use of MR of the marrow in evaluating lymphoma patients will need continued consideration, as diagnostic techniques and treatments evolve and improve. Refinement of MR methods to concomitantly stage the lymph nodes and marrow is on-going, and will help to further define and improve its use in staging and monitoring patients with lymphoma. Techniques of molecular biology, including polymerase chain reaction (PCR), are also beginning to find use in the detection of marrow disease.[19,20] These methods may improve the sensitivity of bone marrow aspiration for the detection of microscopic disease, but in the meantime, MR imaging has a defined role in the evaluation of suspected marrow involvement by lymphoma.

References

(1) Brunning RD, Bloomfield CD, McKenna RW, Peterson L. Bilateral trephine bone marrow biopsies in lymphoma and other neoplastic diseases. *Ann Intern Med* 1975; 82: 365–6.

(2) Coller BS, Chabner BA, Gralnick HR. Frequencies and patterns of bone marrow involvement in non-Hodgkin lymphomas: observations on the value of bilateral biopsies. *Am J Hematol* 1977; 3: 105–19.

(3) Haddy TB, Parker RI, Magrath IT. Bone marrow involvement in young patients with non-Hodgkin's lymphoma: the importance of multiple bone marrow samples for accurate staging. *Med Pediatr Oncol* 1989; 17: 418–23.

(4) Schicha H, Franke M, Smolorz J, Linden A, Waters W, Diehl V. Diagnostic strategies and staging procedures for Hodgkin's lymphoma: bone marrow scintigraphy and magnetic resonance imaging. *Rec Results Cancer Res* 1989; 117: 112–19.

(5) Ferrant A, Rodhain J, Michaux JL, Piret L, Maldague B, Sokal G. Detection of skeletal involvement in Hodgkin's disease: a comparison of radiography, bone scanning, and bone marrow biopsy in 38 patients. *Cancer* 1976; 35: 1346–53.

(6) Shields AF, Porter BA, Churchley S, Olson DO, Appelbaum FR, Thomas ED. The detection of bone marrow involvement by lymphoma using magnetic resonance imaging. *J Clin Oncol* 1987; 5: 225–30.

(7) Olson DO, Shields AF, Scheurich CJ, Porter BA, Moss AA. Magnetic resonance imaging of the bone marrow in patients with leukemia, aplastic anemia, and lymphoma. *Invest Radiol* 1986; 21: 540–6.

(8) Richards MA, Webb JAW, Jewell SE, Amess JAL, Wrigley PFM, Lister TA. Low field strength magnetic resonance imaging of bone marrow in patients with malignant lymphoma. *Br J Cancer* 1988; 57: 412–15.

(9) Stimac GK, Porter BA, Olson DO, Gerlach R, Genton M. Gadolinium-DTPA-enhanced MR imaging of spinal neoplasms: preliminary investigation and comparison with unenhanced spin-echo and STIR sequences. *AJNR* 1988; 9: 839–46.

(10) Döhner H, Gückel F, Knauf W et al. Magnetic resonance imaging of bone marrow in lymphoproliferative disorders: correlation with bone marrow biopsy. *Br J Haematol* 1989; 73: 12–17.
(11) Linden A, Zankovich R, Theissen P, Diehl V, Schicha H. Malignant lymphoma: bone marrow imaging versus biopsy. *Radiology* 1989; 173: 335–9.
(12) Bydder GM, Young IR. MR imaging: clinical use of the inversion recovery sequence. *J Comput Assist Tomogr* 1985; 9: 659–75.
(13) Hoane BR, Shields AF, Porter BA, Shulman HM. Detection of lymphomatours bone marrow involvement with magnetic resonance imaging. *Blood* 1991; 78: 728–38.
(14) Smith SR, Roberts N, Percy DF, Edwards RHT. Detection of bone marrow abnormalities in patients with Hodgkin's disease by T1 mapping of MR images of lumbar vertebral bone marrow. *Br J Cancer* 1992; 65: 246–51.
(15) Longo DL, Devita VT, Jaffe ES, Mauch P, Urba WJ. Lymphocytic lymphomas. In: DeVita VT Jr, Hellman S, Rosenberg SA, eds. *Cancer: principals and practice of oncology*. Philadelphia: JB Lippincott, 1993: 1859–927.
(16) Moormeier JA, Williams SF, Golomb HM. The staging of non-Hodgkin's lymphomas. *Semin Oncol* 1990; 17: 43–50.
(17) Shields AF, Hoane BR, Borrow JW, Porter BA. Comparison of initial lymphoma staging using computed tomography (CT) and magnetic resonance imaging (MR). *Blood* 1992; 80: 37a.
(18) Dawson KL, Moore SG, Rowland JM. Age-related changes in the Pelvis: MR and anatomic findings. *Radiology* 1992; 183: 47–51.
(19) Arnold A, Cossman J, Bakkshi A, Jaffe ES, Waldmann TA, Korsmeyer SJ. Immunoglobulin-gene rearrangements as unique clonal markers in human neoplasms. *N Engl J Med* 1983; 309: 1593–9.
(20) Bregni M, Borrello MG, Siena S et al. Detection of bone marrow minimal disease in non-Hodgkin's lymphoma patients by gene rearrangement analysis. *Haematologica (Pavia)* 1989; 74: 397–400.

Use and interpretation of tumour markers in haematological malignancies, lymphoma and leukaemia

D C AZIZ and R R BARATHUR

Acute leukaemia

B-lineage acute lymphoblastic leukaemia

In acute leukaemia, the diagnostic accuracy of morphological classification is 60–70%; 89% when morphology and cytochemistry are used together and 99% when immunophenotyping is performed by flow cytometry. B-lineage acute lymphoblastic leukaemia (ALL), which comprises 85% of ALLs, is characterized by CD19 or CD22 expression; CD19, expressed in 95%, is the most consistent marker. Six immunophenotypic groups are characterized by the degree of differentiation (Table 1).[1] Surface immunoglobulin-positive (SIg+), usually IgM, B-ALL (Group VI) is associated with the leukaemic phase of American Burkitt-type, non-Hodgkin's lymphoma (FAB L3 ALL). These cells co-express CD19, CD20 and HLA-DR. The SIg−, CD10+, cytoplasmic mu-positive (Cμ+) B-lineage ALL (Group V) can be divided into two subgroups according to the presence or absence of t(1;19). The t(1;19) chromosomal translocation, which is associated with the juxtaposition of *E2A* from chromosome 19 and the *PBX1* gene on chromosome 1, is detectable by Southern blot (SB) or polymerase chain reaction (PCR) in 25% of children with pre-B-ALL (Group V) and is associated with a poorer prognosis.[2] In contrast, children who are Cμ+ (Group V) without the t(1;19) or *E2A–PBX1* gene rearrangement have a prognosis similar to the CD10 (CALLA)+, early pre-B-ALL (Groups III and IV). CD34 is expressed in 70% of childhood ALL and is associated with a superior, event-free, 5-year survival (83% versus 63%).[3] CD45 is

All correspondence to: Dr D Aziz, Specialty Laboratories Inc , 2211 Michigan Avenue, Santa Monica, California 90404, USA.

Cambridge Medical Reviews: Haematological Oncology Volume 4

Table 1. *Proposed classification of B-lineage acute lymphoblastic leukaemia (ALL)*

	Cell markers								
	HLA-DR	CD34	CD19	cCD22	CD10	CD20	Cμ	SIg	Alternate designation
Group I	+	+	−	−	−	−	−	−	undifferentiated
Group II	+	+	+	+	−	−	−	−	early B-precursor ALL
Group III	+	+/−	+	+	+	−	−	−	early B-precursor ALL
Group IV	+	+/−	+	+	+	+	−	−	early B-precursor ALL
Group V	+	−	+	+	+	+	+	−	B-precursor ALL
Group VI	+	−	+	+	+/−	+	−	+	mature B-ALL

expressed in 80% of B-lineage ALL and is associated with a lower failure rate (5% versus 30%).[4]

Numerical abnormalities in ALL include pseudodiploidy, hyperdiploidy (51 to 60 chromosomes which is common in childhood ALL [25%] and associated with a good prognosis) and near haploidy (which has the worst prognosis). Extra copies of chromosome 4 and 10 are associated with the favorable outcome of hyperdiploid ALL. Translocations t(8;14), t(2;8) and t(8;22) involving *MYC* oncogene deregulation are detectable in 90% of ALL-L3 and associated with a poor prognosis. Translocation t(4;11) and 6q- detectable in pre-B and B-cell ALL have an intermediate prognosis.[5, 6]

Surface Ig expression is not detectable until maturation of the B-cell occurs with a functional rearrangement of both Ig heavy chain and Ig light chain. Clonal Ig heavy chain rearrangements occur in virtually all precursor-B-ALL (Groups I–VI). Clonal Ig light chain rearrangements are found in only some of the common ALL (pre-B-cell), pre-B ALL and SIg+ ALL (Groups III–VI) but are specific for B-lineage ALL, because only Ig heavy chain rearrangements can be detected in non-B-cell neo-plasms.[7, 8] Clonal rearrangements of the Ig heavy chain are detectable with PCR, although false-negative results are common.[9] Up to 30% of B-lineage ALL can contain a T-cell receptor (TCR) clonal rearrangement (Fig. 1).[10]

The *BCR/ABL* gene rearrangement (See CML below) is detectable in 20–35% of patients with adult ALL (mostly CD10+ ALL) and 6–17% of children with ALL. Both the *M-bcr* and m-*bcr* forms are detectable by RT–PCR in patients with ALL (Fig. 2).[11,12] Early detection of relapse prior to clinical, haematological or cytogenetic indicators in bone-marrow transplant patients is possible by detecting the *BCR/ABL* gene rearrangement by RT–PCR[13] or Ig heavy chain rearrangements by PCR.[14]

T-lineage acute lymphoblastic leukaemia

CD7 is expressed on all T-lineage ALL which accounts for about 15 to 25% of ALL. Some acute myeloid leukaemia (AML), biphenotypic and undifferentiated acute leukaemia may express CD7, but it is rarely found in B-cell lymphoma or leukaemia. The combination of CD5 and CD7 is 100% sensitive and 94% specific for the diagnosis of T-ALL. Cytoplasmic CD3 (cCD3) is expressed prior to membrane CD3, which is helpful in classifying T-ALL according to the differentiation of the thymocyte (Table 2).[1] The intermediate stages of T-ALL (Stage II and III) are more likely to have a mediastinal mass. Although, the remission induction failure rate is higher in early stage T-ALL, immunophenotype has no impact on event-free survival and outcome among the paediatric T-ALL groups once remission is achieved.[15] In adults, the CD7+CD4-CD8-phenotype is associated with high leukaemia cell count, mediastinal mass, skin lesions and

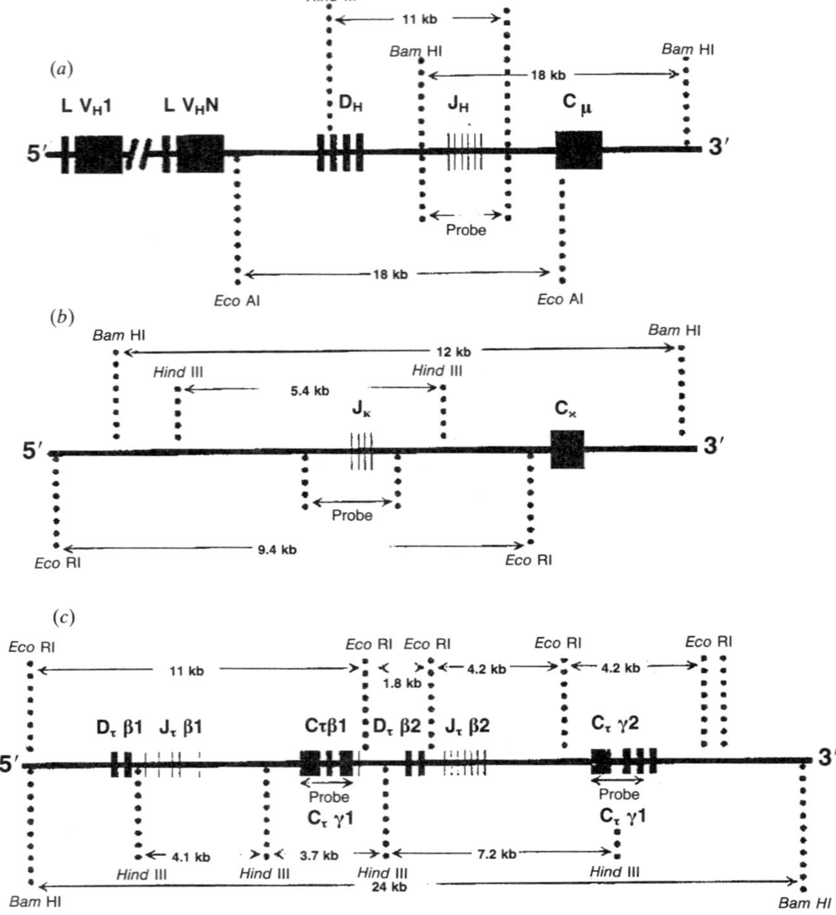

Fig. 1. Genomic organization of: (*a*) immunoglobulin heavy chain; (*b*) immunoglobulin kappa light chain gene; (*c*) T-cell receptor beta chain gene. The DNA is digested with specific restriction endonucleases, such as *Hind* III, *Eco* RI, *Bam* HI, and probed with a specific sequence of probes to the above genes. The expected germline restriction fragment lengths are known from these maps. Monoclonal rearrangement of the gene is diagnosed by the presence of an unexpected restriction fragment band in addition to the restriction fragments shown here. (Adapted from Cossman J *et al.*, *Am J Clin Pathol* 95: 347, 1991, with permission.)

(*a*)

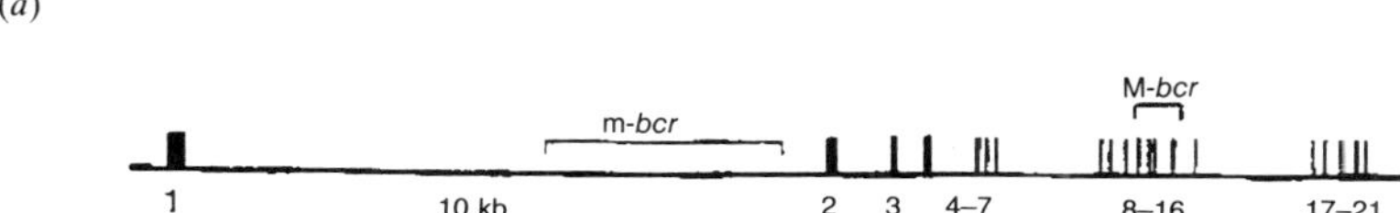

(*b*)

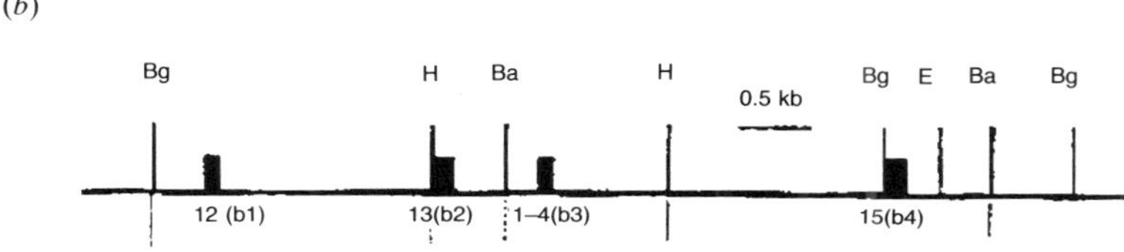

(*c*)

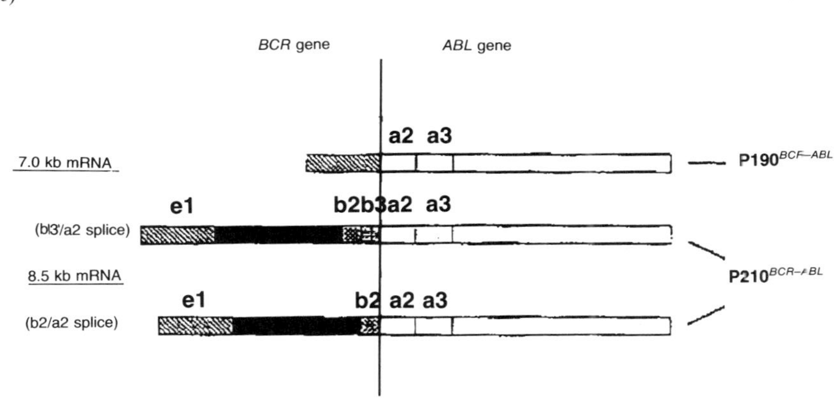

ig. 2. (*a*) Genomic organization of the *BCR* gene on chromosome 22; m-*bcr*, the nor breakpoint cluster region and M-*bcr*, the major breakpoint cluster region, nded in (*b*). (*c*) *BCR* translocation to the *ABL* gene on chromosome 9. M-*bcr* nd in 100% of CML and 50% of Ph^1+ acute leukaemia. M-*bcr* gives rise to kilobase mRNA in which either exon 13(b2) or 14(b3) of *BCR* is spliced (a2) of *ABL* each yielding a $P210^{BCR-ABL}$ protein. m-*bcr* occurring in 50% cute leukaemia results in a 7.0 kilobase mRNA in which exon 1(e1) of iced to exon 2 of *ABL* (a2) yielding a $P190^{BCR-ABL}$ protein. (Adapted A *et al.*, *Blood* 78: 1155, 1991.)

Table 2. *Proposed classification of T-lineage acute lymphoblastic leukaemia (T-ALL)*

	Cell markers								
	TdT	cCD3	CD3	CD7	CD5	CD2	CD4	CD8	CD1
Stage I[a]	+	+	–	+	+ (90%)[b]	+ (75%)[b]	–	–	–
Stage II[a]	+	+	–	+	+	+	+	+	+
Stage III[a]	–	+	+	+	+	+	+	+	+
Stage IV[a]	–	+	+	+	+	+	+/–	+/–	–

[a] Alternate names:

Stage I =early thymocyte type
Stage II =intermediate thymocyte type
Stage III=new subtype
Stage IV=mature T-cell.

[b] Figures in parentheses indicate approximate proportion of positive cells in specimen.

central nervous system disease that is unresponsive to conventional chemotherapy.[16]

Most T-ALL contains a detectable clonal gene rearrangement of TCR-β; whereas, TCR-δ is rearranged more commonly in the early thymocyte stage. Rearrangements of Ig heavy chain (but not light chain) can be detected by SB in some T-ALL.[17]

Acute myeloblastic leukaemia

One or more of the myeloid antigens, CD33, CD13 or CD14 must be present to make a diagnosis of acute myeloblastic leukaemia (AML), particularly in FAB-M0 which is morphologically and cytochemically undifferentiated. CD14 expression is diagnostic of monocytic cells, (FAB-M4 or M5); platelet-specific antigens such as CD41 are detected in FAB-M7. Cases of AML that express CD13 or CD9 have a lower remission rate.[18] CD34 expression correlates with undifferentiated morphology (FAB-M0 or M1), secondary leukaemia and low remission rate.[19] CD7+ AML patients have a significantly lower response rate and poorer prognosis than CD7− AML patients.[20]

Acute promyelocytic leukaemia (APL) or FAB-M3 is characterized by hypergranular myelocytes and abnormalities in coagulation such as disseminated intravascular coagulation (DIC). The t(15;17)(q22;q21) translocation involving juxtaposition of the retinoic acid receptor-α (*RAR*-α) gene on chromosome 17 and *PML* on chromosome 15, is found in essentially 100% of APL patients.[21,22] Tretinoin (all-*trans*-retinoic acid) induces complete remission in 80% of APL and SB analysis of the *RAR*-α gene shows loss of the rearranged band when the patients achieve remission,[23] however, RT–PCR remains positive.[24]

Patients with AML M4Eo, characterized by increased numbers of eosinophils and associated with cytogenetic abnormalities involving band q22 of chromosome 16 [such as inv(16)(pl3q22) and del(16q22)] have high remission rates and long overall survival, but are at increased risk of central nervous system relapse. This translocation creates a fusion protein between the CBF-β and myosin heavy chain genes which should lead to an RT–PCR test specific for this disease.[25]

Clonal cytogenetic abnormalities, detected in 50 to 90% of AML, provide independent prognostic information. The t(8;21)(q22;q22) detected primarily in FAB-M2 associated with chloromas, t(15;17) found exclusively in FAB-M3 (APL) and abnormalities involving 16q22 in FAB-M4Eo are associated with high remission rates and long periods of remission. *AML*13 is the translocated oncogene locus associated with t(8;21).[26] Monosomy 5, monosomy 7, del(5q) and del(7q) are strongly associated with AML occurring after chemotherapy, after exposure to environmental leukaemogenic agents or during myelodysplastic syndrome; patients with these abnormalities have lower remission rates. About 10% of AML contain a clonal rearrangement of TCR or Ig heavy chain and the same proportion express terminal deoxytransferase (TdT). In TdT+AML, Ig and TCR are rearranged in 60%; whereas, in TdT–AML only 5% contain rearrangements in these genes.[27]

Acute undifferentiated and hybrid leukaemia

The term acute hybrid leukaemia refers collectively to acute leukaemia with cells which express two distinct lineages (biphenotypical), consist of two distinct populations (bilineal) or arise from a separate transforming event (biclonal).[28]

The co-expression of T-cell and myeloid antigens (biphenotypic) typically have AML morphology with myeloperoxidase expression, myeloid antigens CD13 and CD11c as well as T-cell antigens CD2, CD7 and cCD3. TCR-β is rearranged in half of cases. These children present with higher leukocyte counts, lymphadenopathy and poor response to AML induction therapy.[29]

Lymphocyte antigen-positive AML frequently has karyotypes commonly seen in AML such as t(8;21)(q22;q22), inv(16)(p13;q22), t(15;17)(q22;q21) or t(9;11)(p22;q23) which are detected in 71% of cases.[30] Adults with AML consisting of blasts with lymphocyte markers (CD2 and CD19) in the absence of other features of lymphocytic leukaemia have a more favourable prognosis than patients without this phenotype.[30]

Approximately, 7% of childhood ALL and 18% of adult ALL express myeloid antigens (My+ ALL).[28] These cases are more frequently B-lineage ALL than T-lineage ALL and are associated with clonal karyotypes involving t(9;22) (Ph^1 chromosome) or bands at 11q23 or 14q32. Adult My+ ALL has a worse prognosis than My− ALL, but in children the prognosis is the same.[28,31]

MLL, the myeloid lymphoid leukaemia oncogene found at 11q23, is associated with the translocations t(9;11)(p22;q23), t(10;11)(p13;q23), t(11;17)(q23;q25), t(11;19)(q23;p13) and del(11)(q23).[32] These changes are detected in both AML, specifically in infants or secondary to epipodophyllotoxin therapy, in FAB–M4 or M5 subtypes and in ALL in infants <6 months of age (70%).[33,34] The projected event-free survival is 15% for infants with rearrangements of *MLL* compared to 80% for those without this abnormality.

Chronic myeloproliferative disorders

Chronic myelogenous leukaemia and myelodysplastic syndromes

Immunophenotypical analysis is not helpful in the differential diagnosis of the chronic myeloproliferative disorders. Both chronic myelogenous leukaemia (CML) and the myelodysplastic syndromes (MDS) express the myeloid antigens CD33, CD13 and CD11c. CD45 and the isoform CD45RO are expressed in CML, but not CD45RA which helps to differentiate CML from AML.[35] Because CML cells express HLA–DR, they can be differentiated from normal bone marrow precursors.[36] Detection of CD34+ cells in the peripheral blood in MDS as well as high HLA–DR and low CD11b expression are associated with a greater likelihood of transformation to AML (CD34+, 40%; CD34−, 0%).[37,28]

Normal chromosomes are detected in 21% of patients with MDS and are associated with long survival; only 12% progress to AML. Deletions at 7q or monosomy 7 detected in 16% of MDS are associated with the shortest survival; 72% progress to AML. Trisomy 8 is a single chromosomal defect found in 8% of patients. Patients with complex chromosomal abnormalities have intermediate to poor prognosis. Deletions at 5q or monosomy 5 are associated with a good to intermediate prognosis.[39] *N-ras* mutations in MDS are associated with an increased likelihood of transformation to AML.[40]

The presence of t(9;22)(q34;q11) or the Philadelphia (Ph^1) chromosome, which is detectable in approximately 95% of CML,[41] is helpful in differentiating CML from MDS. The 'break point cluster region' or *BCR* gene at 22q11 translocates with the *ABL* gene at 9q34 creating Ph^1, which is detectable by Southern blot (SB) using a *BCR* probe, PCR using reverse-transcribed mRNA as a template (RT-PCR) or fluorescent in situ hybridization (FISH) using fluorescent-labelled probes to *BCR* and *ABL*.[42] The Ph^1 chromosome is typically detected by conventional chromosome analysis, but this methodology is expensive and labour intensive and it is rapidly being replaced by molecular methods. RT-PCR can determine the type of breakpoint in the *BCR* gene: either *M-bcr*, the major breakpoint region which is detectable in CML and 50% of Ph^1+ acute leukaemia or m-*bcr*, the minor breakpoint region, which is detectable in 50% of Ph^1+ acute leukaemia but not CML (Fig. 2).[12] Using RT-PCR or SB for the initial diagnosis of CML is more sensitive and has quicker turnaround time and lower costs than karyotypes. Chromosome analysis must be used in CML patients undergoing blast crisis because other numerical (i.e. +8) and structural changes cannot be detected with RT-PCR or SB. The *BCR/ABL* gene rearrangement is detectable in essentially all cases of CML, even in $Ph-^1$ CML, but not MDS. Quantitative RT-PCR post-bone marrow transplant identifies patients prior to overt relapse and is used for minimal disease detection.[43]

Chronic lymphoid leukaemia

Chronic B-lymphoid leukaemia

Chronic lymphocytic leukaemia (CLL), prolymphocytic leukaemia (PLL) and hairy-cell leukaemia (HCL) are all B-cell lymphoproliferative disorders and, therefore, the cells express B-cell antigens, CD19, CD20 in addition to HLA–DR. Restriction of κ and λ light chain expression (i.e. the cells express κ, but not λ or vice versa), is the most important nonmorphological criterion in differentiating a chronic B-cell leukaemia from normal peripheral blood or bone marrow. Co-expression of CD5 with the B-cell antigens (CD19 and CD20) and low-density monotypical surface immunoglobulin (SIg) expression are typical of CLL.[1] CD11c and CD23 may be expressed in CLL and are associated with a poorer prognosis.[44] Conversely, high density or bright SIg, FMC-7 expression and lack of CD23 are typical of PLL. CD5 may or may not be expressed in PLL.[45] HCL typically co-expresses CD25 and CD11c along with B-cell antigens and has bright monoclonal SIg. A rare HCL variant with features intermediate between HCL and PLL is CD25−. The CD5+ B-cells of CLL produce low affinity autoantibodies, although they are unlikely to contribute to the CLL-associated autoimmune disorders.[46]

The most common chromosomal abnormalities in CLL are 14q+ and trisomy− 12 (+12). Using a probe to the centromeric region of chromosome 12, +12 can be detected by FISH[47] which is quicker, more sensitive and less expensive than classical cytogenetics. Metaphase spreads are often difficult to obtain in CLL because the CLL cell is terminally differentiated; however, +12 is detectable in interphase cells by FISH. CLL with +12 is associated with an abnormal morphology and these patients need earlier treatment (Fig. 3).[48–50]

Detection of clonal rearrangements of both Ig heavy chain and Ig κ light chain gene is specific for mature B-cell malignancies such as CLL, PLL and HCL.[51]

Plasma cell disorders

The plasma cell represents terminal differentiation of the B-cell and, therefore, frequently secretes large amounts of monoclonal immunoglobulin. Multiple myeloma (MM), Waldenström macroglobulinaemia (WM) and heavy chain disease are usually associated with serum monoclonal gammopathy which can be detected by electrophoresis and typed by immunoelectrophoresis (IEP) or immunofixation electrophoresis (IFE). Quantitation of these immunoglobulins is best performed by nephelometry. The detection of Bence–Jones proteins or monoclonal free light chains in the urine requires high resolution IEP or IFE; quantitation in a 24-h urine can be used for staging and monitoring the effectiveness of therapy.[52]

WM, a pre-terminal differentiation of the B-cell, weakly expresses the B-cell antigens CD19 and CD20, expresses CD38 and HLA–DR and reacts with the monoclonal antibodies PCA-1 and PC-1. The diagnostic immunophenotypical feature of WM is monotypic expression of surface and cytoplasmic IgM heavy chains.[1,53]

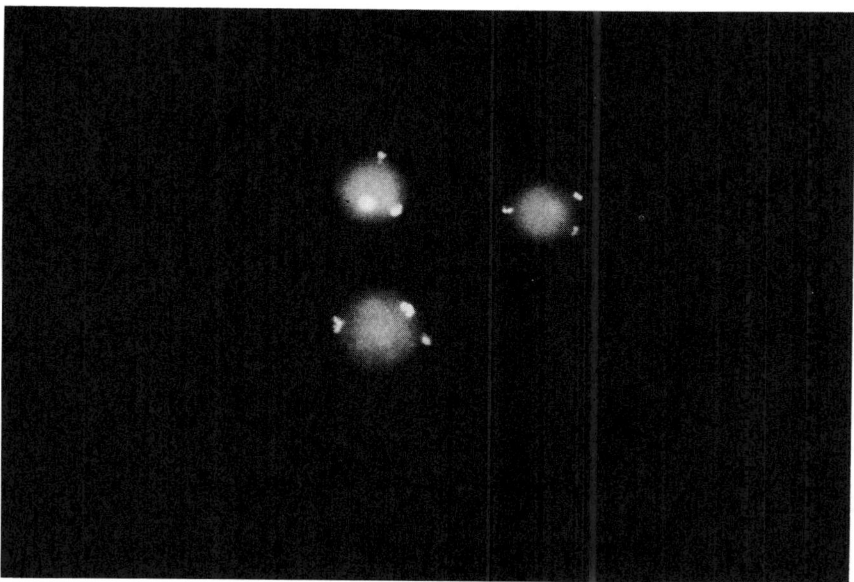

Fig. 3. Fluorescent in situ hybridization FISH of a chromosome 12 centrometric probe labelled with FITC and hybridized to chronic myelogenous leukaemia cells which contain Trisomy-12. The counter stain is properdium iodide. The three dots in each cell indicate Trisomy-12 or three copies of chromosome 12.

Benign and malignant terminally differentiated plasma cells usually lose expression of the B-cell antigens CD19, CD20, CD21, CD22, CD23 and HLA–DR as well as CD45. They lack surface immunoglobulin expression, but express CD24 and CD38 and react with monoclonal antibodies PCA-1 and PC-1.[1] Monotypical expression of cytoplasmic immunoglobulins is diagnostic of a plasma cell disorder such as WM or MM. CD10 is usually negative, but expression of CD10 or other non-lymphoid antigens indicates a poor prognosis.[54,55] CD56 expression is detected in 80% of cases; absence of this antigen is also associated with a poorer prognosis.[56]

The plasma cell labelling index (PCLI) is a measure of the S-phase or DNA synthesis phase of the cell cycle. Essentially all patients with monoclonal gammopathy of undetermined significance (MGUS), smouldering multiple myeloma (SMM) or MM in plateau stage have <10% plasma cells in the bone marrow and a PCLI of 0.0 to 0.8%. Greater than 10% plasma cells in the bone marrow and PCLI $\geqslant$ 1.0% indicate MM; 50% of patients are in this range and have a poor prognosis.[57,58]

Chronic T- and NK-cell leukaemia

Adult T-cell leukaemia • T-cell chronic lymphocytic leukaemia • T-cell prolymphocytic leukaemia • Sezary syndrome • Mycosis fungoides • T-cell large granular lymphocytic leukaemia • NK-cell large granular lymphocytic leukaemia

T-cell leukaemia is diagnosed immunophenotypically by: a) clonal restriction CD4 or CD8 expression (i.e. all of the cells express CD4, but not CD8 or vice versa); b) aberrant expression of T-cell antigens; c) absence of one or more of the T-cell antigens resulting in a phenotype not typical of normal T-cell development or d) co-expression of CD4 and CD8 which are not normally co-expressed in mature T-cells. The immunophenotypic diagnosis of a T-cell neoplasm is less certain than that of a B-cell neoplasm, because other non-clonal conditions may cause abnormal relative numbers of the CD4+ and CD8+ cells. Cells from patients with Sezary syndrome (SS) express T-cell antigens CD2, CD3, CD4 and CD5, but not CD25, CD10 or CD7. Mycosis fungoides (MF), the skin counterpart of SS, has a similar phenotype except CD7 is expressed in 85%. HTLV-I-associated adult T-cell leukaemia/lymphoma (ATL) expresses CD2, CD3, CD4, CD5 and CD25; CD25 (IL-2 receptor) is the diagnostic antigen differentiating HTLV-I from SS, MF and peripheral T-cell lymphoma/leukaemia (Table 3).[1,59] Hypercalcaemia is common in ATL (32%).[60] T-cell prolymphocytic leukaemia (T-PLL) expresses CD2, CD3, CD5 and CD7. In contrast to ATL, T-PLL expresses CD7, is negative for HTLV-I and hypercalcaemia is not overrepresented.[61] Most (65%) T-PLL are CD4+ CD8−, but 13% are CD8+ CD4− and 21% express both antigens.[62]

Large granular lymphocytic (LGL) leukaemia, also known as T-γ lymphoproliferative disease, T-γ lymphocytic leukaemia or T-CLL, can be divided into two immunophenotypical lineages: NK-LGL (15%) and T-LGL (85%). Although the two types of LGL cells are indistinguishable by light microscopy, the immunophenotype of NK-LGL leukaemia is negative for the T-cell antigens, CD3, CD4 and CD8 as well as CD57, but expresses the natural killer (NK) antigens CD56 and CD16; whereas, T-LGL expresses CD3, CD8 and CD57, but is usually negative for CD56.[63–66]

Most chronic T-lymphoproliferative disorders, such as MF, SS, ATL and T-PLL, can be genotyped by TCR-β only. TCR-γ is usually clonally rearranged, but limited diversity of these rearrangements yields false-positive results precluding its routine use.[64] A clonal rearrangement in TCR-β is detectable in 95% of T-LGL, but not in NK-LGL.[63]

Lymphoma

Non-Hodgkin's lymphoma

The basic analytical rationale in evaluating a suspected lymphoma is to determine if it is of lymphoid origin, and, if so, is it benign or malignant?

Table 3. *Immunophenotype of chronic lymphoid leukaemia*

	CD2	CD3	CD4	CD5	CD7	CD8	CD11c	CD19	CD20	CD25	CD57	FMC-7	Ig	PCA-1	CD56 CD16
B-cell															
CLL	–	–	–	+	–	–	±	+	+	–	–	–	s, wk	–	–
PLL	–	–	–	±	–	–	±	+	+	–	–	+	s, bright	–	–
HCL	–	–	–	–	–	–	+	+	+	+	–	±	s, bright	–	–
WM	–	–	–	–	–	–	–	±	±	–	–	–	cy	+	–
MM		–	–	–	–	–	–	±	±	–	–	–	cy	+	+
T-cell															
ATL	+	+	+	+	+	–	–	–	–	+	–	–	–	–	–
T-PLL	+	+	±	+	+	∓	–	–	–	–	–	–	–	–	–
CTCL/SS	+	+	+	+	–	–	–	–	–	–	–	–	–	–	–
MF	+	+	+	+	+*	–	–	–	–	–	–	–	–	–	–
T-LGL	+	+	–	+	–	+	–	–	–	–	+	–	–	–	–
NK–LGL	∓	–	–	–	–	–	–	–	–	–	–	–	–	–	+

* 85%.

CLL: Chronic lymphocytic leukaemia; PLL: Prolymphocytic leukaemia; HCL: Hairy-cell leukaemia; WM: Waldenström macroglobulinaemia; MM: Multiple myeloma; ATL: Adult T-cell leukaemia/lymphoma; T-PLL: T-cell prolymphocytic leukaemia; CTCL: Cutaneous T-cell lymphoma; SS: Sezary syndrome; MF: Mycosis fungoides; T-LGL: T-cell large granular lymphocytic leukaemia; NK–LGL: Natural killer cell large granular lymphocytic leukaemia; s: surface; wk: weak; cy: cytoplasmic.

Is the malignant lymphoma Hodgkin's or non-Hodgkin's? T- cell or B-cell? aggressive or indolent? Histopathological diagnosis is used to classify these neoplasms. Adjunct testing, such as immunophenotyping using flow cytometry and immunohistochemistry, genotyping using SB and PCR and classical cytogenetics, confirms clonality and specific subtypes.

Flow cytometry is useful in determining if a lymphoma is of B-cell or T-cell origin (Table 4). If B-cell lineage is suspected, clonality can be confirmed by proving monotypical light chain expression. Most B-cell lymphoma express CD19 and CD20 and either κ or λ, but not both. Proving T-cell monoclonality in a lymphoma is more difficult, but aberrant antigen expression (such as lack of a normal antigen or expression of a combination of antigens not normally present on mature T lymphocytes) or the presence of aneuploidy are diagnostic. Normal mature T-cells express CD2, CD3, CD5, CD7 and CD4 or CD8. Failure to identify a diagnostic abnormality by flow cytometry (despite suspicious morphology) may be due to sampling error, the presence of a minor clone below the level of sensitivity of the technique or a T-cell neoplasm with a phenotype similar to normal cells. In these cases, additional diagnostic techniques such as immunohistochemistry, SB and cytogenetics are helpful (Fig. 4).

Small lymphocytic lymphoma

The hallmark of a true B-cell lymphoma is expression of pan-B-cell antigens CD19 and CD20 and monoclonal surface immunoglobulin. In small lymphocytic lymphoma (SLL), CD5 is usually co-expressed and monotypic surface immunoglobulin expression is weak, which is immunophenotypically similar to CLL.

Mantle zone lymphoma

Mantle zone lymphoma (MZL) or lymphocytic lymphoma of intermediate differentiation (IDL) is a B-cell lymphoma that co-expresses CD5. CD5 is helpful in differentiating MZL from follicular lymphoma (FL) which is CD5−. Surface immunoglobulin in MZL/IDL is brighter than SLL/CLL and FMC-7 is usually positive, similar immunophenotypically to PLL.[1,67] MZL/IDL frequently contains the t(11;14)(q13;q32) translocation that corresponds to the *BCL*-1 gene (located at the q13 band of chromosome 11) and the immunoglobulin heavy chain gene detectable by SB. Rearrangements in *BCL*-1 are found in 73% of MZL/IDL using a combination of four probes, but not in cases of CLL/SLL or FL.[68,69]

Follicular lymphoma

Nearly all follicular lymphoma (FL) are B-cell and express CD19 and CD20. Unlike SLL/CLL and MZL/IDL, CD5 and CD43 are usually not expressed; whereas, CD10 and CDw75 are frequently positive. By

Table 4. *Immunophenotype and genotype of non-Hodgkin's lymphoma*

Histology	Phenotype	Translocation	Oncogene
SLL	CD19+, CD20+, CD5+, SIg weak, CD10−	t(14;19)(q32;q13)	*BCL*-3
MZL/IDL	CD19+, CD20+, CD5+, CD10−,. SIg bright, FMC-7+	t(11;14)(q13;q32)	*BCL*-1
FL	CD10+, CD20+, CD5−, CD10+, SIg bright	t(14;18)(q32;q21.3)	*BCL*-2
DLCL (B-cell, 80%)	CD19+, CD20+, CD10+ (20%)	t(14;18)(q32;q21.3)	*BCL*-2
	CD19+, CD20+, SIg+	t(3;14)(q27;q32)	*BCL*-6
		t(3;22)(q27;q11)	
		t(2;3)(p12;q27)	
DLCL (T-cell, 20%)	CD2+, CD5+, CD7+, CD4+ (65%)		
LL (B-cell)	CD19+, CD20±, CD10±		
LL (T-cell)	CD7+, TdT+, CD2±, CD3±, CD5±		
ALCL	CD30+ (Ki-1), CD15+, CD25+	t(2;5)(p23;q35)	
BL	CD10+, CD20+, CD22+, CD21±, CD10+, TdT−	t(8;14)(q24;q32)	
		t(2;8)(p12;q24)	c-*MYC*
		t(8;22)(q24;q11)	

SLL: Small lymphocytic lymphoma; MZL: Mantle zone lymphoma; IDL: Lymphocytic lymphoma of intermediate differentiation; FL: follicular lymphoma; DLCL: Diffuse large-cell lymphoma; LL: Lymphoblastic leukaemia; ALCL: Anaplastic large-cell lymphoma; BL: Burkitt's lymphoma.

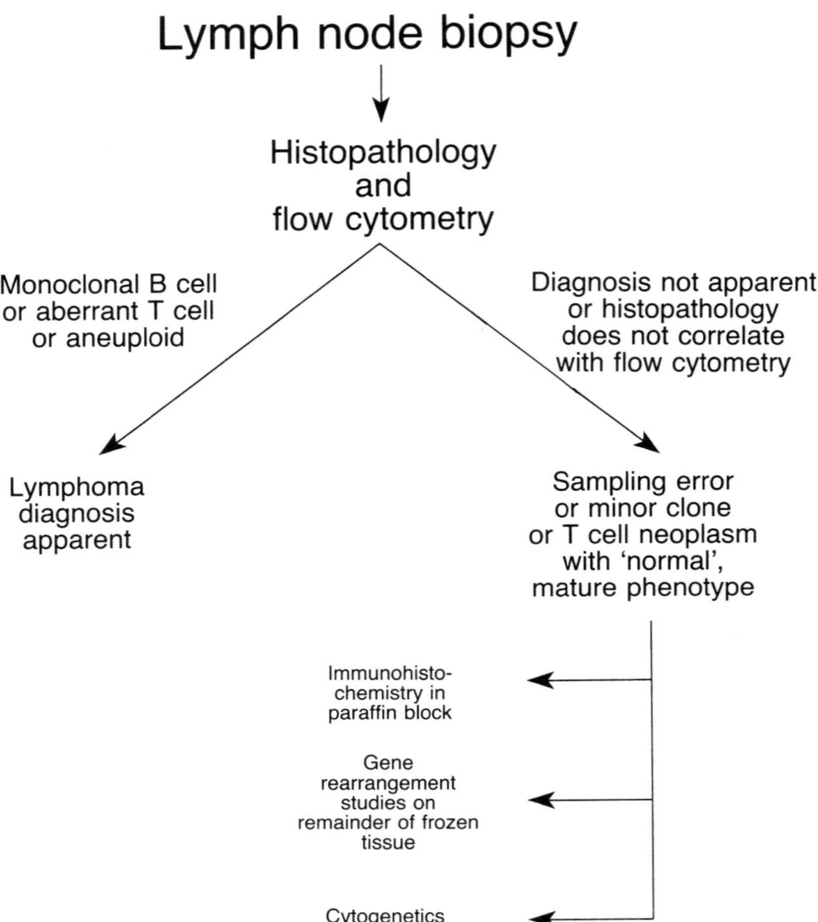

Fig. 4. Strategy for choosing tests for suspected lymphoma. Questions to be answered: What is the cell of origin? Is it a lymphoma? Is it Hodgkin's disease or non-Hodgkin's lymphoma? Is it T-cell or B-cell? What is the biology: aggressive or indolent?

immunohistochemistry, FL has monoclonal, CD10+ germinal centres and CD5− mantle zones; whereas, MZL/IDL has polyclonal germinal centres and monoclonal, CD5+ mantle zones.[69] Demonstration of surface immunoglobulin light chain clonal restriction is paramount in cases where distinction between FL and a reactive lymph node is difficult morphologically.

The characteristic cytogenetic abnormality in FL is the t(14;18)(q32;q21) which is detectable in 90% of FL. This translocation causes the *BCL*-2 gene at 18q21 to move into the proximity of the immunoglobulin heavy chain gene encoded at 14q32, the majority of which can be detected by SB or PCR.[69] *BCL*-2 codes for a protein associated with the inner mitochondrial membrane and its deregulation may prevent programmed B-cell death.[70] The breakpoints commonly occur at two 'hot spots' 20 kilobases apart: the major and the minor breakpoint regions. Transformation of FL to diffuse-type lymphoma is associated with mutations in p53 which is detectable by PCR or immunohistochemistry.[71,72]

Diffuse large-cell lymphoma

Diffuse large-cell lymphoma (DLCL) is of B-cell (80%) or T-cell (20%) immunotype. Most of the B-cell DLCL express SIg, CD19, CD20, HLA-DR and contain clonal immunoglobulin gene rearrangements; CD10 is expressed in about 20%. T-cell DLCL usually contains a clonal gene rearrangement in TCR-β and expresses an aberrant T-cell immunophenotype: CD2, CD3, CD5 and/or CD7; most (65%) are CD4+. The short-term prognosis for patients with T-cell DLCL is significantly worse than for B-cell, although the overall survival is not different. At two years post-diagnosis, no patient with T-cell DCLC remains free of disease; whereas, half of patients with B-cell DCLC are disease free.[73]

About 20% of de novo B-cell DLCL contain the *BCL*-2 gene rearrangement, which is more frequently present as an early-stage, non-mucosal-associated extranodal tumour that is HLA-DR-negative. 5-year, relapse-free survival is poor in *BCL*-2+ cases (11% versus 48%), but overall survival is not much different from B-cell DLCL without the rearrangement because *BCL*-2+ cases tend to respond to either chemotherapy or radiotherapy.[74] *BCL*-6, located at 3q27, translocates with each of the three immunoglobulin genes (heavy, ϰ and λ) in SIg+ B-cell DLCL and may be a specific genetic marker for this disease.[75,76]

Lymphoblastic lymphoma

Most lymphoblastic lymphoma (LL) have an immature T-cell phenotype expressing TdT and CD7 along with any of the other T-cell antigens, similar to T-ALL. B-lineage LL are less common and display a phenotype similar to B-lineage ALL.[77]

Anaplastic large-cell lymphoma

These tumours have a similar morphology to immunoblastic DLCL, but should be considered a distinct group. They may be confused with carcinoma or Hodgkin's disease, but the immunophenotype clarifies the diagnosis. CD30(Ki-1), CD15, CD25, CD71 and HLA-DR are usually positive in anaplastic large cell lymphoma (ALCL). This is the same immunotype as the Reed-Sternberg cell of Hodgkin's disease and this neoplasm may be classified in the Hodgkin spectrum of lymphoma. CD45 may or may not be positive and EMA can be expressed, which leads to confusion when distinguishing this neoplasm from a carcinoma.

ALCL is associated with the t(2;5)(q23;q35) translocation, the genes involved have yet to be cloned.[78]

Burkitt lymphoma

Small, non-cleaved lymphoma (SNCL), both classical Burkitt's lymphoma (BL) and non-Burkitt's variant, express the mature B-cell antigens, CD19, CD20 and CD22. Most cases of African or endemic BL (eBL) are associated with CD21, the Epstein–Barr virus (EBV) and C3d receptor; whereas most non-African (non-endemic) BL are $CD21-^{1}$. CD10 is expressed in all BL, but only 30% of BL-like lymphoma. TdT is usually negative in all SNCL.

The c-*MYC* oncogene located at 8q24 is involved in a reciprocal translocation in 100% of BL.[79] The immunoglobulin heavy chain at 14q32 is involved in 80% of cases, the λ light chain at 21q11 in 15% and the κ light chain at 2p11 in 5%. These translocations are detectable in eBL found in Africa and New Guinea which is associated with EBV infection, sporadic (American) BL (sBL) of no known viral association, and AIDS-associated BL (AIDS–BL). AIDS–BL and eBL have similar breakpoint locations related to c-*MYC*, distinct from sBL. EBV DNA is detectable in all of the tumors with a breakpoint outside of c-*MYC*, but not in those tumours with a breakpoint within c-*MYC*.[80] These rearrangements in c-*MYC* are detectable by SB.

Benign lymphoproliferative disorders

Some histologically benign T-cell lymphoproliferative disorders such as lymphomatoid papulosis or angioimmunoblastic lymphadenopathy have the potential to progress to a malignant lymphoma. Immunophenotypically these disorders contain a proliferation of CD4+ T-cells and clonal rearrangements in the TCR-β. Benign lymphoepithelial proliferation of Sjögren's disease and AIDS-related lymphoproliferative disorders commonly contain immunoglobulin gene rearrangements. These clonal populations frequently regress and the presence of clonal gene rearrangements does not necessarily indicate progression to malignant lymphoma.[81–85]

Hodgkin's disease

The malignant Reed-Sternberg (RS) cell of Hodgkin's disease (HD), which usually expresses CD30, CD15 and CD25, is detectable by flow cytometry or more practically by immunohistochemistry. In lymphocyte-predominant HD, the surrounding lymphocytes are T-cells which are mostly CD4+; RS cells express CD45, but may be negative for CD30, CD15 and CD25.[86]

References

(1) Vaickus L, Ball ED, Foon KA. Immune markers in hematologic malignancies. *Crit Rev Oncol Hematol* 1991; 11: 267.

(2) Crist WM, Carroll AJ, Shuster JJ et al. Poor prognosis of children with pre-B acute lymphoblastic leukemia is associated with the t(1;19)(q23;p13): a pediatric oncology group study. *Blood* 1990; 76: 117.
(3) Pui C–H, Hancock ML, Head DR et al. Clinical significance of CD34 expression in childhood acute lymphoblastic leukemia. *Blood* 1993; 82: 889.
(4) Behm FG, Raimondi SC, Schell MJ et al. Lack of CD45 antigen on blast cells in childhood acute lymphoblastic leukemia is associated with chromosomal hyperdiploidy and other favorable prognostic features. *Blood* 1992; 79 1011.
(5) Schneider NR: Cytogenetic evaluation of childhood neoplasms. *Arch Pathol Lab Med* 1993; 117: 1220.
(6) Cline MJ. The molecular basis of leukemia. *N Engl J Med* 1994; 330: 328.
(7) Little JV, Foucar K, Duncan MH et al. A comparative analysis of cytoplasmic Mu (Cμ) expression in acute lymphoblastic leukemia by molecular and immunologic techniques. *Am J Clin Pathol* 1992; 97: 885.
(8) Dyer MJS, Heward JM, Zani VJ et al. Unusual deletions within the immunoglobulin heavy-chain locus in acute leukemias. *Blood* 1993; 82: 865.
(9) Ramasamy I, Brisco M, Morley A. Improved PCR method for detecting monoclonal immunoglobulin heavy chain rearrangement in B cell neoplasms. *J Clin Pathol* 1992; 45: 770.
(10) Cossman J, Zehnbauer B, Green CT et al. Gene rearrangements in the diagnosis of lymphoma/leukemia. *Am J Clin Pathol* 1991; 95: 347.
(11) Maurer J, Janssen JWG, Thiel E et al. Detection of chimeric PCR-ABL genes in acute lymphoblastic leukaemia by the polymerase chain reaction. *Lancet* 1991; 337: 1055.
(12) Mills KI, Benn P, Birnie GD. Does the breakpoint within the major breakpoint cluster region (M-bcr) influence the duration of the chronic phase in chronic myeloid leukemia? An analytical comparison of current literature. *Blood* 1991; 78: 1155.
(13) Miyamura K, Tanimoto M, Morishima Y et al. Detection of Philadelphia chromosome – positive acute lymphoblastic leukemia by polymerase chain reaction: possible eradication of minimal residual disease by marrow transplantation. *Blood* 1992; 79: 1366.
(14) Brisco MJ, Condon J, Hughes E et al. Outcome prediction in childhood acute lymphoblastic leukaemia by molecular quantification of residual disease at the end of induction. *Lancet* 1994; 43: 196.
(15) Pui CH, Behm FG, Singh B et al. Heterogeneity of presenting features and their relation to treatment outcome in 120 children with T-cell acute lymphoblastic leukemia. *Blood* 1190; 75: 174.
(16) Kurtzberg J, Waldmann TA, Davey MP et al. CD7+, CD4−, CD8− acute leukemia: a syndrome of malignant pluripotent lymphohematopoietic cells. *Blood* 1989; 73: 381.
(17) Liang R, Chan V, Chan TK et al. Rearrangement of immunoglobulin and T cell receptor genes in acute and chronic leukaemias. *Acta Haematol* 1991; 85: 71.
(18) Schwarzinger I, Valent P, Koller V et al. Prognostic significance of surface marker expression on blasts of patients with de novo acute myeloblastic leukemia. *J Clin Oncol* 1990; 8: 423.
(19) Borowitz MJ, Gockerman JP, Moore JO et al. Clinicopathologic and cytogenic

features of CD34 (My 10)-positive acute nonlymphocytic leukemia. *Am J Clin Pathol* 1989; 91: 265.

(20) Kita K, Miwa H, Nakase K et al. Clinical importance of CD7 expression in acute myelocytic leukemia. *Blood* 1993; 81: 2399

(21) Biondi A, Rambaldi A, Alcalay M et al. RAR-alpha gene rearrangements as a genetic marker for diagnosis and monitoring in acute promyelocytic leukemia. *Blood* 1991; 77: 1418.

(22) Grignani F, Fagioli M, Alcalay M et al. Acute promyelocytic leukemia: from genetics to treatment. *Blood* 1994; 83: 10.

(23) Warrell RP, Frankel SR, Miller WH Jr et al. Differentiation therapy of acute promyelocytic leukemia with tretinoin (all-*trans*-retinoic acid). *N Engl J Med* 1993; 324: 1385.

(24) Miller WH Jr, Levine K, DeBlasio A et al. Detection of minimal residual disease in acute promyelocytic leukemia by a reverse transcription polymerase chain reaction assay for the PML/RAR-α fusion mRNA. *Blood* 1993; 82: 1689.

(25) Liu P, Tarle SA, Hajra A et al. Fusion between transcription factor CBFβ/PEBP2β, and a myosin heavy chain in acute myeloid leukemia. *Science* 1993; 261: 1041.

(26) Maseki N, Miyoshi H, Shimizu K et al. The 8;21 chromosome translocation in acute myeloid leukemia is always detectable by molecular analysis using AMLI. *Blood* 1993; 81: 1573.

(27) Foa R, Casorati G, Guibellino C et al. Rearrangements of immunoglobulin and T-cell receptor beta and gamma genes are associated with terminal deoxynucleotidyl transferase expression in acute myeloid leukemia. *J Exp Med* 1987; 165: 879.

(28) Drexler HG, Thiel E, Ludwig W–D. Review of the incidence and clinical relevance of myeloid antigen-positive acute lymphoblastic leukemia. *Leukemia* 1991; 5: 637.

(29) Jensen AW, Hokland M, Jorgensen H et al. Solitary expression of CD7 among T-cell antigens in acute myeloid leukemia: identification of a group of patients with similar T-cell receptor β and δ rearrangements and course of disease suggestive of poor prognosis. *Blood* 1991; 78: 1292.

(30) Ball ED, Davis RB, Griffin JD et al. Prognostic value of lymphocyte surface markers in acute myeloid leukemia. *Blood* 1991; 77: 2242.

(31) Smith FO, Lampkin BC, Versteeg C et al. Expression of lymphoid-associated cell surface antigens by childhood acute myeloid leukemia cells lacks prognostic significance. *Blood* 1992; 79: 24151.

(32) Sorensen PHB, Shen C-S, Smith FO et al. Molecular arrangements of the *MLL* gene are present in most cases of infant acute myeloid leukemia and are strongly correlated with monocytic or myelomonocytic phenotypes. *J Clin Invest* 1994; 93: 429.

(33) Thirman MJ, Gill JH, Burnett RC et al. Rearrangement of the *MLL* gene in acute lymphoblastic and acute myeloid leukemias with 11q23 chromosomal translocation. *N Engl J Med* 1993; 329: 909.

(34) Cleary ML. A promiscuous oncogene in acute leukemia. *N Engl J Med* 1993; 329: 958.

(35) Caldwell CW, Patterson WP, Toalson BD, Yesus YW. Surface and cytoplasmic expression of CD45 antigen isoforms in normal and malignant myeloid cell differentiation. *Am J Clin Pathol* 1991; 95: 180.
(36) Verfaillie CM, Miller WJ, Boylan K, McGlave PB. Selection of benign primitive hematopoietic progenitors in chronic myelogenous leukemia on the basis of HLA-DR antigen expression. *Blood* 1992; 79: 1003.
(37) Sullivan SA, Marsden KA, Lowenthal RM et al. Circulating CD34+ cells: an adverse prognostic factor in the myelodysplastic syndromes. *Am J Hematol* 1992; 39: 96.
(38) Kantarjian HM, Deisseroth A, Kurzrock R et al. Chronic myelogenous leukemia: a concise update. *Blood* 1993; 82: 691.
(39) Yunis JJ, Lobell M, Arnese MA et al. Refined chromosome study helps define prognostic subgroups in most patients with primary myelodysplastic syndrome and acute myelogenous leukaemia. *Br J Haematol* 1988; 68: 189.
(40) Paquette RL, Landaw EM, Pierre RV et al. N-ras mutations are associated with poor prognosis and increased risk of leukemia in myelodysplastic syndrome. *Blood* 1993; 82:590.
(41) Kreipe H, Felgner J, Jaquet K et al. DNA analysis to aid in the diagnosis of chronic myeloproliferative disorders. *Am J Clin Pathol* 1992; 98: 46.
(42) Tkachuk DC, Westbrook CA, Amdreeff M et al. Detection of *bcr–abl* fusion in chronic myelogenous leukemia by in situ hybridization. *Science* 1990; 252: 559.
(43) Cross NCP, Feng L, Chase A et al. Competitive polymerase chain reaction to estimate the number of BCR-ABL transcripts in chronic myeloid leukemia patients after bone marrow transplantation. *Blood* 1993; 82: 1929.
(44) Geisler CH, Larsen JK, Hansen NE et al. Prognostic importance of flow cytometric immunophenotyping of 540 consecutive patients with B-cell chronic lymphocytic leukemia. *Blood* 1991; 78: 1795.
(45) Dighiero G, Travade P, Chevret S et al. B-cell chronic lymphocytic leukemia: present status and future decisions. *J Am Soc Hematol* 1991; 78: 1901.
(46) Kipps TJ, Carson DA. Autoantibodies in chronic lymphocytic leukemia and related systemic autoimmune diseases. *Blood* 1993; 81: 2475.
(47) Le Beau MM. Detecting genetic changes in human tumor cells: have scientists 'gone fishing?' *Blood* 1993; 81: 1979.
(48) Escudier SM, Pereira–Leahy JM, Drach JW et al. Fluorescent in situ hybridization and cytogenetic studies of trisomy 12 in chronic lymphocytic leukemia. *Blood* 1993; 81: 270.
(49) Que TH, Marco JG, Matutes JE et al. Trisomy 12 in chronic lymphocytic leukemia detected by fluorescence in situ hybridization: analysis by stage, immunophenotype, and morphology. *Blood* 1993; 81:571.
(50) Anastasi J, Le Beau MM, Vardiman JW et al. Detection of trisomy 12 in chronic lymphocytic leukemia by fluorescence in situ hybridization to interphase cells: a simple and sensitive method. *Blood* 1992; 79: 1796.
(51) Lenormand B, Ghanem N, Tilly H et al. Rearrangements of immunoglobulin light and heavy chain genes and correlation with phenotypic markers in B-cell chronic lymphocytic leukemia. *Leukemia* 1991; 5:928.

(52) Grogan TM, Tubbs R. Myeloma and related immunoproliferative disorders. *Am J Surg Pathol* 1989; 13: 163.
(53) Deegan MJ. Membrane antigen analysis in the diagnosis of lymphoid leukemias and lymphomas. *Arch Pathol Lab Med* 1989; 113: 606.
(54) Durie BGM, Grogan TM. CALLA-positive myeloma: an aggressive subtype with poor survival. *Blood* 1985; 66: 229.
(55) Epstein J, Xiao H, He X–Y. Markers of multiple hematopoietic-cell lineages in multiple myeloma. *N Engl J Med* 1990; 322: 664.
(56) Van Camp B, Durie BGM, Spier C et al. Plasma cells in multiple myeloma express a natural killer cell-associated antigen: CD56 (NKH-1; Leu-19). *Blood* 1990; 79: 377.
(57) Witzig TE, Gonchoroff NJ, Katzmann JA et al. Peripheral blood B cell labeling indices are a measure to disease activity in patients with monoclonal gammopathies. *J Clin Oncol* 1988; 6: 1041.
(58) Greipp PR, Lust JA, O'Fallon M et al. Plasma cell labeling index and β_2-microglobulin predict survival independent of thymidine kinase and C-reactive protein in multiple myeloma. *Blood* 1993; 81: 3382.
(59) Bennett JM, Catovsky D, Daniel M-T et al. Proposals for the classification of chronic (mature) B and T lymphoid leukeamias. *J Clin Pathol* 1989; 42: 567.
(60) Yamaguchi K: Human T-lymphotropic virus type I in Japan. *Lancet* 343: 213, 1994
(61) Brunning RD: T-prolymphocytic leukemia. *Blood* 1991; 78: 3111.
(62) Matutes E, Brito-Babapulle V, Swansbury J et al. Clinical and laboratory features of 78 cases of T-prolymphocytic leukemia, *Blood* 1991; 78: 3269.
(63) Loughran TP Jr. Clonal diseases of large granular lymphocytes. *Blood* 1993; 82: 1.
(64) McDaniel HL, MacPherson BR, Tindle BH, Lunde JH: Lymphoproliferative disorder of granular lymphocytes. *Arch Pathol Lab Med* 1992; 116: 242.
(65) Chan WC, Gu LB, Masih A et al. Large granular lymphocyte proliferation with the natural killer-cell phenotype. *Am J Clin Pathol* 1992; 97: 353.
(66) Sivakumaran M, Richards SJ, Hunt KM et al. Patterns of CD16 and CD56 expression in persistent expansions of CD3+NKa+ lymphocytes are predictive for clonal T-cell receptor gene rearrangements. *Br J Haematol* 1991; 78: 368.
(67) Carbone A, Gloghini A, Volpe R. Immunohistochemistry of Hodgkin and non-Hodgkin lymphomas with emphasis on the diagnostic significance of the BNH9 antibody reactivity with anaplastic large cell (CD30 positive) lymphomas. *Cancer* 1992; 70: 2691.
(68) Medeiros J, Van Krieken JH, Jaffe ES, Raffeld M. Association of bcl-l rearrangements with lymphocytic lymphoma of intermediate differentiation. *Blood* 1990; 76: 2086.
(69) Weisenburger DD, Chan WC. Lymphomas of follicles. Mantle cell and follicle center cell lymphomas. *Am J Clin Pathol* 1993; 99: 409.
(70) Hockenbery D, Nunez G, Milliman C et al. bcl-2 is an inner mitochondrial membrane protein that blocks programmed cell death. *Nature* 1990; 348: 334.
(71) Lo Coco F, Gaidano G, Louie DC et al. p53 mutations are associated with histologic transformation of follicular lymphoma. *Blood* 1993; 82: 2289.

(72) Sander CA, Yano T, Clark HM et al. p53 mutation is associated with progression in follicular lymphomas. *Blood* 1993; 82: 1994.
(73) Lippman SM, Miller TP, Spier CM et al. The prognostic significance of the immunotype in diffuse large-cell lymphoma: a comparative study of the T-cell and B-cell phenotype. *Blood* 1988; 72: 436.
(74) Jacobson JO, Wilkes BM, Kwiatkowski DJ et al. bcl-2 rearrangements in de novo diffuse large cell lymphoma. *Cancer* 1993; 72: 231.
(75) Baron BW, Nucifora G, McCabe N et al. Identification of the gene associated with the recurring chromosomal translocations t(3;14)(q27;q32) and t(3;22)(q27;qll) in B-cell lymphomas. *Proc Natl Acad Sci USA* 1993; 90: 5262.
(76) Ye BH, Rao PH, Chaganti RSK, Dalla-Favera R. Cloning of bcl–6, the locus involved in chromosome translocation affecting band 3q27 in B-cell lymphoma. *Cancer Res* 1993;r 53: 2732.
(77) Jaffe ES, Raffeld M, Medeiros LJ, Stetler-Stevenson M. An overview of the classification of non-Hodgkin's lymphomas: an integration of morphological and phenotypical concepts. *Cancer Res*(Suppl) 1992; 52: 5447.
(78) Mason DY, Bastard C, Rimokh R et al. CD30-positive large cell lymphomas ('Ki-1 lymphoma') are associated with a chromosomal translocation involving 5q35. *Br J Haematol* 1990; 74: 161.
(79) Croce CM: Molecular biology of lymphomas. *Semin Oncol* 1993; 20:31.
(80) Ratech H. The use of molecular biology in hematopathology. Oncogenes as diagnostic markers in non-Hodgkin's malignant lymphoma. *Am J Clin Pathol* 1993; 99: 381.
(81) Feller AC, Griesser HH, Schilling CV et al. Clonal gene rearrangement patterns correlate with immunophenotype and clinical parameters in patients with angioimmunoblastic lymphadenopathy. *Am J Pathol* 1988; 133: 549.
(82) Weiss LM, Wood GS, Trela M et al. Clonal T-cell populations in lymphomatoid papulosis. Evidence of a lymphoproliferative origin for a clinically benign disease. *N Engl J Med* 1986; 315: 475.
(83) Kadin ME, Vonderheid EC, Sako D et al. Clonal composition of T cells in lymphomatoid papulosis. *Am J Pathol* 1987; 126: 13.
(84) Ainenberg AC: Utility of gene rearrangements in lymphoid malignancies. *Annu Rev Med* 1993; 44: 75.
(85) Casey TT, Olson SJ, Cousar JB, Collins RD. Plastic section immunohistochemistry in the diagnosis of hematopoietic and lymphoid neoplasms. *Clin Lab Med* 1990; 10: 199.
(86) Carbone A, Pinto A, Gloghini A et al. B-zone small lymphocytic lymphoma: a morphologic, immunophenotypic, and clinical study with comparison to 'well-differentiated' lymphocytic disorders. *Hum Pathol* 1992; 23:438.

Index

Page numbers in *italic* refer to figures and/or tables

Index